Principles of Skin Care and the Oncology Patient

Edited by

Marilyn L. Haas, PhD, RN, CNS, ANP-BC
Giselle J. Moore-Higgs, ARNP, PhD(c), AOCN®

Oncology Nursing Society
Pittsburgh, Pennsylvania

ONS Publishing Division
Publisher: Leonard Mafrica, MBA, CAE
Director, Commercial Publishing: Barbara Sigler, RN, MNEd
Managing Editor: Lisa M. George, BA
Technical Content Editor: Angela D. Klimaszewski, RN, MSN
Staff Editor: Amy Nicoletti, BA
Copy Editor: Laura Pinchot, BA
Graphic Designer: Dany Sjoen

Principles of Skin Care and the Oncology Patient

Library of Congress Control Number: 2009935300

ISBN: 978-1-890504-88-5

Publisher's Note

This book is published by the Oncology Nursing Society (ONS). ONS neither represents nor guarantees that the practices described herein will, if followed, ensure safe and effective patient care. The recommendations contained in this book reflect ONS's judgment regarding the state of general knowledge and practice in the field as of the date of publication. The recommendations may not be appropriate for use in all circumstances. Those who use this book should make their own determinations regarding specific safe and appropriate patient-care practices, taking into account the personnel, equipment, and practices available at the hospital or other facility at which they are located. The editors and publisher cannot be held responsible for any liability incurred as a consequence from the use or application of any of the contents of this book. Figures and tables are used as examples only. They are not meant to be all-inclusive, nor do they represent endorsement of any particular institution by ONS. Mention of specific products and opinions related to those products do not indicate or imply endorsement by ONS. Web sites mentioned are provided for information only; the hosts are responsible for their own content and availability. Unless otherwise indicated, dollar amounts reflect U.S. dollars.

ONS publications are originally published in English. Publishers wishing to translate ONS publications must contact the ONS Publishing Division about licensing arrangements. ONS publications cannot be translated without obtaining written permission from ONS. (Individual tables and figures that are reprinted or adapted require additional permission from the original source.) Because translations from English may not always be accurate or precise, ONS disclaims any responsibility for inaccuracies in words or meaning that may occur as a result of the translation. Readers relying on precise information should check the original English version.

Printed in the United States of America

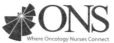

Oncology Nursing Society
Integrity • Innovation • Stewardship • Advocacy • Excellence • Inclusiveness

Ideas are exchanged at oncology meetings, but it is when you return home that ideas become reality. I dedicate this textbook to many of my oncology colleagues who joined me in learning and sharing to promote evidence-based care. To my patients, thank you for sharing your journey as we strive to improve your care. Finally, to my parents, husband, and sons, who understand and love me even when I come home with more adventures.

—Marilyn

I dedicate this to my niece Kelsey, a college freshman who is embarking on her own academic career, and to the patients who have touched my life and taught me so much about caring for others.

—Gigi

Many thanks for the assistance of the ONS Publishing Division, especially Barbara Sigler, Lisa George, and Amy Nicoletti, for their expertise and commitment to this project.

Contributors

Editors

Marilyn L. Haas, PhD, RN, CNS, ANP-BC
Nurse Practitioner
Mountain Radiation Oncology
Asheville, North Carolina
Chapter 14. Complementary Therapies for Oncology Cutaneous Reactions

Giselle J. Moore-Higgs, ARNP, PhD(c), AOCN®
Assistant Director
Clinical Trials Office
University of Florida Shands Cancer Center
Gainesville, Florida
Chapter 3. Benign Skin Disorders: Impact on Cancer Therapy; Chapter 12. Psychological Distress Related to Skin Problems in the Oncology Patient Population

Authors

Elizabeth A. Ayello, PhD, RN, ACNS-BC, ETN, FAPWCA, FAAN
Clinical Associate Editor
Advances in Skin and Wound Care
President
Ayello Harris and Associates
Copake, New York
Chapter 5. Wound Care Products and Treatments

Sharon Baranoski, RN, MSN, CWOCN, APN, DAPWCA, FAAN
President
Wound Care Dynamics, Inc.
Consultant Services
Shorewood, IL
Chapter 5. Wound Care Products and Treatments

Diane Candiotto, BASc, RD
Clinical Dietitian
General Internal Medicine
St. Michael's Hospital
Toronto, Ontario
Canada
Chapter 13. Nutrition Needs for Healing Skin

Sandra Cochran, RN, BSN, CWOCN
Certified Wound, Ostomy, Continence Nurse
Fox Chase Cancer Center
Philadelphia, Pennsylvania
Chapter 4. Malignant Cutaneous Diseases

Vanna M. Dest, MSN, APRN-BC, AOCN®
Oncology Nurse Practitioner
Radiation Oncology Specialists of Southern Connecticut
Hospital of Saint Raphael
New Haven, Connecticut
Chapter 7. Systemic Therapy–Induced Skin Reactions

Dorothy B. Doughty, MN, RN, CWOCN, FAAN
Director
Wound, Ostomy, and Continence Nursing Education Center
Emory University
Atlanta, Georgia
Chapter 11. Skin and Wound Pain: Assessment and Management

Tammy Fansabedian, BASc, RD
Clinical Dietitian
Head and Neck Oncology
Princess Margaret Hospital
University Health Network
Toronto, Ontario
Canada
Chapter 13. Nutrition Needs for Healing Skin

Claudia Ganson, RN, BScN, CETN(c)
Clinical Coordinator
Surgical Oncology
Toronto General Hospital, University Health Network
Toronto, Ontario
Canada
Chapter 9. Impact of Chronic Disease on Wound Healing

Barbara Holmes Gobel, RN, MS, AOCN®
Oncology Clinical Nurse Specialist
Northwestern Memorial Hospital
Adjunct Faculty
Rush University College of Nursing
Chicago, Illinois
Chapter 10. Impact of Systemic and Infectious Skin Disease During Cancer Treatment

William P. Hogle, RN, MSN, OCN®
Clinical Manager
University of Pittsburgh Medical Center, Passavant Cancer Center
Pittsburgh, Pennsylvania
Chapter 1. Overview of Skin Issues Related to the Oncology Patient

Pamela R. Jakubek, MSN, RN, CWOCN
Clinical Nurse Specialist
Certified Wound, Ostomy, Continence Nurse
Fox Chase Cancer Center
Philadelphia, Pennsylvania
Chapter 4. Malignant Cutaneous Diseases

Sarah H. Kagan, PhD, RN, AOCN®
Ralston House Term Professor of Gerontological Nursing, School of Nursing
Clinical Nurse Specialist, Abramson Cancer Center
Secondary Faculty, Department of Otorhinolaryngology: Head and Neck Surgery
University of Pennsylvania
Philadelphia, Pennsylvania
Chapter 15. Special Needs of Gero-Oncology Patients

Theresa M. Latchford, RN, MS, AOCN®
Oncology Clinical Nurse Specialist
Blood and Marrow Transplant
Stanford Hospital and Clinics
Stanford, California
Chapter 8. Cutaneous Effects of Blood and Marrow Transplantation

Maurene McQuestion, RN, BA, BScN, MSc, CON(C)
Advanced Practice Nurse/Clinical Nurse Specialist
Princess Margaret Hospital
University Health Network
Toronto, Ontario
Canada
Chapter 6. Radiation-Induced Skin Reactions

Anna Liza Rodriguez, RN, MSN, MHA, OCN®
Director
Oncology Nursing and Service Line
Mt. Sinai Hospital
Chicago, Illinois
Chapter 10. Impact of Systemic and Infectious Skin Disease During Cancer Treatment

Pamela Savage, RN, MAEd, CON(C)
Clinical Nurse Specialist
Medical Oncology
Princess Margaret Hospital, University Health Network
Toronto, Ontario
Canada
Chapter 9. Impact of Chronic Disease on Wound Healing

Mary Ellyn Witt, RN, MS, AOCN®
Clinical Research Nurse
Radiation Oncology
University of Chicago Medical Center
Chicago, Illinois
Chapter 2. Common Drug Reactions With Cutaneous Manifestations

Melodie Young, MSN, RN, ANP-C, GNPc
Nurse Practitioner
Private Practice
Modern Dermatology
Dallas, Texas
Chapter 2. Common Drug Reactions With Cutaneous Manifestations

Disclosure

Editors and authors of books and guidelines provided by the Oncology Nursing Society are expected to disclose to the participants any significant financial interest or other relationships with the manufacturer(s) of any commercial products.

A vested interest may be considered to exist if a contributor is affiliated with or has a financial interest in commercial organizations that may have a direct or indirect interest in the subject matter. A "financial interest" may include, but is not limited to, being a shareholder in the organization; being an employee of the commercial organization; serving on an organization's speakers bureau; or receiving research from the organization. An "affiliation" may be holding a position on an advisory board or some other role of benefit to the commercial organization. Vested interest statements appear in the front matter for each publication.

Contributors are expected to disclose any unlabeled or investigational use of products discussed in their content. This information is acknowledged solely for the information of the readers.

The contributors provided the following disclosure and vested interest information:

Elizabeth A. Ayello, PhD, RN, ACNS-BC, ETN, FAPWCA, FAAN, 3M Healthcare, Molnlycke, Smith + Nephew, MEDLINE, Healthpoint, Coloplast, Hill-Rom, KCI, speakers bureaus and consultant

Sharon Baranoski, RN, MSN, CWOCN, APN, DAPWCA, FAAN, Wolters Kluwer Health, Lippincott Williams & Wilkins, Molnlycke Healthcare, Hill-Rom, MEDLINE, consultant; American Professional Wound Care Association, board member; Agency for Healthcare Research and Quality, advisory board

Vanna M. Dest, MSN, APRN-BC, AOCN®, Myriad Laboratories, EUSA Pharmaceuticals, speakers bureaus

Pamela Savage, RN, MAEd, CON(C), 3M Healthcare Canada, consultant, presenter; Molnlycke Healthcare, Healthpoint, presenter

Melodie Young, MSN, RN, ANP-C, GNPc, Abbott, Amgen, Centocor, consultant and speaker; Celgene, Basilea, Tolmar, sub-investigator

Contents

Chapter 4. Malignant Cutaneous Diseases   77

Chapter 5. Wound Care Products and Treatments   101

Chapter 6. Radiation-Induced Skin Reactions   115

Chapter 7. Systemic Therapy–Induced Skin Reactions   141

Chapter 8. Cutaneous Effects of Blood and Marrow Transplantation   167

Chapter 9. Impact of Chronic Disease on Wound Healing   195

Chapter 10. Impact of Systemic and Infectious Skin Disease During Cancer Treatment   215

Chapter 11. Skin and Wound Pain: Assessment and Management   237

Chapter 12. Psychological Distress Related to Skin Problems in the Oncology Patient Population   257

Preface

A few minutes after the nurse entered the exam room, the patient's head remained bowed, raising only to utter the words "I feel like I am on fire, and I am not sure I want to finish treatment." The patient just completed his fifth week of chemotherapy and radiation to his head and neck. Knowing the likely cause of the patient's discomfort, the oncology nurse immediately inspected the patient's skin. The treatment field, once pink, was now brightly erythematic, moist in the crease of his neck, and skin taut.

Oncology nurses face this situation every day in their clinical practice. Knowing when to expect skin reactions is easy, but it is the intervention that becomes a challenge. There are no standard guidelines to follow or quick pocket guides that contain algorithms. Often oncology nurses rely on their own clinical pearls to help the patient. In the opening scenario, the oncology nurse searches for the clinical evidence to treat the patient's skin reaction.

Principles of Skin Care and the Oncology Patient begins to address issues of skin care and helps to guide physicians, nurse practitioners/physician assistants, and nurses who care for patients with cancer who develop skin problems. Information about evidence-based principles and practice guidelines in caring for the oncology patient who has developed skin problems is presented. The chapters begin with an in-depth discussion about anatomy and physiology of the skin and accessory organs, including the healing process after injury. Also included is a review of common drug reactions that can cause cutaneous manifestations. Benign and malignant cutaneous diseases are presented. A nursing expert in wound and ostomy care shares clinical decision making when selecting wound care products and treatments. Skin reactions caused by radiation and chemotherapy are highlighted, and manifestations are discussed. A more specific topic of cutaneous effects from blood and marrow transplantation is shared, highlighting acute and chronic graft-versus-host disease. The topics of wound pain, psychological distress, nutritional needs for healing, chronic disease, systemic and infectious diseases, complementary therapies, and special needs of the gero-oncology patient are presented in relation to skin problems.

The following work begins to answer the opening concerns of the oncology nurse: Where is the supportive evidence to treat oncology patients with skin reactions? The efforts of many authors to synthesize scientific information have strengthened the quest to build a foundation of knowledge with the expectation to improve the quality of care for patients with cancer.

CHAPTER 1

Overview of Skin Issues Related to the Oncology Patient

William P. Hogle, RN, MSN, OCN®

Introduction

The skin acts as a tough exterior barrier of protection; it is essentially the body's first line of defense. It also serves as a host to numerous microorganisms and is reactive to innumerable external stimuli, including stress. As a result, patients frequently ask healthcare professionals to assess some variation of rash, abrasion, excoriation, ulceration, pruritus, or inflammatory cutaneous reaction. These common and often benign complaints occur with a high degree of frequency among the general population. When these same complaints occur among patients with cancer, oncology practitioners have much to consider in terms of the cause (treatment-related or from other factors), comorbid conditions, and the potential impact any intervention may have on the reaction. The purpose of this chapter is to provide basic background knowledge about the integumentary system and surrounding soft tissues, as well as a basic understanding of normal tissue healing. A general overview of evidence-based risk factors for poor wound healing is provided, and a brief review of the paradigm of support for wound healing is explored.

On a large scale, the integumentary system consists of skin, sweat and sebaceous glands, hair follicles, and nails. Together, these components function to protect, moderate temperature, and excrete waste. On a smaller scale, the integumentary system consists of water molecules, proteins, lipids, and numerous minerals and chemical components. Skin, the primary component of the integumentary system, is the largest organ of the human body. Often taken for granted, the skin is pliable and water resistant. In an average adult, skin weighs 9–11 pounds and accounts for approximately 7% of total body weight. Skin varies in thickness from 0.05 mm (eyelids) up to 4 mm or more (soles and palms). The skin is divided into three layers: the epidermis, the dermis, and the subcutaneous tissue, also referred to as the hypodermis (Marieb, 2001) (see Figure 1-1).

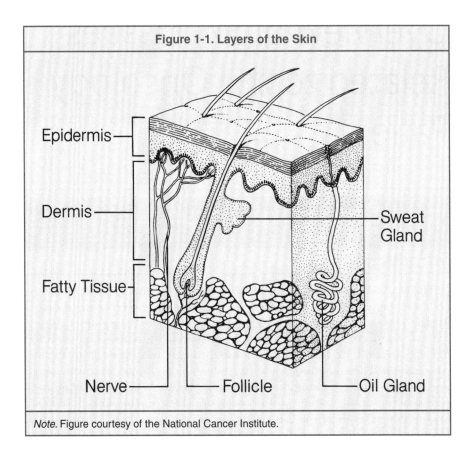

Figure 1-1. Layers of the Skin

Note. Figure courtesy of the National Cancer Institute.

Epidermis

The *epidermis* is the outermost portion of the skin and is a stratified squamous epithelium. Throughout the epidermis, typically four different cell types can be found: *melanocytes*, which synthesize pigment; *Langerhans cells*, which help to activate the immune system; *Merkel cells*, which perform sensory functions; and *keratinocytes*, which gradually mature to serve as the outermost layer of skin. Variations in total skin thickness are determined by the thickness of the epidermis in a given area. Thicker skin consists of all five layers of the epidermis: stratum basale, stratum spinosum, stratum granulosum, stratum lucidum, and stratum corneum. Thinner skin consists of the same layers except for the stratum lucidum, although each layer has less volume (Marieb, 2001; Shier, Butler, & Lewis, 2004).

Stratum Basale

The *stratum basale* is the deepest of all epidermal layers and is attached to the dermis in an uneven, almost wave-like, fashion. This layer consists of the youngest of keratinocytes, which are constantly undergoing rapid division. Melanocytes and Merkel cells also can be seen in the stratum basale. From this layer, keratinocytes continually work their way up to the skin surface while undergoing gradual changes through each successive layer of the epidermis (Shier et al., 2004).

Stratum Spinosum

The *stratum spinosum* consists of web-like filaments that are made up of tension-resisting bundles of pre-keratin filaments. At this level, keratinocytes are flatter than in the stratum basale, are irregular in shape, and are sometimes referred to as *prickle cells*. Melanin and Langerhans cells are abundant in this layer (Shier et al., 2004).

Stratum Granulosum

In the *stratum granulosum*, keratinocytes continue to surface while undergoing further visual change by flattening and acquiring properties that aid in their ability to retain fluid. Glycolipids are acquired by the keratinocyte, and their plasma membrane thickens so as to become more resilient to everyday use and exposure. At this level, the keratinocyte begins to grow beyond capillary extension and begins to die (Shier et al., 2004).

Stratum Lucidum

The *stratum lucidum* is a layer that consists of clear, flat, dead keratinocytes and is seen in the thickened skin of the palms and soles.

Stratum Corneum

The *stratum corneum*, also referred to as the horny layer, makes up approximately 75% of the epidermal thickness and is the outermost layer of the epidermis. At this layer, hardened keratinocytes protect against physical assault, and glycolipids between each cell act to waterproof the entire body (Shier et al., 2004).

Dermis

The *dermis* is the second major skin layer and consists of strong, flexible connective tissue. This layer is made up of a semifluid matrix, which is heavily embedded with collagen, elastin, and reticular fibers. Cells most frequently seen in the dermis are similar to those seen in other connective tissue and include fibroblasts, mast cells, and leukocytes. The dermis also contains numerous nerve fibers and appendages of the integumentary system, such as sweat and sebaceous glands and hair follicles. The dermis consists of two layers, the papillary layer and the reticular layer. Together, these layers act to bind the epidermis to the underlying tissue (Marieb, 2001; Shier et al., 2004).

Papillary Layer

The *papillary layer* of the dermis is a thin superficial layer of connective tissue that contains collagen and elastin fibers and a rich supply of blood vessels. It also contains a number of nerve fibers that are sensitive to light touch (*Meissner corpuscles*) and heavier pressure (*Pacinian corpuscles*), whereas others are sensitive to temperature. Here, dermal ridge patterns begin to form that give way to epidermal ridges, which are one's finger, palm, toe, and sole prints. These epidermal ridges allow people to grip surfaces by means of increased friction (Shier et al., 2004).

Reticular Layer

The deeper *reticular layer* accounts for most of the thickness of the dermis. It consists of dense connective tissue and dense collagen fibers. These collagen fibers provide strength and resiliency to the skin, allowing it to prevent many scrapes and cuts from penetrating into deeper skin and body tissues.

Subcutaneous Layer

The *subcutaneous layer* of skin lies beneath the dermis and consists largely of loose connective and adipose tissue. This layer functions mainly as a heat insulator, keeping heat inside and retarding excessive heat from outside the body. The amount of adipose tissue varies from one person to the next, as does the amount found in different portions of the body. Adipose tissue is thicker in the abdominal region and essentially nonexistent in the eyelids. An individual's nutritional status also influences the amount of adipose tissue found throughout the body (Shier et al., 2004).

Accessory Organs of the Skin

Along with the skin itself, the integumentary system contains a number of accessory organs, sometimes referred to as skin appendages, including sweat and sebaceous glands, hair and hair follicles, and nails.

Sweat Glands

Sweat glands, also referred to as *sudoriferous* glands, can be found in all regions of the body. Some sweat glands, apocrine glands, respond to emotional stress and sexual stimulation. They become active during puberty and are most abundant in the axillary regions, in the groin, and around the nipples. They are usually associated with hair follicles. Other sweat glands, the *eccrine* glands, respond to elevated body temperature from environmental heat or physical exercise. These glands are not associated with hair follicles and are common on the forehead, neck, and back. Fluid secreted by sweat glands is carried to the surface of the skin through the pores. Sweat contains body salts, urea, and uric acid. Thus, the sweat glands function, to a small degree, to remove waste from the body (Shier et al., 2004).

Sebaceous Glands

Sebaceous glands, also referred to as *oil glands*, are found throughout the skin, except on the palms and soles. These glands produce globules of fatty material that accumulate, causing cells to swell and burst. The resulting mixture of cellular debris and fatty material is called *sebum*. When sebum is excreted through hair follicles, as it often is, it helps to maintain pliability and waterproof ability of hair and skin. Sebum sometimes is excreted directly to the skin surface, such as from the lips, corners of the mouth, or external reproductive organs (Shier et al., 2004).

Hair and Hair Follicles

Hair is present on all surface areas of the skin except the palms, soles, lips, nipples, and various parts of the external reproductive organs. Hair may appear very fine and less obvious or rather coarse and apparent. Each hair develops from a group of epidermal cells at the base of a tube-like depression called a *hair follicle*. The hair follicle extends from the surface into the dermis and may pass into the subcutaneous layer. Epidermal cells at the follicle's base receive nourishment from dermal blood vessels. As these epidermal cells grow and divide, older cells are pushed toward the surface, thus becoming keratinized, and die. Therefore, hair is actually composed of dead epidermal cells. Hair color is determined by the pigment produced by epidermal melanocytes at the base of the hair follicles. Dark hair contains an abundance of melanin, whereas blond hair contains an intermediate amount. Albino hair is absent of any pigment, and red hair contains iron pigment, or *trichosiderin*. A mixture of pigmented and unpigmented hair usually results in the appearance of gray hair (Shier et al., 2004).

Nails

Nails are protective coverings on the ends of the fingers and toes. Each nail consists of a *nail plate* that overlies a surface of skin known as the *nail bed*. The nail plate is produced by specialized epithelial cells that are continuous with the epithelium of the skin. The *lunula* is the whitish half-moon–shaped region at the base of each nail plate and is the most active region in terms of growth. The epithelial cells of the nail undergo heavy keratinization as they grow forward, thus giving the nail a hardened horn-like consistency. Nails are useful for scratching and aid in picking up small objects (Shier et al., 2004).

Soft Tissue

In humans, as in all complex organisms, cells are organized into layers or groups called *tissues*. *Soft tissue* is a term that can be used to describe muscle and fascia, or it can be used in a broader sense to include multiple different types of tissues, including but not limited to skin. Although the cells of different tissues vary in size, shape, arrangement, and function, those within a particular tissue are rather similar. The tissues of the human body include the following four major classifications:
- Epithelial tissue
- Connective tissue
- Muscle tissue
- Nervous tissue.

Epithelial Tissue

Epithelial tissue consists mostly of epithelial cells, which were discussed throughout the previous section. Epithelial tissue is widespread and essentially covers all body surfaces. It is the major tissue of the glands. The underside of the epithelial tissue is anchored to connective tissue by a thin, nonliving layer called the *basement membrane.* Generally, epithelial tissue lacks blood vessels and is nourished by underlying connective tissue. Although the cells of some tissues have limited abilities to reproduce, epithelial cells reproduce readily. Thus, injuries to the skin and lining of the gastrointestinal tract heal relatively quickly, as epithelial tissue is quite abundant in these areas. Epithelial tissues are classified according to shape, arrangement, and function (Shier et al., 2004) (see Table 1-1).
- *Simple:* Composed of single layers of cells
- *Stratified:* Those with many layers of cells
- *Squamous:* Those with thin, flattened cells
- *Cuboidal:* Those with cube-like cells
- *Columnar:* Those with elongated cells.

In addition, glandular tissue, or *glandular epithelium,* is also a type of epithelial tissue that is composed of specialized cells that produce and secrete various substances into ducts or body fluids. These glandular cells usually are found in columnar or cuboidal epithelium. Glands that secrete into ducts that open onto an internal or external surface are called *exocrine* glands, and glands that secrete into tissue or blood are called *endocrine* glands.

Table 1-1. Types of Epithelial Tissue			
Type	**Description**	**Function**	**Location**
Simple squamous epithelium	Single layer, flattened cells	Filtration, diffusion, osmosis, covers surface	Alveoli, capillary walls, linings of blood and lymph vessels
Simple cuboidal epithelium	Single layer, cube-shaped cells	Secretion, absorption	Surface of ovaries, linings of kidney tubules, and linings of ducts of certain glands
Simple columnar epithelium	Single layer, elongated cells	Protection, secretion, absorption	Linings of uterus, stomach, and intestines
Pseudostratified columnar epithelium	Single layer, elongated cells	Protection, secretion, movement of mucus and substances	Linings of respiratory passages
Stratified squamous epithelium	Many layers, top cells flattened	Protection	Outer layer of skin, linings of oral cavity, throat, vagina, anal canal
Stratified cuboidal epithelium	2–3 layers, cube-shaped cells	Protection	Lining of the larger ducts of the mammary glands, sweat glands, salivary glands, and the pancreas
Stratified columnar epithelium	Top layer of elongated cells, lower layers of cube-shaped cells	Protection, secretion	Vas deferens, part of the male urethra, parts of the pharynx
Transitional epithelium	Many layers of cube-shaped and elongated cells	Distensibility, protection	Inner lining of urinary bladder, and linings of ureters and part of urethra
Glandular epithelium	Unicellular or multicellular	Secretion	Salivary glands, sweat glands, endocrine glands

Note. From *Hole's Human Anatomy and Physiology* (10th ed., p. 141), by D. Shier, J. Butler, and R. Lewis, 2004, Boston: McGraw-Hill. Copyright 2004 by McGraw-Hill. Reprinted with permission.

Connective Tissue

Connective tissues are present in all parts of the body and act to bind structures together, provide support and protection, store fat, produce blood cells, and assist in repair of damaged tissue. Connective tissues have an abundance of intercellular matrix that consists of fibers and a ground substance whose consistency varies from fluid to semisolid or solid. Some connective tissues, such as bone and cartilage, are quite rigid. Loose, adipose, and fibrous connective tissues are much more flexible (see Table 1-2). Another connective tissue, blood, is mostly liquid in form and sometimes referred to as reticuloendothelial tissue. It is composed of a variety of specialized cells that are widely scattered throughout the body. Although a variety of cells can be found in the more flexible and rigid types of connective tissue, such tissues routinely consist of fibroblasts, macrophages, and mast cells. Other types of white blood cells may be present as well; however, this usually is in response to some type of infection in a particular area (Shier et al., 2004).

Muscle Tissue

Muscle tissues are contractile and consist of fibers that can change shape by becoming shorter and thicker. As muscle fibers contract, they pull at their attached ends, resulting in body movement. The three types of muscle tissue are
- Skeletal
- Smooth
- Cardiac.

Skeletal muscles are attached to bones and can be controlled by conscious effort and therefore are called *voluntary muscles*. These types of muscle are striated in appearance and are responsible for all movements of the head, trunk, and limbs, as well as for chewing, swallowing, and breathing. Smooth muscles are not striated and cannot be stimulated to contract through conscious effort. Smooth muscle tissue is found in the walls of hollow organs and is responsible for moving matter such as blood, digested matter, or urinary waste through a particular part of the body. *Cardiac* muscle tissue is striated and is found only in the heart. It is controlled involuntarily and can continue to function without being stimulated by nerve impulses. This type of muscle tissue makes up the bulk of the heart and is responsible for pumping blood through the heart chambers and into the blood vessels (Shier et al., 2004).

Nervous Tissue

Nervous tissue consists of *neurons*, which are considered highly specialized body cells. Neurons are very sensitive to changes in their environment and respond by transmitting nerve impulses to other neurons or to muscles and glands. Their role is to coordinate and regulate many body functions. In addition to neurons, *neuroglial* cells are present in nervous tissue. These cells bind and support the components of nervous tissue that are active during phago-

Table 1-2. Types of Connective Tissue			
Type	**Description**	**Function**	**Location**
Loose connective tissue	Cells in fluid-gel matrix	Binds organs together, holds tissue fluids	Beneath the skin, between muscles, beneath most epithelial tissues
Adipose tissue	Cells in fluid-gel matrix	Protection, insulation, and storage of fat	Beneath the skin, around the kidneys, behind the eyes, on the surface of the heart
Reticular connective tissue	Cells in fluid-gel matrix	Support	Walls of liver, spleen, and lymphatic organs
Dense connective tissue	Cells in fluid-gel matrix	Binds organs together	Tendons, ligaments, dermis
Elastic connective tissue	Cells in fluid-gel matrix	Provision of elastic quality	Connecting parts of spinal column, in walls of arteries and airways
Hyaline cartilage	Cells in solid-gel matrix	Support, protection, provision of framework	Ends of bones, nose, and rings in walls of respiratory passages
Elastic cartilage	Cells in solid-gel matrix	Support, protection, provision of flexible framework	Framework of external ear and part of larynx
Fibrocartilage	Cells in solid-gel matrix	Support, protection, absorption of shock	Between bony parts of spinal column, parts of pelvic girdle, and knee
Bone	Cells in solid matrix	Support, protection, provision of framework	Bones of skeleton, middle ear
Blood	Cells and platelets in fluid matrix	Transportation of gases, defense against disease, clotting	Throughout the body within a closed system of blood vessels and heart chambers

Note. From *Hole's Human Anatomy and Physiology* (10th ed., p. 150), by D. Shier, J. Butler, and R. Lewis, 2004, Boston: McGraw-Hill. Copyright 2004 by McGraw-Hill. Reprinted with permission.

cytosis and help to supply nourishment to neurons by connecting them to blood vessels. Nervous tissue is only found in the brain, spinal cord, and peripheral nerves (Shier et al., 2004).

Epithelial Tissue Reproduction

The cells of the four types of tissue previously described vary greatly in their abilities to reproduce. Epithelial cells, found in the skin and digestive tract, and connective tissue cells, found in the blood and bone marrow, continuously reproduce. However, striated, cardiac muscle, and nerve cells show little propensity to reproduce after becoming differentiated. Fibroblasts, found primarily in connective tissue, respond rapidly to injuries and are the principal agents of repair. In tissues where fibroblasts are limited, such as cardiac and nerve, healing from assault or degeneration is absent or limited at best.

The Healing Process

Few organs in the body can regenerate and self-heal to the extent that skin can. Normal skin and wound healing in an individual without risk factors for altered wound healing occurs in a series of distinct phases. The time it takes for healing to occur varies widely from person to person. Additionally, all wounds, even if on the same person, do not heal at the same rate. Therefore, predictions as to how long a wound will take to heal in a person without comorbidities are based on knowledge of the skin and wound healing process and clinical experience. A number of conditions can affect wound healing, many of which are described later in this chapter. The process by which damaged skin heals depends largely on the extent of the injury. If a break in the skin is shallow, epithelial cells along its margin are stimulated to reproduce more rapidly than usual, and the newly formed cells simply fill in the defect. If the injury extends into the dermis or subcutaneous layer, then a more intricately detailed and systematic approach to healing occurs (McNees, 2006).

Healing is a natural restorative response to tissue injury. Wound healing has three distinct and highly complex phases, although some literature has described models with four or five phases. This three-phase description combines most of the actions that are addressed in lengthier models:
• Hemostatic/inflammatory phase
• Fibroblastic or proliferation/granulation phase
• Maturation or remodeling phase.

Hemostatic Phase

During the hemostatic phase, the body is essentially attempting to stop or minimize external bleeding while mobilizing agents necessary for later wound healing. Platelets and the agents they secrete are most active during this phase. Platelets begin to clump or accumulate so as to form a clot that acts to seal any nearby bleeding vessels. In addition, as platelets congregate, they secrete substances that aid in the production of *thrombin*, which, in turn, stimulates *fibrin* production. Fibrin then forms a mesh-like structure that works with the actual clot formation to solidify a hemostatic plug at the site of injury. An increased accumulation of prostaglandins, histamine, and vasoactive agents further aids hemostasis. Essentially, enzymes and coagulation factors are stimulated in a sequential manner so as to activate what is referred to as the *coagulation cascade* (see Figure 1-2). A number of inhibitors and control mechanisms keep the clotting reaction local-

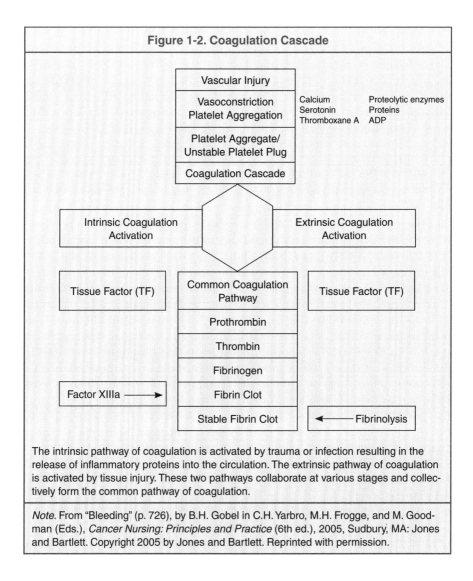

Figure 1-2. Coagulation Cascade

The intrinsic pathway of coagulation is activated by trauma or infection resulting in the release of inflammatory proteins into the circulation. The extrinsic pathway of coagulation is activated by tissue injury. These two pathways collaborate at various stages and collectively form the common pathway of coagulation.

Note. From "Bleeding" (p. 726), by B.H. Gobel in C.H. Yarbro, M.H. Frogge, and M. Goodman (Eds.), *Cancer Nursing: Principles and Practice* (6th ed.), 2005, Sudbury, MA: Jones and Bartlett. Copyright 2005 by Jones and Bartlett. Reprinted with permission.

ized to the site of injury. When these control mechanisms fail, coagulopathy occurs, including thrombocytopenia and disseminated intravascular coagulation (McNees, 2006).

The hemostasis phase of healing also includes an accumulation of leukocytes and monocytes, which is needed to mount an immune response against any invasive pathogen. Thus, the initiation of a humoral immune response takes place during this first phase of wound healing.

Fibroblastic Phase

During the fibroblastic phase, existing fibroblasts are mobilized and their proliferation increases so as to synthesize collagen production. *Fibroblasts*, the most common cell in connective tissue, produce fibers of protein; one such protein is *collagen*. Collagen fibers are only slightly elastic and occur in bundles. Collagen is essential for strengthening the wound site. Fibroblasts also initiate the production of *granulation* tissue, which is vascular connective tissue. This is the initial process of reestablishing microcirculation to a wound to supply needed oxygen and nutrients while removing waste and debris (McNees, 2006; Romo, Pearson, Yalamanchili, & Zoumalan, 2008).

Maturation Phase

The *maturation*, or *remodeling*, phase is the final and most time-intensive phase of the healing process. During maturation, successive collagen replacement occurs many times over. With each successive replacement, the previously damaged tissue is essentially attempting to become successful clones of the cells that were in place prior to any injury. After each replacement, the general appearance improves, and a scar may appear at the site of injury. Additional collagen replacements result in further visual improvements and softening of scar tissue. A scar can form wherever a wound or ulceration has occurred. The scarred epidermis is thin and generally without normal skin lines. If an overgrowth of collagen fibers and capillaries occurs, a *keloid* or *hypertrophic* scar may result. Keloids differ from normal scars in that they tend to increase in dimension over time, grow beyond the border of the original wound, and do not spontaneously regress. Keloids can result in numbness, tingling, itching, pain, and deformity (Robbins, 2007). Hypertrophic scars stay within the original borders of injury and usually resolve spontaneously. Little is known as to the complete etiology of keloids and hypertrophic scars. Abnormalities associated with these irregularities include the following (Romo et al., 2008):

- Abnormal cell migration
- Proliferation
- Inflammation
- Synthesis and secretion of extracellular matrix proteins and cytokines.

If skin loss from a cut, deep abrasion, or burn has occurred, the process of healing previously described involves two other elements: re-epithelialization and wound contracture. Normally, when skin has been removed, epithelial cells migrate across the surface area of the wound. This process begins at the wound edges. If a wound edge is compromised by tissue sloughing or by means of a burn, re-epithelialization can be very slow to occur. In these cases, flaps or grafts may be necessary to close an open wound. Wound contracture, although not dependent on collagen synthesis, occurs at the same time during the fibroblastic phase of healing. *Wound contracture* is defined as the centripetal movement of wound edges that facilitates closure of the wound defect. Maximal wound contraction occurs 5–15 days from initial injury (Romo et al., 2008).

Skin Burns

Depending on its severity, a skin burn can be traumatic and even life threatening. A skin burn does not necessarily result in a break in the integrity of the skin. In such cases, healing occurs through a gradual process of basal and epithelial cell replacement. The erythema initially seen in a burn or burn-like reaction usually is transient and the result of capillary dilation and increased vascular permeability. Subsequent redness from a minor burn is caused by a release of histamine from damaged cells (Sparks, 2007). Other reactions resulting from mild to moderate burns, such as hypo- or hyperpigmentation, desquamation, and fibrosis, are typical reactions to radiation therapy and are covered in Chapter 6.

A burn can result from
- Ultraviolet radiation damage (including solar exposure)
- High-energy x-rays or gamma rays (from megavoltage radiation therapy)
- Thermal damage (fires or exposure to extremely hot surface or liquids)
- Chemical damage (when chemical compounds interact with the skin surface)
- Electrical damage (including electrical accidents and lightning strikes)
- Friction or abrasion.

As with other types of injuries, the skin's response to a burn depends on the amount of damage it sustains. For the purpose of description and treatment, burns are classified according to the depth of tissue damage, regardless of the cause (Johnson & Richard, 2003).

Superficial Burn

Previously characterized as a first-degree burn, a *superficial burn* exists when the skin is only lightly burned. The area of injury may simply become warm and erythematous as dermal capillaries are dilated and histamine is released. Over time, the surface layer of the skin may shed. Superficial burns are considered the least serious of all burns, affect only the epidermis, and usually require little or no treatment. Excessive unprotected sun exposure usually results in a superficial burn to the skin. Long-term tissue damage is rare and usually consists of permanent hypo- or hyperpigmentation (Johnson & Richard, 2003; Morgan, Bledsoe, & Barker, 2000).

Superficial Partial-Thickness Burn

Previously characterized as a second-degree burn, a *partial-thickness burn* involves injury to the epidermis and part of the dermal layer of skin. Partial-thickness burns become intensely erythematous and are characterized by the appearance of blisters caused by fluid escaping from dermal capillaries, which accumulates beneath the outer layers of epidermal cells. When pressure is applied to the reddened area, the area will blanch but will demonstrate a rapid capillary refill upon release of the pressure. Edema may or may not be present, and the site of injury frequently is painful. Recovery from partial-thickness burns usually is complete, and scar tissue typically does not result unless infection occurs. Permanent hypo- or hyperpigmentation may result from a partial-thickness burn (Johnson & Richard, 2003; Morgan et al., 2000).

Deep Partial-Thickness Burn

As with a superficial partial-thickness burn, damage from a deep partial-thickness burn extends beyond the epidermis and into the reticular layer of the dermis. These burns present as mixed erythema/waxy white in appearance. Areas of redness may continue to blanch when pressure is applied, as capillary refill may be absent or sluggish when pressure is released. Blisters usually are absent, although the exposed surface of the wound is likely to appear wet or moist. Edema frequently is present, and sensation is altered with this type of injury (Johnson & Richard, 2003).

Full-Thickness Burn

Previously characterized as third-degree burns, *full-thickness burns* destroy the full thickness of the skin and may also damage subcutaneous and underlying tissues (including muscle and bone). A full-thickness burn affects every body system and organ. This type of burn can be completely painless because nerve tract and nerve endings may be totally burned away. The burn site appears white or charred, and ulceration often occurs as a result of such a serious assault to the skin's integrity. Repair of full-thickness burns often involves skin grafts transplanted from another area of one's body, called an *autograft*, or from a cadaveric donor or synthesized skin substitute, called a *homograft*. Permanent scarring, nerve damage, and contracture are not unusual following full-thickness burns. Patients with full-thickness burns are at risk for overriding sepsis, require aggressive medical support, and often undergo multiple reconstructive surgical procedures (Balasubramani, Kumar, & Babu, 2001; Johnson & Richard, 2003).

Impaired Skin and Wound Healing During Cancer Treatment

Patients receiving cancer treatment are at risk for altered skin integrity. Skin reactions are generally categorized as acute or chronic. *Acute* skin reactions from cancer treatment can be caused or exacerbated primarily as a result of three variables: patient-specific factors, treatment-related factors, and presence of chronic systemic or comorbid disease. *Chronic* skin reactions usually result in an altered appearance and are not typically a disruption of the skin integrity per se; exceptions might include chronic nonhealing wounds present before the initiation of treatment. In the presence of impaired vascularity, peripheral neuropathy, or preexisting collagen vascular disease, wounds can become chronic in nature and represent a significant challenge to the caregiver and patient. The presence of multiple variables will obviously increase one's likelihood for developing a disruption in skin integrity during cancer therapy. Therefore, careful assessment before initiation of treatment is important.

Patient-Related Factors

Patient-related factors that affect skin reactions include age (older patients are at increased risk), compromised nutritional status, low performance status, anatomic location of treatment area (skinfolds and body contour, especially with radiation therapy), degree of previous sun or radiation exposure, smoking, and one's individual degree of sensitivity to chemotherapy or radiation therapy (Maher, 2005; Pearce, 2005; Porock, Kristjanson, Nikoletti, Cameron, & Pedler, 1998). Patient-specific factors that influence skin and wound care are addressed in greater detail later in this chapter.

Treatment-Related Factors

At times, modalities used to treat malignancy can actually cause or impact the degree of disruption in one's skin integrity. Most chemotherapeutic toxicity profiles include the potential for some type of cutaneous reaction, including
- Pruritus
- General erythematous rash
- Hyperpigmentation
- Photosensitivity
- Alopecia
- Nail changes.

More serious reactions include urticaria, a sign of cutaneous hypersensitivity reaction, and *acral erythema*, also known as *palmar-plantar erythrodysesthesia* (hand-foot syndrome). Acral erythema is painful scaling and sloughing, along with erythema, of the palms and soles, followed by desquamation and reepithelialization of the skin (Camp-Sorrell, 2005). It is believed that acral erythema is a result of direct toxic effect on the epidermis and dermal vasculature or possibly an accumulation of chemotherapeutic agent in the eccrine glands, which are present in the palms and soles (Eich, Scharffetter-Kochanek, Eich, Tantcheva-Poor, & Krieg, 2002; Remlinger, 2003). Monoclonal antibodies that act as epidermal growth factor receptor (EGFR) inhibitors have been associated with skin toxicities, including acneform rash, folliculitis, skin dryness, pruritus, fissuring, and nail changes. The etiology of skin toxicity associated with the administration of EGFR inhibitors is unclear, but preclinical studies have demonstrated that it results from EGFR expression in normal skin (Perez-Soler & Saltz, 2005). The incidence of rash reported in numerous studies of EGFR inhibitors ranges from 37%–90% and is typically mild to moderate (grade 1 or 2), with severe (grade 3 or 4) rash uncommon (Oishi, 2008).

Some chemotherapeutic agents (5-fluorouracil, methotrexate, paclitaxel, and doxorubicin) and monoclonal antibodies, when given concurrently with radiation therapy, act synergistically. These agents may increase the severity of radiation skin reactions, cause them to occur at a lower dose of radiation, and possibly prolong the reaction (Maher, 2005; Oishi, 2008; Sparks, 2007).

Radiation therapy is known to cause a number of temporary skin reactions, including erythema, pruritus, and dry or moist desquamation. More permanent yet less common skin effects from radiation include the following (Chiao & Lee, 2005; D'Haese et al., 2005; Haas, 2005; Porock & Kristjanson, 1999):

• Fibrosis
• Telangiectasia
• Ulceration
• Necrosis.

Ionizing radiation inhibits the mitotic ability of stem cells within the basal layer, thus preventing the process of repopulation and weakening the integrity of the skin (Archambeau, Pezner, & Wasserman, 1995). The severity of skin reactions from radiation therapy is influenced by the

• Dose delivered with each treatment (fraction)
• Total cumulative dose
• Volume of tissue treated
• Type of radiation used (electrons and lower-energy photons produce higher skin doses and, thus, increased risk for skin reactions)
• Use of bolus material on the skin itself, which increases the total dose (D'Haese et al.; Haas; Porock et al., 1998).

Normal anatomic skinfolds in areas such as the axilla, inframammary region, groin, and perineum are at increased risk for adverse skin reactions secondary to radiation therapy (Haas). Obese patients are at even greater risk because obesity usually results in larger skinfold areas, which are more prone to increased moisture and friction.

Patients may experience *radiation recall*, which is an inflammatory skin reaction at a previously irradiated site subsequent to the administration of a number of pharmacologic agents, including anthracyclines, alkylating agents, antimetabolites, and taxanes. Such a reaction can occur days to years following radiation. The precise mechanism of action for radiation recall is poorly understood. Skin reactions commonly seen with radiation recall are erythema, maculopapular eruptions, vesicle formation, and desquamation of the affected areas. The reactions can range from mild rash to severe skin necrosis (Azria et al., 2005; Sparks, 2007).

Chronic Disease

Patients with cancer also may be affected by one or many states of chronic disease. Because of the very nature of chronic disease, its impact is eventually manifested in every body system. Although epidermal and dermal changes may take longer to occur, they can develop into alterations ranging from pruritus, erythema, or edema to discomfort, formation of lesions, cellulitis, or chronic ulceration. The following is a brief review of selected disease states and conditions and the effects they have on the integumentary system. For a more thorough and detailed review of how chronic, systemic, and infectious skin diseases affect the integumentary system, refer to Chapters 9 and 10.

Cardiovascular disease is a serious and complex state that can encompass a wide variety of systemic disorders. Peripheral obstructive arterial and venous conditions can result in increased intravascular pressure and reduced blood flow, or *stasis*. Stasis then may lead to vascular leak syndrome and possibly skin ulceration and thrombosis. Signs of decreased vascular flow include
• Skin discoloration
• Hyperpigmentation
• Pain
• Neuropathy
• Cyanosis.
Patients who have arterial stenosis or occlusion may develop *critical limb ischemia* (CLI), which occurs when basal requirements for tissue oxygenation cannot be met. Patients with diabetes mellitus are known to have diffuse and sometimes severe CLI. Ischemic ulcers, characteristic of CLI, are very painful and usually appear at the end of one's toes or over a bony prominence. Gangrene can result in end-stage CLI. These patients require aggressive debridement, antimicrobial therapy, and revascularization. Patients with venous insufficiency may develop ulcers from mechanisms similar to arterial insufficiency: increased pressure, leading to edema and tissue necrosis. *Stasis dermatitis* is a common dermatologic finding in patients with congestive heart failure (CHF). Dysfunction of the deep peripheral venous system, caused by CHF, leads to venous stasis and edema. Continued pressure from edema causes reduced oxygenation of the surrounding tissues and overlying skin. The result is localized pigmentation changes of the skin and possibly venous stasis ulceration (Englert, 2003; Jaff, 2001).

Lymphedema, whether primary or secondary in nature, is defined as chronic swelling caused by impairment in the lymphatic system drainage. When an obstruction develops in the lymphatic system, the flow of lymphatic fluid is circumvented into the surrounding interstitial tissue, thus causing an accumulation of a highly concentrated, protein-filled fluid in an area distal to the blockage. The fluid accumulation results in inflammation leading to skin changes and fibrosis. Skin affected by stage II or III lymphedema may leak or ooze fluid and is at increased risk for cellulitis, infection, or ulceration (Holcomb, 2006; Lawenda, Mondry, & Johnstone, 2009; Marrs, 2007). For more information about the stages of lymphedema, see Table 1-3.

Some pulmonary diseases can have cutaneous manifestations. These usually are not seen as primary characteristics of respiratory illness, and diagnosis typically is made long before symptoms are present. *Erythema multiforme* and *erythema nodosum* can be seen in bacterial pneumonia and sarcoidosis, respectively. Papules and skin nodules may be present in cases of bronchogenic carcinoma, and patients with tuberculosis may develop destructive skin lesions known as *lupus vulgaris* (Murray, 2000).

Chronic renal disease often results in varying degrees of pruritus, muscle weakness, and spontaneous tendon rupture. Pruritus in these patients is believed to be a result of high systemic levels of calcium and phosphorus (Martin, Gonzalez, & Slatopolsky, 2004). Other bone and soft-tissue disorders, such as erosive arthritis, joint effusions, and amyloidosis, also may exist in this patient population. In many cases, a parathyroidectomy can correct these abnormalities (Martin et al.). Another dermatologic effect of renal disease reported in up to 40% of patients is a condition known as *half-and-half nails* (HHNs).

Table 1-3. Stages of Lymphedema		
Stage	**Characteristics**	**Assessment Parameters**
Stage 0 Latency stage	Subclinical in nature	Asymptomatic, or mild heaviness of limb
Stage I Reversible lymphedema	Soft and pitting in nature without fibrosis	Prolonged elevation can lead to complete resolution.
Stage II Spontaneously irreversible lymphedema	Intradermal fibrosis, decreased suppleness, and decreased ability to pit, although pitting is possible.	Not reversible with elevation; skin on back of fingers and toes cannot be lifted or is lifted with difficulty. Pitting, if present, is measured on a 0–3+ scale.
Stage III Lymphostatic elephantiasis	Increase in severity of fibrosis and tissue volume; formation of cysts, fistulas, and papillomas more likely; adipose tissue can replace fluid in limbs.	As above in stage II, and skinfolds at wrist and ankles deepen.
Note. Based on information from Lawenda et al., 2009.		

Characterized by a dark distal band that occupies 20%–60% of the nail bed and by a white proximal band, HHNs typically disappear after successful renal transplantation. Pathophysiology for this condition is related to the proximal half of the nail appearing white because of edema associated with a dilated capillary network and the other half of the nail bed appearing normal (Headley & Wall, 2002; Martin et al.).

Patients with chronic liver disease may develop skin reactions. Palmar erythema is seen in 23% of patients with liver cirrhosis and is caused by abnormally high levels of serum estradiol, which typically is metabolized by the liver (Serrao, Zirwas, & English, 2007). Another cutaneous manifestation of chronic liver disease, spider angioma, also is believed to result from elevated serum estradiol levels. Spider angiomas usually appear on the trunk and consist of a central arteriole from which radiate numerous small branching vessels. Pruritus is another fairly common symptom of hepatobiliary disease. It may or may not be associated with jaundice. It is believed that pruritus is caused by a build-up of bile acid and its derivatives (Khopkar & Pande, 2007). Jaundice can occur when the liver is stressed or damaged from either acute injury or chronic disease, such as hepatitis or cirrhosis. Jaundice results when bilirubin is produced in excess or when the liver is unable to excrete circulating bilirubin into the intestinal tract. As a result, bilirubin continues to circulate throughout the body and eventually is deposited into tissue and skin.

Autoimmune disorders such as systemic lupus erythematosus (SLE) and rheumatoid arthritis also can affect overall skin, joint, and soft-tissue health. Symptoms from autoimmune disease may vary over time and from patient to patient. Inflammation resulting from the autoimmune response leads to arthralgia and swollen joints. The dermatologic manifestations of SLE include (Myers & Allen, 2001)

- Butterfly rash
- Photosensitivity
- Mucosal ulcers
- Alopecia
- Pruritus
- Bruising.

Although not a disease state but rather a symptom of many disease states, peripheral neuropathy can predispose one to skin ulceration. Peripheral neuropathy is the end result of peripheral, motor, sensory, and autonomic neuron damage. Peripheral neuropathy can be categorized into three different types. The first is acquired—caused by environmental factors such as illness (including diabetes, renal disease, and nutritional deficiencies), infection, trauma, or chemical absorption, including chemotherapy-induced. The other two types are hereditary and idiopathic. The chemotherapeutic agents most frequently associated with peripheral neuropathy are platinum compounds, taxanes, vinca alkaloids, thalidomide, and bortezomib. Peripheral neuropathy can progress to *polyneuropathy* when numerous peripheral nerves become damaged or malfunction. Patients with chronic polyneuropathy may lose the ability to sense temperature and pain, often resulting in thermal burns or open wounds from prolonged pressure or friction (Cavaletti & Zanna, 2002; Visovsky, Collins, Abbott, Aschenbrenner, & Hart, 2007).

Patients with diabetes mellitus, in addition to having peripheral neuropathy, are at further risk for wound ulceration caused by atherosclerosis of the arteries and capillary system. Atherosclerosis prevents adequate transfer of oxygen and nutrients between the vascular system and surrounding tissues, leading to an ischemic state, which increases the likelihood of tissue breakdown. Patients with diabetes also frequently have inadequate collateral circulation to compensate for existing diseased vasculature (Mousley, 2007).

Impaired Wound Healing in Non-Comorbid Disease

In addition to comorbid disease, a number of variables influence one's ability to heal. These variables include those on which one can exert influence, such as nutrition, tobacco use, and, to some degree, body type and psychological distress. Other variables that are not completely within one's control but can certainly influence overall skin health and ability to heal include age, immune response, and the presence of foreign matter.

Age

With advanced age come increased chances of developing diabetes, cardiovascular disease, rheumatoid arthritis, and a number of other medical ailments that leave one susceptible to altered skin and delayed wound healing. In addition, as age increases, physical changes occur in the structure of the dermis and at the dermal-epidermal junction. These changes alter the appearance of the skin and predispose one to partial-thickness skin injuries, such as lateral skin tears (Gosain & DiPietro, 2004). Aging also results in a gradual decrease in the production of collagen and elastin, resulting in fine wrinkles, thinning of the skin, and loss of underlying fat (Pittman, 2007). Lastly, the three phases of healing, as previously discussed in this chapter, exhibit characteristic changes with aging. Decreased levels of growth factors, diminished cell proliferation and migration, and diminished extracellular matrix secretion have been demonstrated (Gosain & DiPietro). Detailed information regarding skin and healing issues in older adult patients with cancer can be found in Chapter 15.

Nutrition

Individuals with certain types of cancer are at increased risk for malnutrition. Those with Hodgkin lymphoma and cancers of the upper respiratory and digestive tracts are at increased risk for weight loss and malnutrition from disease state, mechanical obstruction, and physiologic dysfunction resulting from local tumor progression (Bloch & Charuhas, 2002). Additionally, all cancer therapies can cause nutritional deficiencies, the degree of which depends on the area of treatment, type of treatment, number of therapeutic modalities utilized, dosage of therapy, and length of treatment (Cunningham & Huhmann, 2005).

Nutrition has long been examined as a variable in postoperative wound healing. A significant amount of literature supports this, with numerous studies reporting on the negative effects of poor nutrition, or malnourishment, in patients who have undergone dental, orthopedic, and amputation procedures. In many cases, patients with decreased serum albumin levels, or those categorized as malnourished, did not fare as well when compared to nonmalnourished patients with regard to postamputation wounds and fractured hips (Foster, Heppenstall, Friedenberg, & Hozack, 1990; Kay, Moreland, & Schmitter, 1987; Marin, Salido, Lopez, & Silva, 2002; Pedersen & Pedersen, 1992). For detailed information about nutrition and its impact on wound healing, refer to Chapter 13.

Smoking

The significance of smoking relates to the reduced ability of cells to reoxygenate during cancer treatment, as well as the adverse effects of nicotine on wound healing and cutaneous vasoconstriction (Wells & MacBride, 2003). Smoking has long been associated with a number of dermatologic conditions, such as poor wound healing, premature skin aging, squamous cell carcinoma, melanoma, oral cancer, psoriasis, and hair loss. Smoking also has an impact on the skin lesions observed in patients with diabetes and lupus. In vitro studies suggest that tobacco smoke impairs the production of collagen and increases the production of tropoelastin and matrix metalloproteinases, which degrade matrix proteins (Freiman, Bird, Metelitsa, Barankin, & Lauzon, 2004; Morita, 2007). Numerous studies have suggested a link between smoking and poor wound healing in the postoperative setting. Recently, Artioukh, Smith, and Gokul (2007) identified smoking as a risk factor for impaired perineal wound healing following resection for rectal carcinoma. Furthermore, patients who smoked while undergoing hyperbaric oxygen therapy for chronic wounds had a poor response, despite receiving treatment known to improve the healing potential of chronic wounds (Oubre, Roy, Toner, & Kalns, 2007).

Body Type

Obesity has been cited as a risk factor for many diseases and is known to increase the rate of complications following surgery. Obese patients are at risk for impaired mobility, which directly affects the likelihood of developing pressure ulcers. With extreme obesity comes the risk of lower extremity edema, thromboembolic disease, skin compression, fungal infections, and venous stasis ulcers (Gates, Davis, & Evans, 2005). Surgical wounds are more prone to dehiscence and evisceration in obese patients because of increased tension on the edges of the fascia at the time of wound closure (Hahler, 2006). Derzie, Silvestri, Liriano, and Benotti (2000) reported a 15% postoperative complication rate among morbidly obese patients, including seroma formation, wound dehiscence, and wound infections. Obese patients were found to have higher rates of complications including flap loss, hematoma, delayed wound healing, and donor site hernia when compared to normal weight or overweight patients following transverse rectus abdominis myocutaneous flap reconstructions (Spear, Ducic, Cuoco, & Taylor, 2007).

Emaciated or extremely thin patients are also at risk for skin alterations or impaired wound healing. This may be partly because these individuals are malnourished and thus are at increased risk for a number of systemic complications. In addition, immobile patients with little or no body weight are at increased risk for pressure ulcers, particularly near a bony prominence.

Patients who have a stoma are at risk for skin excoriation or localized infection, usually candidal in nature. Factors leading to skin alterations secondary to stoma include improper anatomic location, appliance failure, or poor stoma care. A stoma should be constructed so that it is visible to the patient and located away from the umbilicus, skin creases, scars, and bony prominences. Areas damaged by radiation therapy or altered by skin grafts should be avoided. Localized skin irritations around the stoma can result from prolonged contact with fecal or urinary waste or from an allergic reaction to a portion of the appliance itself. Local skin care and patient or caregiver education usually resolve problems with ill-fitting appliances and poor hygiene practices (Lavery & Erwin-Toth, 2004; Minkes, McLean, Mazziotti, & Langer, 2008).

Infection/Immune Response

Open skin wounds do not have the protective defense mechanisms of intact skin, and all are colonized with microbial organisms. *Wound contamination* is defined as the presence of nonreplicating organisms within that wound. *Colonization* is defined as the presence of replicating microorganisms adherent to the wound in the absence of tissue damage. Colonization alone does not interfere with the wound healing process. In fact, chronic wounds support the existence of a diverse microbial flora. Subinfective levels of bacteria within a wound are important in determining the degree of inflammation and appear to accelerate wound healing and formation of granulation tissue, with increased infiltration of neutrophils, monocytes, and macrophages. Inflammation is a normal component of the immune response. However, an excessive inflammatory response can prolong the repair and healing process. A number of variables have been shown to influence whether colonizing wounds progress to wound infection and subsequently delay healing. These variables include the following (Bucknall, 1980; Davies et al., 2007; Dow, Browne, & Sibbald, 1999; Edwards & Harding, 2004; Konturek et al., 2001; Laato, Niiniko-ski, Lundberg, & Gerdin, 1988; Wysocki, 2002):

- Present bacteria level less than 10^5 per gram of tissue
- Virulence and pathogenicity of the organism
- Presence of four or more bacterial species in a given wound
- Ability of the host to mount an effective immune response.

The ability to mount an immune response is a key issue to the oncology patient population. Neutropenia and neutrophil dysfunction in conjunction with radiation therapy, steroids, and microvascular disease are found to pre-dispose patients with cancer to bacterial infection and have been associated with delayed wound healing (Meuli et al., 2001). Many of the treatment reg-imens used in oncology can cause mild to severe neutropenia. A number of studies have examined rates of infection among neutropenic patients. Elihu and Gollin (2007) conducted a retrospective review of children with low abso-lute neutrophil counts and patients who had a central venous catheter insert-ed. This study reported that placement of a central venous catheter in neutro-penic children was associated with substantial infectious morbidity and one death. However, a review of 18 published series in adults showed that neutro-penia on the day of catheter insertion was not associated with infectious com-plications (Press, Ramsey, Larson, Fefer, & Hickman, 1984). This is contrary to the findings by Howell, Walters, Donowitz, and Farr (1995), who conclud-ed that neutropenia was an independent risk factor for infection related to long-dwelling tunneled central venous catheters.

Marin et al. (2002) looked at patients outside of the oncology realm and examined those receiving a hip or knee prosthetic. The researchers reported that the patient's preoperative lymphocyte count (when less than 1,500 cells/mm^3) was associated with a delay in postoperative wound healing.

Psychological Distress

Stress has a documented influence on the immune system. Chronic stress, in general, has immunosuppressive effects, whereas acute stress has stimula-tory effects on immune function (Bauer-Wu & Post-White, 2005). People un-dergoing treatment for cancer not only have an altered immune system, but they often are also subject to feelings of psychological distress. Psychological stressors are experienced along the continuum of cancer, beginning prior to diagnosis, continuing through primary prevention activities to tertiary care strategies related to treatment, survivorship, and palliative care (Zichi-Cohen & Carlson, 2005). Studies performed outside the oncology population have demonstrated that acute psychological stress delays skin barrier function, re-covery, and healing (Altemus, Rao, Dhabhar, Ding, & Granstein, 2001; Garg et al., 2001; Robles, 2007). Furthermore, depressive symptoms were also pre-dictive of delayed mucosal wound healing in healthy young adults (Bosch, Engeland, Cacioppo, & Marucha, 2007). A detailed review of how psycholog-ical distress affects skin and wound healing is provided in Chapter 12.

Foreign Matter

Any material foreign to the body, once impregnated or retained within, can cause an acute reaction resulting in local and potentially systemic complications. If not removed, foreign objects can cause prolonged inflammation, infection, ulceration, fistula, and possibly necrosis. Foreign objects can include

- Debris (e.g., gravel, wood, glass) or shrapnel from a traumatic injury
- Ingestion of nonfood materials (e.g., magnets, coins, pins, small toys)
- A retained object from a surgical procedure (e.g., sponge, needles, instruments).

The medical literature is scattered with reports of retained surgical material from days, months, and even years after one's original date of surgery. Although many of these cases do not necessarily result in complications, some have resulted in nonhealing fistulous wounds, hematomas, obstructions, and abscess formation (Abdul-Karim, Benevenia, Pathria, & Makely, 1992; Gencosmanoglu & Inceoglu, 2003; Lone, Bhat, Tak, & Garcoo, 2005).

Occasionally, a foreign body such as a subcutaneous port, defibrillator, or pacemaker placed for therapeutic purposes may result in skin erosion or fistula tract formation (Camp-Sorrell, 2004; Kolker, Redstone, & Tutela, 2007; Nathan, Piccione, Kumar, Attanasio, & Schaer, 2006). Implantable subcutaneous ports, placed in the subclavicular area or in the arm used for chemotherapy administration and venous access, are known to erode through the skin surface. The incidence of this occurring is quite low, with only a handful of anecdotal cases reported (Almhanna, Pelley, Budd, Davidson, & Moore, 2008; Camp-Sorrell, 2004; Lersch et al., 1999). Port erosion can occur as a result of wound dehiscence, repeated access in the same location, loss of viable tissue over the portal body, and poor healing of the wound insertion site. In addition, the frequent use of topical anesthetic sprays, such as ethyl chloride, can be a cause of skin breakdown (Beheshti et al., 1998; Camp-Sorrell, 1992; Lersch et al.; Moureau & Zonderman, 2000; Whitman, 1996).

Paradigm of Support for Wound Healing

As with any adverse or damaging effect, an underlying cause must be recognized and stopped before complete repair and healing can begin. The medical literature has identified a number of factors that inhibit wound healing. Most are in some way related to external trauma (including radiation or chemical burns) or pressure, vascular insufficiency, infection, comorbid disease, or adverse effects of medication or treatment. It is perceivable that removal of the causative factor may not always be possible (e.g., with permanent edema, chronic disease, incurable malignancy) and, thus, complete healing may never occur or may occur on a very gradual basis over a prolonged period of time. However, in most cases, even chronic wounds can be healed given adequate nutrition and aggressive intervention.

Keast and Orsted (1998) proposed the following three fundamental principles that underlie wound care:
- Identification and, if possible, control of underlying causes
- Support of patient-centered concerns
- Optimization of local wound care.

The identification and control of underlying causes is relatively self-explanatory and includes removing environmental causes of injury and minimizing the impact of comorbid factors. Support of patient-centered concerns entails including patients in the plan of care and gaining their support for that plan and each specific intervention. It also means being cognizant of any quality-of-life issues that may exist, such as difficulty with transportation for clinic visits, financial burdens, or acute or chronic pain that can affect one's degree of fatigue, compliance, and, possibly, nutritional status. Consideration should be given to any cultural influences that may affect wound care and management. Optimization of local wound care involves appropriate utilization of myriad medications, dressings, and treatment techniques that exist. For specific interventions and wound care products, see Chapters 5 and 11.

McNees (2006) suggested the following five basic factors that guide the wound management process.
- If indicated, gentle cleansing of the wound using products supported by evidence-based research. Specific products known to impede wound healing should be avoided.
- If necrotic tissue is present, debridement by autolytic, enzymatic, or surgical means is to be strongly considered. *Autolytic debridement* involves the degradation and dissipation of devitalized tissues by using naturally occurring body fluids and enzymes from within the wound itself. This method requires a moist wound environment, thus often requiring some type of primary or cover dressing over the existing wound. *Enzymatic debridement* involves the addition of selective enzymes to the wound so as to expedite debridement. *Surgical debridement* involves the expeditious and manual surgical removal of devitalized tissue. When necrotic tissue is infected, surgical debridement should be a strong consideration.
- Caregivers should assess for factors that might impede or prevent healing, such as tunneled sinus tracts or calloused or rolled wound edges.
- If a wound cavity exists, the defect should be filled with a primary dressing including foam, hydrofibers, or gels, depending on the indication for each.
- Wounds should be covered, regardless of whether a cavity is present. Most wounds can be adequately covered with a moisture-retentive dressing. Highly exudative wounds may necessitate an absorbent dressing.

More recently Knox, Datiashvili, and Granick (2007) proposed that two parallel yet divergent management systems for chronic wounds have evolved. The medical approach uses a variety of dressings, topical enzymes, and local and systemic medications, including antibiotics, to promote healing by secondary intention or by optimizing the wound for subsequent surgical reconstruction. Medical management consists of using debridement techniques similar to those described by McNees (2006) as well as mechanical debridement or biologic therapy. Mechanical debridement includes the use of traditional wet-to-dry gauze dressings to essentially tear necrotic tissue from the wound, which, at times, can be quite painful. Furthermore, this technique randomly removes areas of necrotic tissue as well as tissue needed for granulation, thus resulting in tissue reinjury. Additionally, maintenance of a traditional moist gauze dressing requires changing it two to three times daily. Lawrence (1994) demonstrated that bacteria were capable of infiltrating up to 64 layers of gauze. Thus, the efficacy of mechanical debridement via dressing changes has been questioned.

Biologic therapy involves application of blow-fly maggots (*Phaenicia sericata*) directly to the wound surface. This type of intervention can be an effective debridement method, especially for patients whose medical comorbidities preclude surgical intervention. Maggots secrete an enzyme that acts to dissolve necrotic tissue into a nutrient-rich food source while sparing normal, healthy tissue. The debridement process itself is painless, but some patients feel the movement of the larvae. Although effective, the use of maggots for wound debridement and subsequent healing has a powerful psychosocial effect on some and therefore may not be utilized (Attinger et al., 2006; Courtenay, Church, & Ryan, 2000; Knox et al., 2007).

The surgical management of chronic wounds, as proposed by Knox et al. (2007), has remained the gold standard. Early surgical intervention is used to prepare the wound for reconstruction in a timely manner while promoting the healing process. Surgical debridement is the most efficient means of wound bed preparation by minimizing the bioburden of the wound. Necrotic tissue serves as a substrate for bacteria, which compete for the same nutrients and oxygen required for wound healing. Therefore, it is imperative that necrotic, insensate, nonblanching, nonbleeding skin be excised without delay. Such tissue is continually removed until definitive bleeding occurs from within the dermis. Subcutaneous tissue should be removed until shiny yellow fat is present. Once the wound bed is sufficiently prepared through surgical debridement, further healing can proceed by means of topical therapy with dressings or negative pressure therapy. The ultimate form of surgical debridement, amputation, is reserved for digits and limbs that are no longer viable or not functionally salvageable (Barrett & Herndon, 2003; Knox et al.).

The medical and nursing literature contains numerous proposals for chronic and acute wound management and countless anecdotal reports of wound care techniques, dressings, and topical therapy. Unfortunately, significant variations regarding chronic wound management, despite evidence-based recommendations, have been reported (Jones, Fennie, & Lenihan, 2007). Upon a general review of the wound management literature, consistent themes emerge and include some or all of the following.

- Cleansing of an open wound and, if necessary, removal of any foreign bodies present within
- Use of topical and/or systemic antibiotics

- Pain management
- Debridement of excessive amounts of necrotic, nonviable tissue
- Use of supportive topical therapy, including suspensions, colloids, and gelatinous agents that assist in the healing and debridement process
- Use of moisture-retentive dressings to contain most wounds that are not heavily exudative
- Use of vacuum-assisted closure technology
- Compression therapy, if appropriate
- Improved nutritional intake

Evidence-based complementary and alternative therapies also deserve consideration, as well as novel approaches, such as the use of growth factors and stem cells. However, caregivers must use extreme caution if implementing these interventions in the oncology patient population. For specialized wound management, interventions such as radiation therapy, topical chemotherapy, phototherapy, and hyperbaric oxygenation are available.

Conclusion

The skin, its accessory organs, and the soft tissue beneath its surface comprise a detailed and interrelated network that serves to protect, regulate, and support humans throughout the life span. Under normal, healthy conditions, the skin has an amazing ability to heal and regenerate. The healing process is a complex mechanism that involves hemostasis and the initiation of an immune response, collagen synthesis and the production of granulation tissue, and maturation or remodeling of the area of injury. Interventions for acute and chronic wound management are meant to supplement or expedite the normal healing process. Comorbid disease, individual risk factors, or treatment for malignancy can compromise normal healing. At times, this may result in infection, radical surgical intervention, or the need for chronic wound management.

Chronic wound care can result in significant anxiety for patients and caregivers. In addition to concerns for the patient's obvious physical state of health, provisions must be made for ongoing medical and nursing support, such as outpatient or home care, and for financial aspects related to chronic wound management, such as medical care, supplies, and lost wages. Depending on the type and severity of the wound, psychosocial issues may arise related to feeling ill, disabled, isolated, or disfigured or having a highly odiferous wound. In such cases, the multidisciplinary team caring for this patient population should involve behavioral medicine and social services.

Just as every patient is an individual with an individualized plan of care, so too are skin ailments and chronic nonhealing wounds. Careful assessment is important to ascertain contributing factors to the patient's condition such as comorbid disease, the type of treatment received, or patient-specific considerations, such as the location of one's stoma, surgical wound, skin crease or fold, or position of an implantable device. Patients and practitioners should agree upon an individualized treatment plan in an effort to achieve maximal healing potential. In some cases, this may require allowing the patient's skin or wound to gradually heal itself or preparing the site for intensive surgical and medical intervention.

References

Abdul-Karim, F.W., Benevenia, J., Pathria, M.N., & Makley, J.T. (1992). Case report 736: Retained surgical sponge (gossypiboma) with a foreign body reaction and remote and organizing hematoma. *Skeletal Radiology, 21*(7), 466–469.

Almhanna, K., Pelley, R.J., Budd, G.T., Davidson, J., & Moore, H.C. (2008). Subcutaneous implantable venous access device erosion through the skin in patients treated with anti-vascular endothelial growth factor therapy: A case series. *Anticancer Drugs,19*(2), 217–219.

Altemus, M., Rao, B., Dhabhar, F.S., Ding, W., & Granstein, R.D. (2001). Stress-induced changes in skin barrier function in healthy women. *Journal of Investigations in Dermatology, 117*(2), 309–317.

Archambeau, J.O., Pezner, R., & Wasserman, T. (1995). Pathophysiology of irradiated skin. *International Journal of Radiation Oncology, Biology, Physics, 31*(5), 1171–1185.

Artioukh, D.Y., Smith, R.A., & Gokul, K. (2007). Risk factors for impaired healing of the perineal wound after abdominoperineal resection of rectum for carcinoma. *Colorectal Disease, 9*(4), 362–367.

Attinger, C.E., Janis, J.E., Steinberg, J., Schwartz, J., Al-Attar, A., & Couch, K. (2006). Clinical approach to wounds: Debridement and wound bed preparation including the use of dressing and wound healing adjuvants. *Plastic and Reconstructive Surgery, 117*(Suppl. 7), 72S–109S.

Azria, D., Magne, N., Zouhair, A., Castadot, P., Culine, S., Ychou, M., et al. (2005). Radiation recall: A well recognized but neglected phenomenon. *Cancer Treatment Reviews, 31*(7), 555–570.

Balasubramani, M., Kumar, T.R., & Babu, M. (2001). Skin substitutes: A review. *Burns, 27*(5), 534–544.

Barrett, J.P., & Herndon, D.N. (2003). Effect of burn wound excision on bacterial colonization and invasion. *Plastic and Reconstructive Surgery, 111*(2), 751–752.

Bauer-Wu, S.M., & Post-White, J. (2005). Immunology. In C.H. Yarbro, M.H. Frogge, & M. Goodman (Eds.), *Cancer nursing: Principles and practice* (6th ed., pp. 26–39). Sudbury, MA: Jones and Bartlett.

Beheshti, M.V., Protzer, W.R., Tomlinson, T.L., Martinek, E., Baatz, L.A., & Collins, M.S. (1998). Long-term results of radiologic placement of a central venous access device. *American Journal of Roentgenology, 170*(3), 731–734.

Bloch, A., & Charuhas, P. (2002). Cancer and cancer therapy. In M.M. Gottschlich (Ed.), *The science and practice of nutrition support: A case-based core curriculum* (pp. 643–661). Dubuque, IA: Kendall/Hunt.

Bosch, J.A., Engeland, C.G., Cacioppo, J.T., & Marucha, P.T. (2007). Depressive symptoms predict mucosal wound healing. *Psychosomatic Medicine, 69*(7), 597–605.

Bucknall, T.E. (1980). The effect of local infection upon wound healing: An experimental study. *British Journal of Surgery, 67*(12), 851–855.

Camp-Sorrell, D. (1992). Implantable ports: Everything you always wanted to know. *Journal of Intravenous Nursing, 15*(5), 262–273.

Camp-Sorrell, D. (2004). Implanted ports: Skin erosion. *Clinical Journal of Oncology Nursing, 8*(3), 309–310.

Camp-Sorrell, D. (2005). Chemotherapy toxicities and management. In C.H. Yarbro, M.H. Frogge, & M. Goodman (Eds.), *Cancer nursing: Principles and practice* (6th ed., pp. 412–457). Sudbury, MA: Jones and Bartlett.

Cavaletti, G., & Zanna, C. (2002). Current status and future prospects for the treatment of chemo-therapy-induced peripheral neurotoxicity. *European Journal of Cancer, 38*(14), 1832–1837.

Chiao, T.B., & Lee, A.J. (2005). Role of pentoxifylline and vitamin E in attenuation of radia-tion induced fibrosis. *Annals of Pharmacotherapy, 39*(3), 516–521.

Courtenay, M., Church, J.C., & Ryan, T.J. (2000). Larva therapy in wound management. *Journal of the Royal Society of Medicine, 93*(2), 72–74.

Cunningham, R.S., & Huhmann, M.B. (2005). Nutritional disturbances. In C.H. Yarbro, M.H. Frogge, & M. Goodman (Eds.), *Cancer nursing: Principles and practice* (6th ed., pp. 761–790). Sudbury, MA: Jones and Bartlett.

Davies, C.E., Hill, K.E., Newcombe, R.G., Stephen, P., Wilson, M.J., Harding, K.G., et al. (2007). A prospective study of the microbiology of chronic venous leg ulcers to reevaluate the clinical predictive value of tissue biopsies and swabs. *Wound Repair and Regeneration, 15*(1), 17–22.

Derzie, A.J., Silvestri, F., Liriano, E., & Benotti, P. (2000). Wound closure technique and acute wound complications in gastric bypass surgery for morbid obesity: A prospective randomized trial. *Journal of the American College of Surgeons, 191*(3), 238–243.

D'Haese, S., Bate, R., Claes, S., Boone, A., Vanvoorden, V., & Efficace, F. (2005). Manage-ment of skin reactions during radiotherapy: A study of nursing practice. *European Journal of Cancer Care, 14*(1), 28–42.

Dow, G., Browne, A., & Sibbald, R.G. (1999). Infection in chronic wounds: Controversies in diagnosis and treatment. *Ostomy/Wound Management, 45*(8), 23–40.

Edwards, R., & Harding, K.G. (2004). Bacteria and wound healing. *Current Opinion in Infec-tious Disease, 17*(2), 91–96.

Eich, D., Scharffetter-Kochanek, K., Eich, H.T., Tantcheva-Poor, I., & Krieg, T. (2002). Acral erythrodysesthesia syndrome caused by intravenous infusion of docetaxel in breast cancer. *American Journal of Clinical Oncology, 25*(6), 599–602.

Elihu, A., & Gollin, G. (2007). Complications of implanted central venous catheters in neutropenic children. *American Surgeon, 73*(10), 1079–1082.

Englert, K. (2003). Stasis dermatitis in the patient with CHF. *Dermatology Nursing, 15*(6), 552.

Foster, M.R., Heppenstall, R.B., Friedenberg, Z.B., & Hozack, W.J. (1990). A prospective assessment of nutritional status and complications in patients with fractures of the hip. *Journal of Orthopedic Trauma, 4*(1), 49–57.

Freiman, A., Bird, G., Metelitsa, A.I., Barankin, B., & Lauzon, G.J. (2004). Cutaneous effects of smoking. *Journal of Cutaneous Medicine and Surgery, 8*(6), 415–423.

Garg, A., Chren, M., Sands, L.P., Matsui, M.S., Marenus, K.D., Feingold, K.R., et al. (2001). Psychosocial stress perturbs epidermal permeability barrier homeostasis. *Archives of Dermatology, 137*(1), 53–59.

Gates, J., Davis, J.M., & Evans, E. (2005). Venous stasis ulcers in the patient who is obese. *Journal of Wound, Ostomy, and Continence Nursing, 32*(6), 421–426.

Gencosmanoglu, R., & Inceoglu, R. (2003, September 8). An unusual case of small bowel obstruction: Gossypiboma-case report. *BMC Surgery, 3,* 6.

Gosain, A., & DiPietro, L.A. (2004). Aging and wound healing. *World Journal of Surgery, 28*(3), 321–326.

Haas, M.L. (2005). Skin reactions. In D.W. Bruner, M.L. Haas, & T.K. Gosselin-Acomb (Eds.), *Manual for radiation oncology nursing practice and education* (3rd ed., pp. 49–52). Pittsburgh, PA: Oncology Nursing Society.

Hahler, B. (2006). An overview of dermatological conditions commonly associated with the obese patient. *Ostomy/Wound Management, 52*(6), 34–36, 38, 40.

Headley, C.M., & Wall, B. (2002). ESRD-associated cutaneous manifestations in a hemodi-alysis population. *Journal of Nephrology Nursing, 29*(6), 525–527, 531–539.

Holcomb, S.S. (2006). Identification and treatment of different types of lymphedema. *Advances in Skin and Wound Care, 19*(2), 103–108.

Howell, P.B., Walters, P.E., Donowitz, G.R., & Farr, B.M. (1995). Risk factors for infection of adult patients with cancer who have tunneled central venous catheters. *Cancer, 15*(6), 1367–1375.

Jaff, M.R. (2001). Severe peripheral arterial disease and critical limb ischemia: Incidence, pathophysiology, presentation, methods of diagnosis. In A.T. Hirsch (Ed.), *Primary care series: Peripheral arterial disease and intermittent claudication* (pp. 53–58). Bridgewater, NJ: Excerpta Medica.

Johnson, R.M., & Richard, R. (2003). Partial-thickness burns: Identification and management. *Advances in Skin and Wound Care, 16*(4), 178–189.

Jones, K.R., Fennie, K., & Lenihan, A. (2007). Evidence-based management of chronic wounds. *Advances in Skin and Wound Care, 20*(11), 591–600.

Kay, S.P., Moreland, J.R., & Schmitter, E. (1987, April). Nutritional status and wound healing in lower extremity amputations. *Clinical Orthopaedics and Related Research, 217,* 253–256.

Keast, D.H., & Orsted, H. (1998). The basic principles of wound care. *Ostomy/Wound Management, 44*(8), 24–31.

Khopkar, U., & Pande, S. (2007). Etiopathogenesis of pruritus due to systemic causes. *Indian Journal of Dermatology, Venereology, and Leprology, 73*(4), 215–217.

Knox, K.R., Datiashvili, R.O., & Granick, M.S. (2007). Surgical wound bed preparation of chronic and acute wounds. *Clinics in Plastic Surgery, 34*(4), 633–641.

Kolker, A.R., Redstone, J.S., & Tutela, J.P. (2007). Salvage of exposed implantable cardiac electrical devices and lead systems with pocket change and local flap coverage. *Annals of Plastic Surgery, 59*(1), 26–29.

Konturek, P.C., Brzozowski, T., Konturek, S.J., Kwiecien, S., Dembinski, A., & Hahn, E.G. (2001). Influence of bacterial lipopolysaccharide on healing of chronic experimental ulcer in rat. *Scandinavian Journal of Gastroenterology, 36*(12), 1239–1247.

Laato, M., Niinikoski, J., Lundberg, C., & Gerdin, B. (1988). Inflammatory reaction and blood flow in experimental wounds inoculated with *Staphylococcus aureus. European Surgical Research, 20*(1), 33–38.

Lavery, I.C., & Erwin-Toth, P. (2004). Stoma therapy. In A.A. Cataldo & J.M. MacKeigan (Eds.), *Intestinal stomas: Principles, techniques, and management* (2nd ed., pp. 65–90). New York: Marcel Dekker.

Lawenda, B.D., Mondry, T.E., & Johnstone, P.A. (2009). Lymphedema: A primer on the identification and management of a chronic condition in oncologic treatment. *CA: A Cancer Journal for Clinicians, 59*(1), 8–24.

Lawrence, J.C. (1994). Dressings and wound infection. *American Journal of Surgery, 167*(Suppl. 1A), 21S–24S.

Lersch, C., Eckel, F., Sader, R., Paschalidis, M., Zeilhofer, F., Schulte-Frohlinde, E., et al. (1999). Initial experience with Healthport miniMax® and other peripheral arm ports in patients with advanced gastrointestinal malignancy. *Oncology, 57*(4), 269–275.

Lone, G.N., Bhat, A.H., Tak, M.Y., & Garcoo, S.A. (2005). Transdiaphragmatic migration of forgotten gauze sponge: An unreported entity of lung abscess. *European Journal of Cardiothoracic Surgery, 28*(2), 355–357.

Maher, K.E. (2005). Radiation therapy: Toxicities and management. In C.H. Yarbro, M.H. Frogge, & M. Goodman (Eds.), *Cancer nursing: Principles and practice* (6th ed., pp. 283–314). Sudbury, MA: Jones and Bartlett.

Marieb, E.N. (2001). *Human anatomy and physiology* (5th ed.). San Francisco: Benjamin Cummings.

Marin, L.A., Salido, J.A., Lopez, A., & Silva, A. (2002). Preoperative nutritional evaluation as a prognostic tool for wound healing. *Acta Orthopaedica Scandinavica, 73*(1), 2–5.

Marrs, J. (2007). Lymphedema and implications for oncology nursing practice. *Clinical Journal of Oncology Nursing, 11*(1), 19–21.

Martin, K.J., Gonzalez, E.A., & Slatopolsky E. (2004). Renal osteodystrophy. In B.M. Brenner (Ed.), *Brenner & Rector's the kidney* (7th ed., Vol. 2, pp. 2255–2304). Philadelphia: Saunders.

McNees, P. (2006). Skin and wound assessment and care in oncology. *Seminars in Oncology Nursing, 22*(3), 130–143.

Meuli, M., Liu, Y., Liggitt, D., Kashani-Sabet, M., Knauer, S., Meuli-Simmen, C., et al. (2001). Efficient gene expression in skin wound sites following local plasmid injection. *Journal of Investigative Dermatology, 116*(1), 131–135.

Minkes, R.K., McLean, S.E., Mazziotti, M.V., & Langer, J.C. (2008, October). *Stomas of the small and large intestine.* Retrieved February 5, 2009, from http://www.emedicine.com/ped/topic2994.htm

Morgan, E.D., Bledsoe, S.C., & Barker, J. (2000). Ambulatory management of burns. *American Family Physician, 62*(9), 2015–2026, 2029–2030, 2032.

Morita, A. (2007). Tobacco smoke causes premature skin aging. *Journal of Dermatology Science, 48*(3), 169–175.

Moureau, N., & Zonderman, A. (2000). Does it always have to hurt? Premedications for adults and children for use with intravenous therapy. *Journal of Intravenous Nursing, 23*(4), 213–219.

Mousley, M. (2007). Understanding diabetic foot ulcers. 1: Pathophysiology. *Nursing Times, 103*(31), 28–29.

Murray, J.F. (2000). History and physical examination. In J.F. Murray & J.A. Nadel (Eds.), *Textbook of respiratory medicine* (3rd ed., Vol. 1, pp. 585–605). Philadelphia: Saunders.

Myers, S.A., & Allen, M.H. (2001). Cutaneous manifestations of lupus: Can you recognize them all? *Women's Health in Primary Care, 4*(1), 71–83.

Nathan, S., Piccione, W., Kumar, A., Attanasio, S., & Schaer, G.L. (2006). Erosion of an extrapericardial implantable cardioverter defibrillator patch through the gastric fundus with fistulous tract formation. *Cardiology Review, 14*(6), e21–e23.

Oishi, K. (2008). Clinical approaches to minimize rash associated with EGFR inhibitors. *Oncology Nursing Forum, 35*(1), 103–111.

Oubre, C.M., Roy, A., Toner, C., & Kalns, J. (2007). Retrospective study of factors affecting non-healing of wounds during hyperbaric oxygen therapy. *Journal of Wound Care, 16*(6), 245–250.

Pearce, J.D. (2005). Alterations in mobility, skin integrity, and neurologic status. In J.K. Itano & K.N. Taoka (Eds.), *Core curriculum for oncology nursing* (4th ed., pp. 245–258). St. Louis, MO: Elsevier Saunders.

Pedersen, N.W., & Pedersen, D. (1992). Nutrition as a prognostic indicator in amputations. A prospective study of 47 cases. *Acta Orthopaedica Scandinavica, 63*(6), 675–678.

Perez-Soler, R., & Saltz, L. (2005). Cutaneous adverse effects with HER1/EGFR-targeted agents: Is there a silver lining? *Journal of Clinical Oncology, 23*(22), 5235–5246.

Pittman, J. (2007). Effect of aging on wound healing. *Journal of Wound, Ostomy, and Continence Nursing, 34*(4), 412–415.

Porock, D., & Kristjanson, L. (1999). Skin reactions during radiotherapy for breast cancer: The use and impact of topical agents and dressings. *European Journal of Cancer Care, 8*(3), 143–153.

Porock, D., Kristjanson, L., Nikoletti, S., Cameron, F., & Pedler, P. (1998). Predicting the severity of radiation skin reactions in women with breast cancer. *Oncology Nursing Forum, 25*(6), 1019–1029.

Press, O.W., Ramsey, P.G., Larson, E.B., Fefer, A., & Hickman, R.O. (1984). Hickman catheter infections in patients with malignancies. *Medicine, 63*(4), 189–200.

Remlinger, K.A. (2003). Cutaneous reactions to chemotherapy drugs. *Archives of Dermatology, 139*(1), 77–81.

Robbins, M.A. (2007). Nonmalignant tumors. In M.L. Haas, W.P. Hogle, G.J. Moore-Higgs, & T.K. Gosselin-Acomb (Eds.), *Radiation therapy: A guide to patient care* (pp. 319–324). St. Louis, MO: Mosby.

Robles, T. (2007). Stress, social support, and delayed skin barrier recovery. *Psychosomatic Medicine, 69*(8), 807–815.

Romo, T., III, Pearson, J.M., Yalamanchili, H., & Zoumalan, R.A. (2008, February 18). *Wound healing, skin.* Retrieved February 5, 2009, from http://www.emedicine.com/ent/topic13.htm

Serrao, R., Zirwas, M., & English, J.C. (2007). Palmar erythema. *American Journal of Clinical Dermatology, 8*(6), 347–356.

Shier, D., Butler, J., & Lewis, R. (2004). *Hole's human anatomy and physiology* (10th ed.). Boston: McGraw-Hill.

Sparks, S.G. (2007). Radiodermatitis. In M.L. Haas, W.P. Hogle, G.J. Moore-Higgs, & T.K. Gosselin-Acomb (Eds.), *Radiation therapy: A guide to patient care* (pp. 511–522). St. Louis, MO: Mosby.

Spear, S.L., Ducic, I., Cuoco, F., & Taylor, N. (2007). Effect of obesity on flap and donor-site complications in pedicled TRAM flap breast reconstruction. *Plastic and Reconstructive Surgery, 119*(3), 788–795.

Visovsky, C., Collins, M., Abbott, L., Aschenbrenner, J., & Hart, C. (2007). Putting evidence into practice: Evidence-based interventions for chemotherapy-induced peripheral neuropathy. *Clinical Journal of Oncology Nursing, 11*(6), 901–913.

Wells, M., & MacBride, S. (2003). Radiation skin reactions. In S. Faithful & M. Wells (Eds.), *Supportive care in radiotherapy* (pp. 135–159). Edinburg, United Kingdom: Churchill Livingstone.

Whitman, E. (1996). Complications associated with the use of central venous access devices. *Current Problems in Surgery, 33*(4), 311–378.

Wysocki, A.B. (2002). Evaluating and managing open skin wounds: Colonization versus infection. *AACN Clinical Issues, 13*(3), 382–397.

Zichi-Cohen, M., & Carlson, E. (2005). Cancer-related distress. In C.H. Yarbro, M.H. Frogge, & M. Goodman (Eds.), *Cancer nursing: Principles and practice* (6th ed., pp. 623–638). Sudbury, MA: Jones and Bartlett.

CHAPTER 2

Common Drug Reactions With Cutaneous Manifestations

Mary Ellyn Witt, RN, MS, AOCN®, and Melodie Young, MSN, RN, ANP-C, GNPc

Introduction

Oncology patient care is complicated because of preexisting comorbidities, complex cancer treatments, and numerous prescribed medications from various providers. Patients often are referred to as experiencing *polypharmacy*, or consuming multiple prescription and over-the-counter medications. This increases a patient's risk of developing drug reactions. Drug reactions can vary from simple gastrointestinal distress or muscular discomfort to mild or severe cutaneous reactions. *Cutaneous reactions* to drugs are drug-induced changes of the skin and/or mucous membranes. Overall, exanthems (measles-like eruptions) account for approximately 75%–95% of all skin reactions attributed to medications. *Urticaria* (hives) represent an additional 5%–6% of all skin reactions (James, Berger, & Elston, 2006).

The use of epidermal growth factor receptor inhibitors in patients with cancer will change the epidemiology of reported skin reactions. Prior to their use, commonly prescribed medications with the highest risk of developing skin reactions are sulfonamides; the penicillins, especially the aminopenicillins; and the cephalosporins (Stern, 1997; Svensson, Cowen, & Gaspari, 2001).

Some factors can increase an individual's risk for developing a cutaneous drug reaction, including (James et al., 2006)

- Age
- Gender
- The medication itself
- The patient's immunity
- Hereditary genes.

The incidence increases among older adults and patients who take two or more medications. Females are 1.5 times more likely than males to develop drug eruptions (James et al.). The nature and composition of the medication can affect the risk for developing a skin reaction. For example, nonsteroidal anti-inflammatory drugs (NSAIDs) have a reaction rate of about 1 in 200 (James et al.). In contrast, cutaneous reaction rates for digoxin, lidocaine, prednisone, codeine, and acetaminophen are less than 1 in 1,000 (James et al.). The immune status of a patient may strongly determine the risk for developing certain drug eruptions. Patients with HIV infection or Epstein-Barr virus infections have dramatically increased rates of exanthematous reactions to certain antibiotics. Other patients may have been born with a hypersensitivity syndrome that is associated with genetic differences in the ability of the patient to metabolize a specific medication or a toxic metabolite of the medication (James et al.).

Oncology nurses need to be knowledgeable about the cutaneous reactions caused by oncology drug regimens. Knowledge about the non-oncology medications and risks for cutaneous reactions will enable oncology nurses to use a holistic approach in caring for patients with cancer who present with a skin reaction. This chapter will describe classifications, physiology, and appearances of cutaneous drug reactions. A discussion of common medications causing cutaneous reactions also will be presented. Later in the chapter, special needs of patients with cancer will be highlighted with suggestions for nursing interventions.

Classifications and Physiology of Cutaneous Drug Reactions

Drug eruptions can mimic virtually all of the morphologic expressions in dermatology and should be the first consideration in the differential diagnosis of a suddenly appearing cutaneous eruption. Cutaneous drug reactions can be classified as an immunologically mediated response to a medication or as a nonimmunologic drug reaction (Fitzpatrick, Johnson, Wolff, & Suurmond, 2001).

An immunologic response is an allergic-type reaction classified by Gell and Coombs in 1963. The classification is widely used today and is based on the immune reaction to a causative drug and the clinically observed cutaneous reaction (Gell & Coombs). The classification includes

- Type I: Immunoglobulin (Ig) E (IgE)-mediated hypersensitivity reactions that produce an immediate reaction ranging from mild urticaria to angioedema and anaphylaxis
- Type II: Result in cell lysis producing hemolysis that presents clinically as petechiae/purpura and drug-induced pemphigus. *Pemphigus* is a bullous eruption (diagnosed by skin biopsies) that is more likely to occur as a cuta-

neous drug eruption in a patient on sulfonamides, penicillins, NSAIDs, and antiseizure medications. *Bullae* (fluid-filled blisters) appear rapidly and usually require immediate discontinuation of the offending agent.

- Type III: IgG or IgM responses to drugs producing immune complexes, which can affect small vessels as vasculitis, serum sickness, urticaria, or angioedema
- Type IV: Cell-mediated delayed hypersensitivity reactions in which sensitized lymphocytes react with the drug, releasing cytokines and thus producing an inflammatory response of the skin. Fixed drug eruptions, exanthems, photoallergic cutaneous rashes, and the most serious of reactions, Stevens-Johnson syndrome (SJS) and toxic epidermal necrolysis (TEN), are examples.

SJS and TEN are generalized, life-threatening, painful, usually drug-induced reactions of the skin and mucosa. The lesions have a target-like appearance but then become confluent, are erythematous, show a crinkled surface, and become bullous. If the lesions are touched, the epidermis will tear easily and produce erosions (*Nikolsky sign*). The skin and mucosa are painful, as erosions and sloughing of the epidermis, mouth, anogenital area, palms, soles, and even nails may occur. The duration of the progression is brief, less than four days, and prognosis can be poor, with 5% mortality for SJS and 30% mortality for TEN (Fitzpatrick et al., 2001; Gell & Coombs, 1963; Goodheart, 2003).

Nonimmunologic drug reactions are more commonly seen and can be classified into the following categories.

- Idiosyncrasy sensu strictiori: These reactions occur because of hereditary enzyme deficiencies. For example, patients with a glucose-6-phosphate deficiency have an enzyme deficiency that can make certain medications intolerable.
- Cumulation: Reactions that are drug dose–dependent based on the total amount of drug absorbed, for example, pigmentation changes caused by amiodarone or minocycline
- Photosensitivity: Reactions caused by a combination of drug plus ultraviolet irradiation. A molecule within the drug initiates the sunburn-like reaction when exposed to the source of light.
- Irritancy/toxicity of a topically applied drug: Expected skin responses when a medication is applied directly to the skin. For example, topical 5-fluorouracil may cause redness, soreness, scaling, or peeling of the skin (University of Utah Hospital and Clinics, 2007).
- Individual idiosyncrasy or a mechanism not yet known (Fitzpatrick et al., 2001; Goodheart, 2003)

Most drug-induced eruptions appear within the first week after the drug therapy is started, and attributing an eruption to a specific drug is often straightforward. Antibiotics and allopurinol are well-known exceptions to this rule and may induce rashes up to two weeks after initial therapy. However, determining which specific medication is causing the eruption often is difficult when the patient is taking multiple drugs (Bigby, 2001).

Description of the Cutaneous Reaction and Clinical Manifestations

A vital part of the nursing assessment is to describe skin reactions (color, appearance, raised, size, drainage) and distribution of the reaction, and to know the clinical manifestations. Table 2-1 describes common types of lesions with descriptions.

The most common findings and distribution with cutaneous reactions include (Fitzpatrick et al., 2001; Goodheart, 2003)

- Exanthems: Measles-like lesion, diffuse or coalescing, symmetric on trunk, thighs, upper arms, and face
- Urticaria: Hive-like wheals or papules, visible anywhere on the body
- Acneform eruptions: Pustules in atypical areas

Table 2-1. Common Types of Skin Lesions	
Type of Lesion	**Description**
Bulla	Vesicle > 0.5 cm
Cyst	Firm, raised encapsulated lesion, filled with liquid or semisolid material; may become infected
Macule	Circumscribed, flat change in color of skin; < 1 cm diameter
Nodule	Circumscribed, raised, firm lesion; > 0.5 cm; may have started as a papule
Papule	Raised solid lesion; < 0.5 cm diameter. Papules may become confluent and form plaque.
Patch	Circumscribed, flat lesion (large macule); > 1 cm diameter
Plaque	Circumscribed, raised superficial lesion with flat surface; > 0.5 cm diameter
Pustule	Circumscribed, raised lesion containing purulent exudate that may be cloudy, white, yellow, or hemorrhagic; size varies
Tumor	Large papule or nodule; usually > 1 cm diameter
Vesicle	Circumscribed, raised lesion, filled with liquid or semisolid material; may become infected
Wheal	Firm, raised, pink or red swelling of the skin; size and shape varies; usually itchy; lasts < 24 hours

Note. From "The Necessary Elements of a Dermatologic History and Physical Evaluation," by J. Cole and D. Gray-Miceli, 2002, *Dermatology Nursing, 14*(6), p. 378. Copyright 2002 by Jannetti Publications, Inc. Adapted with permission.

- Photodistribution rash: Erythema or eczema that occurs on the face and dorsal forearms and in a V pattern on the neck and chest
- Purpura: Excessive bleeding that occurs on the lower extremities
- Erythema nodosum: Painful red lesions of lower legs
- Bullous eruptions: Fluid-filled blisters
- Vascular eruptions: Palpable purpura or vasculitis
- Contact dermatitis: Localized pruritic, scaly rash; the distribution most often corresponds to the area of initial insult to the skin.
- Fixed drug eruptions: Plaques or blistering at the same location with each exposure, occurring most often on the extremities or trunk
- Erythema multiforme: Erythroderma, pain, mucosal erosions, and skin necrosis; can be widespread.

Besides describing what is seen, oncology nurses need to consider clinical manifestations during the care of patients. Most drug eruptions are mild and self-limited, resolving after discontinuation of the offending agent. Pruritus is a common complaint and does not have to be accompanied by a visible manifestation. Acute urticarial lesions usually appear shortly after the onset of drug therapy and resolve rapidly with withdrawal of the drug. When drug eruptions cause vasculitis, the vasculitis typically begins 7–21 days after the onset of drug therapy. A patient with vasculitis may have fever, myalgias, arthritis, and abdominal pain. A complete blood count drawn during the time the patient is experiencing a cutaneous reaction may show eosinophilia (Goodheart, 2003). Other clinical manifestations include cardiovascular collapse, urticaria, laryngeal or upper airway edema, wheezing, and hypotension (Riedl & Casillas, 2003). More serious symptoms include presence of fever, mucous membrane lesions, lymphadenopathy, joint tenderness and swelling, and pulmonary symptoms (Riedl & Casillas).

Cutaneous Reactions From Common Drugs

When a patient with cancer appears to have measles, the oncology nurse needs to first assess the patient for a cutaneous reaction related to common drugs. Exanthem, otherwise known as a maculopapular or morbilliform drug reaction, is often symmetric and noted on the trunk, thighs, upper arms, and face. It is likely to be seen with antibiotics, particularly penicillin-related antibiotics, but also can develop with use of tetracyclines, erythromycins, barbiturates, sulfonamides, or NSAIDs (Goodheart, 2003; Hall, 2006).

Urticaria, with or without angioedema, is the second most common drug reaction and is likely to develop abruptly after exposure to the offending agent. Aspirin, NSAIDs, antibiotics, radiocontrast media, angiotensin-converting enzyme inhibitors, and pain medications including codeine and opiates are the most common causative agents (Goodheart, 2003; Hall, 2006).

Photosensitivity from drugs or chemicals develops when a photoallergen initiates a reaction in the presence of ultraviolet light (UVL) from the sun or artificial sources. A sunburn-like reaction in a UVL-exposed pattern will be clinically evident with confluent erythema of exposed skin and well-demarcated unaffected areas where unexposed. Photoallergic drug-induced photosensitivity also can present as an eczematous, hyperpigmented rash that can be difficult to differentiate from contact dermatitis. A classic reaction may include erythema of the forearms. Erythema can appear on the face and neck, giving the appearance of a "V," and can be seen in all races and skin types. Common causative agents include furosemide, hydrochlorothiazide and triamterene, chlorothiazide, amiodarone, chlorpromazine, prochlorperazine, doxycycline, demeclocycline, nalidixic acid, sparfloxacin, lomefloxacin, piroxicam, naproxen, and nabumetone (Fitzpatrick et al., 2001).

Tables 2-2 and 2-3 are provided as a guide for the oncology nurse. Table 2-2 lists drugs and the common skin reactions seen with them. Table 2-3 describes the reactions and common drugs that may cause them.

Table 2-2. Drugs and Associated Dermatoses	
Drug	**Dermatoses/Comments**
Accutane® (Roche)	See *Isotretinoin*
Acetaminophen (Tylenol®, McNeil-PPC, Inc.)	Infrequent cause of drug eruption; urticaria and erythematous eruptions are noted. Also fixed drug eruption.
Adrenocorticotropic hormones (ACTH, prednisone, IM triamcinolone)	Cushing's syndrome, hyperpigmentation, acneiform eruptions, rosacea, striae, perioral dermatitis, seborrheic dermatitis-like eruptions, and hirsutism
Allopurinol (Zyloprim®, Prometheus)	Erythema, maculopapular rash, and severe bullae
Amantadine	Livedo reticularis
Aminosalicylic acid	Scarlatiniform or morbilliform rash, fixed drug eruption, and nummular eczema-like rash
Amiodarone	Photosensitivity reaction and blue-gray discoloration of skin
Amphetamine	Coldness of extremities; redness of neck and shoulders; increased itching in LSC
Ampicillin	See *Antibiotics*; flare of morbilliform eruption in over half of patients with infectious mononucleosis
ACE inhibitors	Maculopapular eruption with eosinophilia, pemphigus, a bullous pemphigoid-like eruption, angioedema, rosacea, urticaria, and possibly flare of psoriasis
	(Continued on next page)

Table 2-2. Drugs and Associated Dermatoses *(Continued)*

Drug	Dermatoses/Comments
Antabuse® (Odyssey Phar-maceuticals)	Redness of face and acne
Antibiotics	Various agents have different reactions, but in general: *candida overgrowth* in oral, genital, and anal orifices results in pruritus ani, pruritus vulvae, and generalized pruritus; candida skin lesions may spread out from these foci. Urticaria, morbilliform and erythema multi-forme-like eruptions, particularly from penicillin. Ampicillin: generalized maculopapular rash, very common in patients with infectious mononucleosis Sulfa derivatives: particular problem in HIV+ patients. See *Streptomycin* and later section on photosensitivity reactions.
Anticoagulants	Coumadin and heparin: severe hemorrhagic skin infarction and necrosis
Antihistamines (in Coricidin® [Schering-Plough Health-Care Products, Inc.], NyQuil® [Procter & Gamble], and many other preparations)	Urticaria, eczematous dermatitis, and pityriasis rosea-like rash
Antineoplastic agents	Skin and mucocutaneous reactions, including alopecia, stomatitis, radiation recall reaction, and erythema
Antitoxin	Immediate reaction: pruritus, urticaria, and sweating Delayed serum sickness reaction: urticaria, redness, purpura
Apresoline	See *Hydralazine*
Aspirin and salicylates (a multitude of cold and anti-pain remedies; e.g., Pepto-Bismol® [Procter & Gamble])	Urticaria, purpura, bullous lesions
Atabrine hydrochloride	Universal yellow pigmentation; blue macules on face and mucosa; lichen planus–like eruption
Atropine	Scarlet fever–like rash
Barbiturates	Urticarial, erythematous, bullous, or purpuric eruptions; fixed drug eruptions
β-blockers	Alopecia; psoriasis flare

(Continued on next page)

Table 2-2. Drugs and Associated Dermatoses *(Continued)*

Drug	Dermatoses/Comments
Bleomycin sulfate injection	Antitumor antibiotic: gangrene, erythema, sclerosis, nail changes, characteristic striate lesions
Captopril	Pemphigus-like eruption; see *ACE inhibitors*
Cetuximab (monoclonal antibody that binds epidermal growth factor receptor)	Follicular eruption (one-third of patients); acneiform eruptions, seborrheic eruptions, nail bed changes
Chemotherapy agents	See *Antineoplastic agents*; also see specific drug
Chloral hydrate	Urticarial, popular, erythematous, and purpuric eruptions
Chloroquine (Aralen®, Sanofi-Aventis U.S. LLC)	Erythematous or lichenoid eruptions, with pruritus and urticaria ocular retinal damage from long-term use of chloroquine and other antimalarials can be irreversible
Chlorothiazide diuretics	Petechial and purpuric eruptions, especially of legs; see section on photosensitivity reactions
Chlorpromazine (Thorazine®, GlaxoSmithKline)	Maculopapular rash, increased sun sensitivity, purpura with agranulocytosis, and icterus from hepatitis Long term therapy: slate-gray to violet discoloration of the skin
Cimetidine	Dry, scaly skin
Codeine and morphine	Erythematous, urticaria, or vesicular eruption
Collagen (bovine) injected	Skin edema, erythema, induration, and urticaria at implantation sites
Contraceptive drugs	Chloasma-like eruption, erythema nodosum, hives; some cases of acne are aggravated
Cortisone and derivatives	Allergy (rare); see *ACTH*
Coumadin® (Bristol-Myers Squibb)	See *Anticoagulants*
Cyclosporine	Hypertrichosis, sebaceous hyperplasia, acne, folliculitis, epidermal cysts, Kaposi's sarcoma, skin precancers and cancers, gingival hyperplasia, follicular keratosis, palmoplantar paresthesias, and dysesthesias associated with temperature change
Dapsone	Red, maculopapular, vesicular eruption with agranulocytosis occurs occasionally resembling erythema nodosum

(Continued on next page)

Table 2-2. Drugs and Associated Dermatoses *(Continued)*

Drug	Dermatoses/Comments
Dextran (used in peritoneal dialysis)	Urticarial reactions
Diethylpropion hydrochloride (Tenuate, Tepanil® oral [3M Pharmaceuticals])	Measles-like eruption
Dilantin® (Pfizer Inc.)	See *Phenytoin*
Docetaxel	Cutaneous reactions: up to 70% incidence beginning usually 2–4 days after treatment with 80% pain or itching; purple-red macules or plaques, often acral, that may peel in 3–4 weeks; if worse with repeated doses, this drug may have to be stopped; local hypothermia may be ameliorative, extravasation necrosis, nail loss, supravenous discoloration, subungual abscesses, skin sclerosis
Doxorubicin (Doxil® [Ortho Biotech]; polyethylene glycol-coated liposomal doxorubicin hydrochloride)	Acral erythrodysesthesia with desquamation; in a few weeks; may worsen each episode and may limit dosage Diffuse: (10%) mild scaly erythema with follicular accentuation; does not necessarily recur Intertrigo eruption: due to friction from clothing; loose-fitting clothes may help Melanotic macules: on trunk or extremities; stomatitis; radiation and sunburn recall To ameliorate reactions: 99% DMSO four times a day, oral antioxidants (vitamins E, C, A, and selenium) and oral misoprostol (prostaglandin E_1 analog)
Estrogenic substances	Edema of legs with cutaneous redness progressing to exfoliative dermatitis
Feldene® (Pfizer Inc.)	See *Piroxicam*
Flagyl® (Pfizer Inc.)	See *Metronidazole*
Gold	Bullous hemorrhagic eruption Eczematous dermatitis of hands, arms, and legs or a pityriasis rosea-like eruption; also, seborrheic-like eruption, urticaria, and purpura
Heparin	See *Anticoagulants*
Hydralazine (Apresoline®, Novartis)	SLE-like reaction

(Continued on next page)

Table 2-2. Drugs and Associated Dermatoses *(Continued)*

Drug	Dermatoses/Comments
Hydroxyurea	Dermopathy mimicking cutaneous findings of dermatomyositis; atrophic, erythematous dermatitis over the back of the hands that may be photoinduced; leg ulcers; hyperpigmentation, especially nails (longitudinal bands) and palms
Ibuprofen (Motrin® [McNeil-PPC, Inc.], Advil® [Wyeth Consumer Healthcare])	Bullous eruptions, including erythema multiforme, Stevens-Johnson syndrome, toxic epidermal necrolysis, urticaria, photosensitivity, fixed drug reactions, morbilliform reactions
Icodextran (used in peritoneal dialysis)	Psoriasiform dermatosis, acute generalized exanthematous pustulosis
Imipramine	Slate-gray discoloration of skin
Insulin	Urticaria with serum sickness symptoms; fat atrophy at injection site
Iodides	Popular, pustular, ulcerative, or granulomatous lesions mainly on acne areas or legs; administration of chloride hastens recovery
Isoniazid	Erythematous and maculopapular, generalized, purpuric, bullous, and nummular eczema-like; acne aggravation
Isotretinoin	Dry red skin and lips (common); alopecia (rare)
Lasix® (Sanofi-Aventis U.S. LLC)	See *Furosemide*
Lamotrigine	At least 10% with cutaneous drug reactions; may be similar to phenytoin cutaneous drug reactions
Lithium	Acne-like lesions on the body; psoriasis exacerbation
Meclizine HCl (Antivert®, Pfizer Inc.)	Urticaria
Meprobamate	Small purpuric lesions; erythema multiforme-like eruption
Metronidazole (Flagyl)	Urticaria, pruritus
Minocycline	Skin (muddy skin syndrome), teeth, and scar discoloration Rare: hypersensitivity, sickness-like reaction, drug-induced lupus erythematosus, SLE-like syndrome, autoimmune hepatitis, *p*-ANCA-positive cutaneous polyarteritis nodosa Rare syndrome: hepatitis, exfoliative dermatitis, fever, lymphadenopathy, eosinophilia, lymphocytosis

(Continued on next page)

Table 2-2. Drugs and Associated Dermatoses *(Continued)*	
Drug	**Dermatoses/Comments**
Morphine	See *Codeine*; lichen planus–like eruption; fixed drug eruption, photosensitivity
Nevirapine	Unusually high incidence of potentially life-threatening Stevens-Johnson syndrome
NSAIDs (e.g., ibuprofen [Motrin], naproxen [Naprosyn®, Roche], indomethacin [Indocin®, Merck], piroxicam [Feldene], diclofenac [Voltaren®, Novartis], celecoxib [Celebrex®, Pfizer Inc.], meloxicam [Mobic®, Boehringer Ingelheim])	Urticaria, erythema multiforme–like eruption, toxic epidermal necrolysis
Penicillin	See *Antibiotics*
Penicillamine	Lupus-like rash, lichen planus–like rash, pemphigus foliaceous
Phenolphthalein (found in 4-way cold tablets, Ex-Lax® [Novartis Consumer Health], bile salts, and pink icing on cakes)	Fixed drug eruption: hyperpigmented or purplish, flat or slightly elevated, discrete, single or multiple patches
Phenothiazine group	See section on photosensitivity reactions
Phenytoin (Dilantin)	Hypertrophy of gums, erythema multiforme–like eruption; pseudolymphoma syndrome, morbilliform reaction Fetal hydantoin syndrome: organ defects plus nail hypoplasia Note: one of the most common causes of toxic epidermal necrolysis or Stevens-Johnson syndrome along with other antiseizure medications
Procainamide	SLE-like reaction
Propranolol (Inderal®, Wyeth)	Rare: drug eruption; see β-blockers
Psoralens	See section on photosensitivity reactions
Quinidine	Edema, purpura, scarlatiniform eruption; may progress to exfoliative dermatitis
Quinine	Diffuse eruption (any kind)
Rauwolfia alkaloids (reserpine)	Urticaria, photosensitivity reactions, petechial eruptions

(Continued on next page)

Table 2-2. Drugs and Associated Dermatoses *(Continued)*	
Drug	**Dermatoses/Comments**
Rifampin	Pruritus, urticaria, acne, bullous pemphigoid, mucositis, exfoliative erythroderma, red urine, reddened soft contact lenses
Salicylates	See *Aspirin*
Streptomycin	Urticaria, erythematous, morbilliform, and purpuric eruptions
Sulfonamides	Urticaria, scarlatiniform eruption, erythema nodosum, eczematous flare of exudative dermatitis, erythema multiforme–like bullous eruption, fixed eruption; see later section on photosensitivity reactions, morbilliform reaction AIDS patients: develop allergic drug eruptions quite often; one of the most common causes of toxic epidermal necrolysis and Stevens-Johnson syndrome See *Sulfonamides* and section on photosensitivity reactions
Sulfonylureas (suramin)	Cutaneous reaction (80%), especially morbilliform, UV light recall, (skin eruptions at the site of previous UV exposure), urticaria, "suramin keratoses"
Taxanes (paclitaxel, docetaxel)	Scleroderma-like skin changes, fixed drug, onycholysis, acral erythema, erythema multiforme, pustular eruptions
Testosterone and related drugs	Acne-like lesions, alopecia in scalp, hirsutism
Tetracycline	Fixed drug eruption, photosensitivity, serum sickness-like reaction < 8 years: teeth staining; see *Antibiotics*
Thalidomide	Erythroderma, pustulosis, toxic epidermal necrolysis
Thiazides	See section on photosensitivity reactions
Trimethoprim (Trimpex®, Roche)	Rarely incriminated drug eruptions
Vitamin A	Long-term, high-dose therapy: scaly, rough, itchy skin with coarse dry, scant hair growth, systemic changes including liver toxicity
Vitamin D	Skin lesions rare, but headache, nausea, diarrhea, increased urination, and sore gums and joints

(Continued on next page)

Table 2-2. Drugs and Associated Dermatoses (Continued)

Drug	Dermatoses/Comments
Vitamin B group	Urticaria, pruritic redness, and even anaphylactic reactions occur after IM or IV administration Nicotinic acid: red flush (common—warn patient to eliminate unnecessary alarm), pruritus (common), hives (rare, within 15–30 minutes after oral ingestion of 50–100 mg)
Warfarin sodium	See *Anticoagulants*

ACE—angiotensin-converting enzyme; ACTH—adrenocorticotropic hormone; AIDS—acquired immunodeficiency syndrome; DMSO—dimethyl sulfoxide; LSC—lichen simplex chronicus; NSAID—nonsteroidal anti-inflammatory drug; SLE—systemic lupus erythematosus; UV—ultraviolet

Note. From "Dermatologic Allergy" (pp. 95–99), by J. Hall in *Sauer's Manual of Skin Diseases* (9th ed.), 2006, Philadelphia: Lippincott Williams & Wilkins. Copyright 2006 by Lippincott Williams & Wilkins. Adapted with permission.

Table 2-3. Dermatoses and the Drugs That Cause Them

Dermatosis	Drugs	Comments
Acne-like or pustular lesions	Bromides, iodides, lithium, testosterone, corticosteroids	–
Acral erythema	Redness, pain, and swelling of the hands and feet associated with various chemotherapeutic agents including cyclophosphamide, cytosine arabinoside, docetaxel, doxorubicin, fluorouracil, hydroxyurea, mercaptopurine, methotrexate, and mitotane	Most commonly cytarabine, doxorubicin, and fluorouracil
Actinic keratosis inflammation	First described with fluorouracil; also doxorubicin, cisplatin, fludarabine, dactinomycin, dacarbazine, vincristine sulfate	Chemotherapy can be continued or briefly interrupted with use of topical corticosteroids
Alopecia	Amethopterin (methotrexate) and other antineoplastic agents; colchicine, clofibrate, testosterone and other androgens; tricyclic antidepressants; β-blockers; heparin; progesterone derivatives, coumarin derivatives, isotretinoin	–

(Continued on next page)

Table 2-3. Dermatoses and the Drugs That Cause Them *(Continued)*		
Dermatosis	**Drugs**	**Comments**
Angioedema	Aspirin, NSAIDs, ACE inhibitors	–
Baboon syndrome	Mercury (most often); also ampicillin, amoxicillin, nickel, erythromycin, heparin, and food additives	Systemic contact dermatitis owing to ingestion, inhalation, or percutaneous absorption; symmetric diffuse acute light red exanthema on buttocks, anogenital area, major flexural areas of extremities and peaks at day 2–5 of exposure to the involved drug; resolves within 1 week
DIDMOHS (drug-induced delayed [3–6 weeks] multi-organ hypersensitivity syndrome of Sontheimer and Houpt; also called *DRESS* [drug rash with eosinophilia and systemic symptoms of Bocquet and Roujeau])	Dapsone, carbamazepine, phenobarbital, minocycline, trimethoprim, sulfamethoxazole, procarbazine, allopurinol, terbinafine	Exanthematous or papulopustular febrile eruption with hepatitis (also possible lung, renal, thyroid involvement), lymphadenopathy, and eosinophilia
Eczematous eruption	Quinine, antihistamines, gold, mercury, sulfonamides, penicillin, organic arsenic	–
Erythema multiforme–like eruption	Penicillin and other antibiotics, sulfonamides, phenolphthalein, barbiturates, phenytoin, meprobamate	–
Erythema nodosum–like eruption	Sulfonamides, iodides, salicylates, oral contraceptives, dapsone	–
Exfoliative dermatitis	Particularly owing to arsenic, penicillin, sulfonamides, allopurinol, barbiturates	In the course of any severe generalized drug eruption
Fixed drug eruption	Phenolphthalein, acetaminophen, barbiturates, organic arsenic, gold, salicylates, sulfonamides, tetracycline, many others	Fixed drug eruption: hyperpigmented or purplish, flat or slightly elevated, discrete, single or multiple patches, occurs at the same sites on drug challenge
		(Continued on next page)

Table 2-3. Dermatoses and the Drugs That Cause Them *(Continued)*

Dermatosis	Drugs	Comments
Hyperpigmentation	Contraceptives, chloroquine, minocycline, chlorpromazine, amiodarone, bismuth and gold, silver salts, ACTH, estrogen, Adriamycin® (Bedford Laboratories), AZT, methotrexate	–
Hypertrichosis	Oral minoxidil, phenytoin, cyclosporine Less severe: oral contraceptives, systemic corticosteroids, psoralens, streptomycin sulfate	–
Keratoses and epitheliomas	Arsenic, mercury, PUVA therapy, immunosuppressive agents	–
Lichen planus–like eruption	Atabrine, arsenic, naproxen, gold, others	–
Lupus erythematous	Minocycline, hydralazine, procainamide, isoniazid, chlorpromazine, diltiazem, quinidine	–
Linear IgA bullous dermatosis	Vancomycin (most common), furosemide, captopril, lithium, amiodarone, diclofenac, cefamandole, somatostatin, rifampin, topical iodine, phenytoin, trimethoprim-sulfamethoxazole, penicillin G, IL-2, interferon	–
Lipoatrophies from injections	Corticosteroids (e.g., triamcinolone), insulin, vasopressin, human growth hormone, iron dextrin, DTP	–
Lipodystrophy	Partial: proteinase inhibitors used to treat AIDS: Indinavir or ritonavir plus saquinavir causes decreased subcutaneous fat on the face (cadaveric or cachectic faces) and extremities (pseudomuscular appearance) with increased prominence of the superficial veins; central adiposity with increased abdominal girth (pseudo-obesity), enlargement of breasts, increased dorsal-cervical fat pads (buffalo hump or pseudo-Cushing's syndrome)	Increased triglyceride and LDL cholesterol and low HDL cholesterol also occurs

(Continued on next page)

Table 2-3. Dermatoses and the Drugs That Cause Them *(Continued)*

Dermatosis	Drugs	Comments
Measles-like eruption	Barbiturates, arsenic, sulfonamides, quinine, many others	–
Mucous membrane lesions	Pigmentation: bismuth Hypertrophy: phenytoin Erosive lesions: sulfonamides, antineoplastic agents, many other drugs	–
Nail changes	Onycholysis (distal detachment): tetracycline, apparently owing to a phototoxic reaction	–
Neutrophilic eccrine hidradenitis	Bleomycin, chlorambucil, cyclophosphamide, cytarabine, doxorubicin, lomustine, mitoxantrone	–
Nicolau syndrome (embolia cutis medicamentosa)	Diclofenac, ibuprofen, iodine, benzathine, penicillin, vitamin K, DTP immunizations, antihistamines, interferon α, corticosteroids	At IM injection site
Nummular eczema–like eruption	Combination of isoniazid and p-amino-salicylic acid	–
Necrosis of the skin	Localized: coumarin and heparin derivatives; recombinant γ interferon Distant: coumarin and heparin derivatives	–
Ochronosis, exogenous	Topical phenol, quinine injections, topical resorcinol With prolonged use: topical hydroquinone, mainly in dark-skinned patients at the site of application only	–
Pemphigoid-like lesions	Furosemide, penicillin, sulfasalazine, ibuprofen	–
Pemphigus-like lesions	Rifampin, penicillamine, captopril, pyrazolone derivatives	–

(Continued on next page)

Table 2-3. Dermatoses and the Drugs That Cause Them *(Continued)*

Dermatosis	Drugs	Comments
Photosensitivity reaction	Sulfonamides: sulfonylurea Hypoglycemics: tolbutamide (Orinase®, Pfizer Inc.), chlorpropamide (Diabinese®, Pfizer Inc.) Antibiotics: demethylchlortetracycline (Declomycin®, Stiefel Laboratories), doxycycline (Doryx® [Mayne Pharma], Monodox® [Watson Pharmaceuticals], Vibramycin®, Pfizer Inc.), griseofulvin (Fulvicin® [Schering], Grifulvin® [OrthoNeutrogena], Gris-PEG® [Pedinol]), Maxaquin® [Pharmacia] (lomefloxacin), nalidixic acid (NegGram® [Sanofi-Aventis U.S. LLC]), tetracycline Benzofurans: amiodarone Chlorothiazine diuretics: chlorothiazide (Diuril®); hydrochlorothiazide; methyclothiazide Phenothiazines: chlorpromazine (Thorazine); prochlorperazine (Compazine); promethazine (Phenergan) Psoralens: methoxsalen (Oxsoralen®); trioxsalen (Trisoralen®) Oxicams: piroxicam (Feldene®)	Several of the newer drugs and some of the older ones cause dermatitis on exposure to sunlight. These skin reactions can be urticarial, erythematous, vesicular, or plaquelike. The mechanism can be either phototoxic or photoallergic, but this distinction can be difficult to ascertain.
Pityriasis rosea-like eruption	Bismuth, gold, barbiturates, antihistamines	–
Porphyria cutanea tarda exacerbation	Estrogen, iron, ethanol ingestion, hexachlorobenzene, chlorinated phenols, polychlorinated biphenyls, possibly pravastatin	–
Pseudolymphoma	Antidepressants, diphenylhydantoin, α antagonists, ACE inhibitors, anticonvulsants, antihistamines, benzodiazepine, β blockers, calcium-channel blockers, lipid-lowering agents, lithium, NSAIDs, phenothiazines, procainamide, estrogen, progesterone	–

(Continued on next page)

Table 2-3. Dermatoses and the Drugs That Cause Them *(Continued)*		
Dermatosis	**Drugs**	**Comments**
Pseudoporphyria cutanea tarda (PCT)	NSAIDs (naproxen, nabumetone, oxaprozin, ketoprofen, mefenamic acid, diflunisal), nalidixic acid, tetracycline, chlorthalidone, furosemide, hydrochlorothiazide/triamterene, Isotretinoin, etretinate, cyclosporine, 5-fluorouacil, pyridoxine, amiodarone, flutamide, dapsone, aspirin	Skin findings but no biochemical abnormalities. May persist for months after offending drug stopped, mimics skin finding and skin biopsy of PCT
Psoriasis exacerbation	Lithium, β-blockers, ACE inhibitors, antimalarials, NSAIDs, terbinafine	–
Purpuric eruptions	Barbiturates, salicylates, meprobamate, organic arsenic, sulfonamides, chlorothiazide diuretics, corticosteroids (long-term use)	–
Pustulosis, acute generalized erythematous (aged or toxic pustulosis)	Antibiotics (mainly β-lactam); many others	–
Scarlet fever–like eruption or "toxic erythema"	Arsenic, barbiturates, codeine, morphine, mercury, quinidine, salicylates, sulfonamides, others	–
Seborrheic dermatitis–like eruption	Gold, ACTH	–
Stevens-Johnson syndrome	Lamotrigine, valproic acid, penicillin, barbiturates, diphenylhydantoin, sulfonamides, rifampin, NSAIDs, salicylates	–
Subacute cutaneous lupus erythematosus	Hydrochlorothiazide, ACE inhibitors, calcium channel blockers, interferons, statins	–
Urticaria	Penicillin, salicylates, serums, sulfonamides, barbiturates, opium group, contraceptive drugs, *Rauwolfia* alkaloids, ACE inhibitors	–
Vesicular or bullous eruptions	Sulfonamides, penicillin, mephenytoin	–

(Continued on next page)

Table 2-3. Dermatoses and the Drugs That Cause Them *(Continued)*		
Dermatosis	**Drugs**	**Comments**
Whitening of hair	Chloroquine, hydroxychloroquine	In blonde- or red-haired people

ACE—angiotensin-converting enzyme; ACTH—adrenocorticotropic hormone; AIDS—acquired immunodeficiency syndrome; DTP—diphtheria-tetanus-pertussis; HDL—high-density lipoprotein; IL—interleukin; IM—intramuscular; LDL—low-density lipoprotein; NSAID—nonsteroidal anti-inflammatory drug; PUVA—psoralens and ultraviolet light

Note. From "Dermatologic Allergy" (pp. 100–103), by J. Hall in *Sauer's Manual of Skin Diseases* (9th ed.), 2006, Philadelphia: Lippincott Williams & Wilkins. Copyright 2006 by Lippincott Williams & Wilkins. Adapted with permission.

Nursing Evaluation of a Cutaneous Drug Reaction

When a patient appears to have a cutaneous drug reaction, the oncology nurse needs to evaluate the patient using a history and physical format, which focuses on the skin manifestations. The nurse should triage the patient with questions and simultaneously perform a brief physical assessment. The oncology nurse's ability to recognize and accurately describe lesions can lead to prompt diagnosis and treatment, as well as help the patient to avoid discomfort and a serious complication (Cole & Gray-Miceli, 2002).

The history should begin with the chief complaint in the patient's own words. Asking specific questions will help to determine onset, location, duration, characteristics, relieving factors, timing, severity, and a history of medications (Cole & Gray-Miceli, 2002). Refer to Figure 2-1 for a list of example triage questions.

The physical examination should be performed in a room that is warm and preferably lighted with diffuse bright daylight. Artificial light, including fluorescent lighting, changes the appearance of the skin and lesions. Cole and Gray-Miceli (2002) advocate having an observant eye, a sensitive touch (gloved hands), a small, flexible, metric ruler, and a small flashlight available.

The nurse should complete the examination in an orderly manner to ensure that important diagnostic clues are not missed. Particular attention should be given to the hair, nails, and mouth. The nurse should use specific terminology to describe the characteristics of the skin lesions (color, configuration, distribution, type of lesion, and lesion pattern), which can then be documented (Johannsen, 2005).

Not only should oncology nurses be able to describe a lesion, but they also should be able to describe the location, distribution, and related symptoms. The general assessment should include vital signs, palpation of the joints for arthralgia, and an assessment for adenopathy. When all of this information is gathered, nurses then face the challenge of determining whether the skin manifestation is a reaction to a medication or is associated with other disease processes. Nursing care management begins simultaneously.

Figure 2-1. Sample of Triage Questions for Assessing Cutaneous Manifestations From Drugs

- When did the skin reaction start?
- How long has the skin reaction been present?
- Does the skin itch?
- What did the reaction first look like?
- Has the skin reaction changed?
- Does the skin reaction come and go?
- Have you recently started any changes in your daily medications?
- Have you recently started any new medications?
- Have you changed soap, detergents, lotions, etc., before you noticed the skin reaction?
- Any history of similar symptoms?
- Have you used or tried anything that seems to make the reaction better or worse?

Note. From "Skin Assessment," by L. Johannsen, 2005, *Dermatology Nursing, 17*(2), p. 166. Copyright 2005 by Jannetti Publications, Inc. Reprinted with permission.

Nursing Management

It can be stated, almost without exception, that any drug systemically administered is capable of causing a drug eruption (Hall, 2006). Nursing management revolves around the following three goals (Hockett, 2004).
- Eliminate the drug.
- Recommend comfort measures for skin discomfort.
- Provide fluid management and support, infection control, and pain management in life-threatening reactions (e.g., SJS, TEN).

A thorough nursing history is a critical contribution to the management of a cutaneous drug reaction. The nursing history can lead to identifying the medication that is causing the manifestation. Often the first line of treatment is to eliminate the drug that is causing the reaction. This simple procedure may be delayed because a careful history was not taken. If the eruption is mild, and the drug is necessary, then discontinuation of the drug may not be mandatory (Hall, 2006). Further therapy depends on the seriousness of the eruption. Most barbiturate-induced measles-like eruptions subside without intervention. An itching drug eruption should be treated to relieve the pruritus. Cases of exfoliative dermatitis or severe erythema multiforme–like lesions require treatment with a corticosteroid and other supportive therapy (Hall). Pruritus (itch) is uncomfortable to live with and can lead to poor sleep, agitation, difficulty with concentration, and infection from scratching. Several modalities may be attempted before total, or even partial, relief is achieved. In addition to using the oral and topical antipruritic medication available, patients can take some simple measures to reduce the intensity of the itch (Yosipovitch & Hundley, 2004).

Emollients are the first-line therapy for pruritus. Although they are generally not considered antipruritics, emollients can help to reduce itch, particularly in patients with dry skin. Water normally evaporates quickly from the skin surface, but emollients contain lipids and other substances that seal in moisture. They should be applied immediately after bathing to promote hydration of the skin by preventing transepidermal water loss (Wahlgren, 1999; Yosipovitch & Hundley, 2004).

Other topical recommendations for pruritus include low-pH cleansers and moisturizers, cooling agents, topical antihistamines, and topical corticosteroids. The low-pH products are useful in maintaining the acidic pH of the skin surface, which helps to preserve its barrier function. Cooling agents usually contain menthol, camphor, or phenol. These substances stimulate nerve fibers that transmit the sensation of cold, thereby masking the itch sensation. Topical antihistamines can be effective antipruritics because they block H_1 receptors. Topical corticosteroids may indirectly provide relief of itch but are not intended for long-term use. Potential side effects of long-term application of topical steroids include skin atrophy, cutaneous eruptions, and dryness (Fleischer, 2000; Yosipovitch & Hu, 2003). Refer to Figure 2-2 for suggestions to reduce itching.

SJS and TEN are severe skin toxicities that may occur in any patient with cancer. They are caused by infection or a drug reaction and can result in sepsis, severe ocular complications, and even death. Skin lesions usually are preceded by prodromal flu-like symptoms. A rash with subsequent blistering and denudation follows (Hockett, 2004). Improving the outcome for patients with SJS and TEN depends on early recognition as well as appropriate interventions. Prompt withdrawal of the suspected offending agent should occur, which means stopping all but life-sustaining drugs to eliminate the suspected agent (Stern, 2000).

Figure 2-2. Measures to Reduce Itch*

- Restrict time in the shower or bathtub.
- Bathe in cool or lukewarm water rather than hot water, which can be drying.
- Use mild soaps.
- Use low-pH cleansers and moisturizers.
- Avoid cleansers containing alcohol.
- Apply moisturizer immediately after bathing to help maintain moisture from the shower/bath.
- Use a humidifier, especially in the winter.
- Wear light clothing.
- Maintain cool ambient temperature.
- Avoid rapid changes in environmental humidity.
- Avoid hot or spicy foods and alcoholic beverages, which can induce histamine secretion.
- Keep fingernails short to prevent skin damage if patients cannot resist the urge to scratch.

* Recommendations not supported by research

Note. From "Practical Guidelines for the Relief of Itch," by G. Yosipovitch and J.L. Hundley, 2004, *Dermatology Nursing, 16*(4), p. 327. Copyright 2004 by Jannetti Publications, Inc. Adapted with permission.

The cornerstone of treatment for patients with SJS and TEN is meticulous skin care, fluid management, nutritional support, pain management, and surveillance for and treatment of infection. Skin, eye, and mouth care are a priority. Oral mucositis may be severe enough to inhibit swallowing. Mucositis and scarring can affect the patient's ability to absorb fluids, nutrients, and medications, resulting in fluid and electrolyte imbalance and altered medication delivery. SJS or TEN can cause permanent loss of vision from severe dryness or necrosis of conjunctiva. These patients often are transferred to burn units. Burn units are specifically prepared to handle the multisystem organ involvement with a multidisciplinary team approach that employs specialized wound care protocols and equipment (Hockett, 2004; Stern, 2000).

Compounding Factors

Evaluating a patient with cancer for a cutaneous reaction requires nurses to be astute in assessment and cognitive of the multiple problems that oncology patients experience on and off therapy. Patients often are in poor health, immunosuppressed, experiencing polypharmacy, and using complementary and alternative medicines (CAM) and may be victims of duplicate prescriptions. These are all factors that should be considered when a patient with cancer develops a cutaneous reaction.

Patients with cancer are susceptible to drug interactions. The most prevalent reason is multiple medication orders. Many of the patients are receiving antineoplastic agents as well as drugs to treat comorbid conditions. Therefore, patients may take medications to treat both therapy-induced toxicity and cancer-related syndromes, such as pain, seizures, and venous thrombosis. The risk of drug interactions is further heightened because the patient's pharmacokinetic parameters may be altered. The change in pharmacokinetic parameters may be caused by a number of factors, such as impaired drug absorption because of mucositis and malnutrition; variation in a drug's systemic distribution because of edema or a reduced levels of proteins; or renal or hepatic dysfunction (Riechelmann et al., 2007). Drug reactions that present as cutaneous manifestations often are the result of an increase or decrease of the plasma concentration of a drug in the bloodstream. Determining the cause or causes for an eruption may avoid the pitfalls of discontinuing medicines that may be needed or altering the course of the patient's treatment (Koppel & Boh, 2006).

Nurses should not ignore the use of CAM by patients with cancer. Vapiwala et al. (2006) reported that 48% of patients with cancer who were being treated with chemotherapy and radiation were using CAM treatment, and a majority (75%) did not tell their doctor, even while they were on conventional treatment. Eighty-eight percent reported using vitamin, herbal, and botanical supplements. Patterson et al. (2002) reported that patients who underwent multiple therapies (chemotherapy, radiation, surgery) were twice as likely to use alternative medicine for cancer treatment or symptom management as compared to those who had surgery alone. When assessing a cutaneous manifestation, oncology nurses need to be aware of any complementary therapies that a patient is using, whether herbs or active therapy such as massage or acupuncture. Nurses must keep in mind that CAM treatment may contribute to an unexplained skin manifestation in a patient.

The Oncology Nursing Society (ONS) position on the use of CAM supports the following (ONS, 2006).

- Oncology nurses should develop an awareness of CAM therapies that potentially can interfere with the outcome of other cancer treatments.
- Oncology nurses should establish evidence-based practice in these areas by synthesizing present knowledge with regard to safety, efficacy, concurrent use with conventional therapy, and long-term use.

Multiple physicians and multiple prescriptions put patients with cancer at risk for duplicate prescriptions. *Duplicate prescribing* is present when two or more drugs from the same class are prescribed to treat the same condition (e.g., morphine and codeine prescribed as routine orders for pain) or different conditions (e.g., corticosteroids to prevent delayed nausea and anti-inflammatory agents). Not only are patients at risk for complications of being overmedicated, but the probability of side effects also increases (Riechelmann et al., 2007).

Conclusion

Caring for patients with cancer is complicated for multiple reasons. Disruption of the patient's skin integrity, the body's first line of defense against microorganisms, can leave a patient feeling uncomfortable for a few days or infected and septic. The most vital nursing function is a thorough nursing assessment with the goal of identifying the drug that is causing the reaction. Observing the patient until the reaction resolves, providing nursing interventions during the reaction, and reassuring the patient are the backbone of the nursing care.

References

Bigby, M. (2001). Rates of cutaneous reactions to drugs. *Archives of Dermatology, 137*(6), 765–770.

Cole, J., & Gray-Miceli, D. (2002). The necessary elements of a dermatologic history and physical evaluation. *Dermatology Nursing, 14*(6), 377–382.

Fitzpatrick, T., Johnson, R., Wolff, K., & Suurmond, D. (2001). *Color atlas and synopsis of clinical dermatology* (4th ed.). New York: McGraw-Hill.

Fleischer, A.B. (2000). *The clinical management of itching.* New York: Parthenon Publishing Group.

Gell, P.G.H., & Coombs, R.R.A. (Eds.). (1963). *Clinical aspects of immunology.* Philadelphia: Davis.

Goodheart, H. (2003). *Goodheart's photoguide of common skin disorders—diagnosis and management* (2nd ed.). Philadelphia: Lippincott Williams & Wilkins.

Hall, J.C. (Ed.). (2006). *Sauer's manual of skin diseases* (9th ed.). Philadelphia: Lippincott Williams & Wilkins.

Hockett, K.C. (2004). Stevens-Johnson syndrome and toxic epidermal necrolysis: Oncologic considerations. *Clinical Journal of Oncology Nursing, 8*(1), 27–30.

James, W.D., Berger, T., & Elston, D. (2006). *Andrews' diseases of the skin: Clinical dermatology* (10th ed.). Philadelphia: Elsevier Saunders.

Johannsen, L. (2005) Skin assessment. *Dermatology Nursing, 17*(2), 165–166.

Koppel, R., & Boh, E. (2006). Cutaneous reactions to chemotherapeutic agents. *American Journal of the Medical Sciences, 321*(5), 327–335.

Oncology Nursing Society. (2006). *The use of complementary, alternative, and integrative therapies in cancer care* [Position statement]. Retrieved December 14, 2007, from http://www.ons.org/Publications/Positions/ComplementaryTherapies.shtml

Patterson, R.E., Neuhouser, M.L., Hedderson, M.M., Schwartz, S.M., Standish, L.J., Bowen, D.J., et al. (2002). Types of alternative medicine used by patients with breast, colon, or prostate cancer: Predictors, motives, and cost. *Journal of Alternative and Complementary Medicine, 8*(4), 477–485.

Riechelmann, R., Tannock, I., Wang, L., Saad, E., Taback, N., & Krzyzanowska, M. (2007). Potential drug interactions and duplicate prescriptions among cancer patients. *Journal of the National Cancer Institute, 99*(8), 592–600.

Riedl, M.A., & Casillas, A.M. (2003). Adverse drug reactions: Types and treatment options. *American Family Physician, 68*(9), 1781–1790.

Stern, R.S. (1997). Cutaneous drug reactions. In K.A. Arndt, B.U. Wintroub, J.K. Robinson, & P.E. LeBoit (Eds.), *Primary care dermatology* (pp. 85–89). Philadelphia: Saunders.

Stern, R.S. (2000). Improving the outcome of patients with toxic epidermal necrolysis and Stevens-Johnson syndrome. *Archives of Dermatology, 136*(3), 410–411.

Svensson, C.K., Cowen, E.W., & Gaspari, A.A. (2001). Cutaneous drug reactions. *Pharmacological Reviews, 53*(3), 357–379.

University of Utah Hospital and Clinics. (2007). *Cancer chemotherapy manual.* St. Louis, MO: Facts and Comparisons.

Vapiwala, N., Mick, R., Hampshire, M.K., Metz, J.M., & DeNittis, A.S. (2006). Patient initiation of complementary and alternative medical therapies (CAM) following cancer diagnosis. *Cancer Journal, 12*(6), 467–474.

Wahlgren, C.F. (1999). Itch and atopic dermatitis: An overview. *Journal of Dermatology, 26*(11), 770–779.

Yosipovitch, G., & Hu, J. (2003). The importance of skin pH. *Skin and Aging, 11*(3), 89–93.

Yosipovitch, G., & Hundley, J.L. (2004). Practical guidelines for the relief of itch. *Dermatology Nursing, 16*(4), 325–328.

CHAPTER 3

Benign Skin Disorders: Impact on Cancer Therapy

Giselle J. Moore-Higgs, ARNP, PhD(c), AOCN®

Introduction

Benign skin disease is common, particularly in adults. As the largest organ of the human body, the skin serves as the crucial mediator between the inner body and the external environment and, therefore, reflects the status of the body's internal health. Although surface irritants can be the source of many isolated skin diseases, a significant number of skin symptoms reflect a more generalized systemic (e.g., cirrhosis) or genetic disease (e.g., albinism). In addition to the disease-related symptoms, symptoms also occur that are related to the treatment of the disease (e.g., drug rash). As a result, it is not unusual for patients with cancer to present with one or more benign skin disorders that may have a direct or indirect impact on their cancer treatment. Healthcare providers need to have an understanding of the most common skin disorders and the potential impact that cancer treatment may have on the disorder.

The understanding of the etiology and pathogenesis of the vast number of skin lesions described in the literature are enhanced by advances in immunopathology and molecular biology, making timely diagnosis and treatment more practical than in the past. Despite these advances, the classification of individual skin disease remains confusing and can result in the delay of a diagnosis and treatment. Accurate physical diagnosis hinges on the ability of clinicians to properly classify the type of lesion or lesions seen on the skin. Four major features of skin lesions or eruptions allow skin disease to be placed in diagnostic categories that facilitate specific diagnosis:

- Morphologic appearance of the individual lesions (see Table 3-1)
- Distribution of lesions over the body surface

- Arrangement of the lesions
- Number of lesions present.

This information also enables healthcare providers to determine whether the lesions are primary or secondary in nature. *Primary lesions* are defined as

Table 3-1. Morphology-Based Classification of Major Skin Disorders		
Group	**Clinical Morphology**	**Example of Diseases in the Group**
Eczematous dermatitis	Erythematous macules, papules, vesicles, lichenification, fine scaling, excoriations, crusting	Contact dermatitis, atopic dermatitis, stasis dermatitis, photodermatitis, exfoliative dermatitis
Maculopapular eruptions	Macules, erythema, papules	Viral exanthems, drug hypersensitivity reactions, Kawasaki disease, vasculitic, purpuric eruptions
Papulosquamous dermatoses	Papules, plaques, erythema with scales	Psoriasis, Reiter's syndrome, pityriasis rosea, lichen planus, seborrheic dermatitis, ichthyosis, secondary syphilis, mycosis fungoides
Vesiculobullous diseases	Vesicles, bullae, erythema	Herpes simplex and zoster, hand-foot-and-mouth disease, insect bites, bullous impetigo, scalded skin syndrome, pemphigus, bullous pemphigoid, dermatitis herpetiformis, porphyria cutanea tarda, erythema multiform
Pustular diseases	Pustules, cysts, erythema	Acne vulgaris rosacea, pustular psoriasis, folliculitis
Urticaria and cellulitis	Wheals and figured, raised erythema, scaling	Urticaria, erythema annulare centrifugum and erysipelas
Nodular lesions	Nodules and tumors, some associated with erosions and ulceration	Benign and malignant tumors—basal cell cancer, squamous cell cancer, rheumatoid nodules, xanthomas
Telangiectasia, atrophic scarring, ulcerative diseases	Atrophic, sclerotic telangiectasia, ulcerative changes	Connective tissue diseases, radiation dermatitis, lichen sclerosis et atrophicus, vascular insufficiency (arterial and venous), pyoderma gangrenosum
Hypermelanosis and hypomelanosis	Increased and decreased melanin deposition in skin	Acanthosis nigricans, café au lait spots, vitiligo, tuberous sclerosis, xeroderma pigmentosum, melasma, freckles

Note. From "Examination of the Skin and Approach to Diagnosing Skin Diseases" (p. 2453), by C. Armstrong in L. Goldman and D. Ausiello (Eds.), *Cecil Textbook of Medicine* (22nd ed.), 2004, Philadelphia: Saunders. Copyright 2004 by Saunders. Reprinted with permission.

those that represent the initial pathologic change, whereas *secondary lesions* result from external forces, such as scratching or infection of primary lesions.

This chapter will provide a review of the most common benign skin disorders that an oncology healthcare provider may see in clinical practice. Disease entities that will be discussed include skin infections, benign tumors, pigment disorders, inflammatory disorders, and collagen vascular disorders of the skin. Although early recognition and treatment are often key to a successful outcome, patient and family education also plays an important role in reducing the potential for a serious and sometimes fatal complication.

Skin Infections

Bacterial Infections

Bacterial infections of the skin and underlying soft tissues (SSTIs) are one of the most common reasons that patients present to an emergency room or office-based medical practice. In a recent U.S. study, nearly a threefold increase in the annual number of emergency department visits for SSTIs was observed, with 3.4 million such visits recorded in 2005 (Pallin et al., 2008). SSTIs occur in different body sites that have been compromised or injured by foreign body, trauma, ischemia, malignancy, or surgery. Common community-acquired SSTIs include

- Cellulitis
- Folliculitis
- Furunculosis
- Impetigo
- Erysipelas
- Infectious gangrene
- Secondary bacterial infections
- Trauma-related wound infections.

Other types of SSTIs include paronychia; anorectal, pilonidal, and perirectal abscesses; infected epidermal cysts; hidradenitis suppurativa; and pustular acne. The increased use of invasive medical procedures (i.e., surgery) and the rising number of immunocompromised patients (immunosuppressive drug therapy, cancer, organ transplant surgery, and HIV/AIDS) have dramatically increased the incidence of complicated SSTIs. In addition, the increased use of tattoos, piercings, and other forms of self-provoked body modifications also has increased the number of SSTIs (Kazandjieva & Tsankov, 2007; Panconesi, 2007).

In general, most SSTIs produce only mild to moderate symptoms, which may be treated on an outpatient basis. However, some infections, particularly in patients with comorbidities (e.g., cancer, diabetes mellitus, ischemic ulceration, chronic lymphedema) or those who have developed bacteremia (e.g., immunocompromised patients), can be classified as complicated and may even be life-threatening (e.g., necrotizing fasciitis) and require hospitalization. SSTIs can progress rapidly; therefore, early recognition and proper management is the cornerstone of therapy.

Incision and drainage constitutes the primary therapy for most SSTIs, including furuncles, abscesses, and septic joints, and should be performed routinely (Gorwitz et al., 2006). If a clinician is unsure whether pus is present in a lesion, an attempt can be made to aspirate fluid from the lesion using an adequately sized needle and syringe (e.g., a 16- to 19-gauge needle on a 10 cc syringe). For small furuncles not amenable to incision and drainage, or collection of material for culture, moist heat may be satisfactory to promote drainage. Cultures should be obtained from the wound to guide the clinician's choice in antibiotic therapy. Although many patients with drainable lesions can be cured with surgical intervention alone, effective antibacterial therapy may improve cure rates, especially among patients with large abscesses or cellulitis.

Historically, *Staphylococcus (S.) aureus* and *Streptococcus* species (spp.), especially *Streptococcus pyogenes*, have been the predominant pathogens, although for skin infections, *Corynebacterium* spp., *Pasteurella* spp., and *Enterobacteriaceae* also are frequently found. Strains resistant to beta-lactams, known as methicillin-resistant *S. aureus* (MRSA), began to emerge in the 1960s and were found predominantly in patients in healthcare facilities. This changed when new "community-associated" strains emerged in the mid-1990s, and community-acquired MRSA is now the leading identifiable cause of SSTIs. The majority of uncomplicated SSTIs can be treated with oral agents targeted against susceptible gram-positive agents, such as a first-generation cephalosporin, a macrolide, or a penicillinase-stable penicillin. Complicated SSTIs usually require aggressive IV antibiotics such as linezolid, quinupristin/dalfopristin, daptomycin, and newer-generation carbapenems and fluoroquinolones designed to primarily cover gram-positive pathogens.

In the oncology patient population, prevention, early recognition, and intervention of SSTIs are key to successful treatment. The ability to resist infection is much lower in this patient population as a result of either the malignancy or the treatment. Individuals undergoing intensive chemotherapy may experience a profound impairment of their cellular and humoral immune system, resulting in a much higher risk of infectious complications with associated significant morbidity and mortality. These patients can develop SSTIs around drain sites, around central line insertion sites, in surgical or traumatic wounds, or around body piercings. Early recognition and immediate referral to a surgeon for management is recommended.

Unfortunately, SSTIs may result in delaying oncologic treatment to allow for healing. It is not generally recommended that patients receive chemotherapy while an active infection is present, as it may increase the risk of further immunosuppression. Radiation therapy (RT) can proceed if the site of infection is not in the treatment field and the treatment area does not include a large volume of bone marrow, which may increase the risk of immunosuppression. However, each patient's situation should be carefully evaluated to weigh the risks versus benefits of treatment. If a delay is necessary, patients and families may require psychosocial support to address their concerns of disease progression and frustration.

Patients and families must receive education in meticulous wound care to enhance healing and prevent further delays. This includes cleansing and dressing changes and instructions regarding signs and symptoms to report. Additional resources such as home health assistance and supplies may be needed in the outpatient setting.

Fungal Infections

Fungal infections of the skin are emerging as another important dermatologic issue in patients with cancer. Many of the infections found in patients with cancer look similar to infections in patients without cancer. However, in some cases, they can become more extensive and even life threatening. Skin fungal infections known under the heading of *dermatomycoses* are the most common forms of fungal disease. Basically, these disorders encompass two main distinct conditions with strikingly different outcomes. On one hand, some of them are primary cutaneous skin infections that most often remain superficial. On the other hand, the lesions may represent a cutaneous manifestation of invasion from a superficial lesion or a deeper site, or from fungaemia (Quatresooz, Pierard-Franchimont, Arrese, & Pierard, 2008).

Debilitated and/or severely immunocompromised patients with cancer are at particular risk for select fungal infections. In general, dermatomycoses remain confined to the stratum corneum and cutaneous appendages. Some subcutaneous mycoses and cutaneous infections also are associated with deep mycoses (Quatresooz et al., 2008). Patients with lymphoma and leukemia are most susceptible for deep fungal infections during periods of severe neutropenia following chemotherapy or bone marrow transplantation. Other predisposing conditions for risk of fungal infection include (Mays & Cohen, 2006)

- Long-term placement of vascular and urinary catheters
- Alteration of the gastrointestinal and oropharyngeal mucosa by chemotherapy
- Administration of broad-spectrum antibiotics
- High-dose corticotherapy or other immunosuppressive therapies
- Advanced age
- Systemic diseases (i.e., diabetes mellitus).

The dermatomycoses found in patients with cancer can be classified in four broad groups: primary superficial dermatophytoses, primary superficial yeast infections, opportunistic mold infections with distinct potential for dissemination, and secondary cutaneous manifestations of fungaemia (Quatresooz et al., 2008). Occasionally, more than one fungus is found inside a given skin lesion. The diagnosis usually relies on three basic laboratory approaches including microbiology, immunology, and histopathology. One of the quickest and most reliable ways to diagnose an invasive mycosis is by the unequivocal demonstration and identification of the agent in histopathologic sections. The common causative agents in oncology patients are *Candida, Aspergillus, Fusarium, Mucor,* and *Rhizopus.*

In patients without neutropenia, cutaneous fungal infections usually respond well to appropriate antifungal therapy applied directly to the lesion or lesions. However, in patients with neutropenia, these infections often are very resistant to aggressive antifungal therapy and may result in one of the following outcomes: the infection may clear; the infection may progress locally and invade into the subcutaneous tissue, muscle, and/or bone; or the infection may disseminate widely (Mays & Cohen, 2006). The main treatment is antifungal therapy, and patients with neutropenia may require weeks of systemic therapy. Debridement may be necessary for deep-seated skin infections but should be undertaken with caution, particularly in patients with neutropenia.

The impact of such a fungal infection on the patient with cancer can be devastating. Each patient should be evaluated and an individualized plan of care developed. Chemotherapy and RT may be given in some patients with a small superficial cutaneous *Candida* infection, whereas this may not be reasonable in a patient with a more advanced infection. In addition to a potential delay in treatment, the patient and family also face the possibility of disseminated disease and the associated morbidity and mortality. These patients often have prolonged or multiple hospitalizations, have protracted treatment plans, and risk further complications that result from being immunocompromised. They require tremendous psychosocial support as well as education to address their needs.

Parasitic Skin Infections

The ectoparasites scabies and pediculosis pubis are common causes of skin rash and pruritus worldwide. They are transmitted primarily by person-to-person contact and generally are associated with low morbidity. However, secondary bacterial infections can occur in patients with infestation, which can further complicate cancer treatment.

Scabies is caused by the mite *Sarcoptes scabiei* variety (var.) *hominis.* The mite is an obligate human parasite that lives in burrowed tunnels in the stratum corneum of the epidermis. Certain populations are at high risk for developing severe or crusted scabies. Patients receiving systemic or potent topical glucocorticoids, organ transplant recipients, physically incapacitated individuals, HIV-infected or human T-lymphotropic virus 1–infected individuals, and individuals with various hematologic malignancies are at risk for developing crusted scabies. Compared with normal scabies, crusted scabies is highly infectious and is characterized by a much higher burden of mites in the infested individual.

Patients with scabies usually complain of pruritus that is most severe at night. Occasionally, patients are asymptomatic. Skin lesions most commonly involve the interdigital spaces and the flexor surfaces of the wrist, axillae, waist, feet, and ankles. In women, the area around the nipple of the breast may be affected, as can the scrotum and penis in men. The initial infection is asymptomatic, with symptoms developing after three to six weeks in association with the development of an immune response to mites and their excrement. The most characteristic lesion of scabies infestation is the burrow, the excavated tunnel in which the mite lives. These burrows are usually thin, curvy, elevated tracts that measure 1–10 mm. Other skin manifestations include papules, blisters, eczematous changes, and nodules.

A presumptive diagnosis of scabies is based on the clinical presentation of pruritus with skin lesions and identification of a characteristic burrow. Definitive diagnosis requires microscopic identification of mites or their eggs or feces. This usually is achieved by obtaining skin scrapings at the site of a burrow or under the fingernails. The preferred treatment for scabies generally has been topical agents such as permethrin 5%. Recently, ivermectin has demonstrated good efficacy in the treatment of scabies, and it may be of particular use in institutional outbreaks or in communities in which scabies is endemic. Combination treatment with topical agents and oral ivermectin may be necessary for crusted scabies. Treating all close contacts and housemates of people with scabies and washing bedding, towels, and clothing in warm to hot water generally are recommended. Items that cannot be washed should be isolated from use for at least three days.

Lice are blood-sucking insects that primarily infest the head (*Pediculus humanus* var. *capitis*), the body (*Pediculus humanus* var. *corporis*), or the pubic region (*Phthirus pubis*). Head lice are the most common lice. The diagnosis is made by the identification of live lice or viable nits in the hair. Malathion, specifically in the formulation containing isopropyl alcohol and terpineol, is the favored first-line agent for the treatment of head lice (Lebwohl, Clark, & Levitt, 2007) and should be used on day 0 and day 7. A patient infected with head lice at any given time will have lice existing at different points in the life cycle, and malathion is the only therapy that will ensure eradication. However, this agent is flammable (keep wet hair away from heat sources) and should not be used in women who are pregnant. Other therapies include lindane 1% and permethrin 1% applied to the scalp or affected body area; however, the literature has shown evidence of resistance (Lebwohl et al., 2007).

Because both of these parasites are highly transmittable, early recognition and treatment are imperative to avoid an epidemic in the oncology setting. If a diagnosis is made, clinicians should follow their institution's infectious disease policy for notifying other patients who may have come in contact with the infected individual. All equipment and furnishings the individual has had contact with should be cleaned and disinfected according to institutional policy to avoid transmission to other patients, particularly those who are immunocompromised. A delay in cancer treatment may be necessary for 7–10 days until the parasitic disease has responded to treatment. Patients and families may require some emotional support in light of the diagnosis, which often is associated with the stigma of poor hygiene.

Benign Tumors

Epidermoid Cysts

Epidermoid cysts, also known as *inclusion cysts* and *epidermal inclusion cysts*, are very common lesions that, with rare exceptions, arise from the infundibular epithelium of the hair follicle (Vicente & Vazquez-Doval, 1998). They are round and mobile, ranging in size from a few millimeters to several centimeters. Histopathologically, epidermoid cysts are lined by stratified squamous epithelia containing a granular layer with a basket weave to laminated stratum corneum and are filled with keratin (Luba, Bangs, Mohler, & Stulberg, 2003). These cysts are commonly found on the face, back, or chest and communicate with the skin through a small, round, keratin-filled plug. They may remain small for years or may grow rapidly. Indications for excision include cosmesis, pain, and recurrent infection (Luba et al.).

Although epidermoid cysts are benign, a number of coexistent pathologic processes have been reported, including squamous cell carcinoma, basal cell carcinoma, seborrheic keratosis-like changes, melanophagic proliferation, melanoma, basal cell layer hyperpigmentation, clear-cell changes, cornoid lamellation, epidermolytic hyperkeratosis, Darier disease–like changes, pyogenic granuloma, Paget disease, mycosis fungoides, Bowen disease, metastatic adenocarcinoma, molluscum contagiosum, and human papillomavirus changes (Swygert, Parrish, Cashman, Lin, & Cockerell, 2007). Routine histologic examination of all excised cutaneous cysts is recommended to exclude a hidden malignancy. Additionally, any child or adult with epidermoid cysts in uncommon areas may have Gardner syndrome (Luba et al., 2003).

No specific recommendations exist for the management of epidermoid cysts in patients with cancer. An increased risk of inflammation of the cyst may occur if the lesion is in the field of radiation, depending on the dose and type of radiation given (electrons versus photons). Acutely inflamed, fluctuant cysts should be incised and drained (Luba et al., 2003). Antibiotics may or may not be necessary. RT may need to be delayed to allow the tissue to heal. Chemotherapy should not have a direct effect on a cyst; however, if the cyst is inflamed, it should be incised and drained and allowed to heal before chemotherapy to reduce the risk of local cellulitis. Immunosuppression may increase the risk of the development of an infected cyst, and patients should be educated to look for changes in the cyst, including redness, warmth to the touch, drainage, and onset of pain.

Lipomas

Lipomas are the most common soft-tissue tumor with a wide spectrum of clinical presentations (Luba et al., 2003; Rydholm & Berg, 1983). Benign musculoskeletal lipomas are found in both soft tissue and bone. They are subclassified according to the anatomic site of the fat cells as dermal, subcutaneous, and subfascial lipomas; or tumors directly related to muscle, bone, synovium, or nerve. The World Health Organization's Committee for the Classification of Soft Tissue Tumors categorizes lipomas into the following nine entities (Fletcher, Unni, & Mertens, 2002):

- Lipoma
- Lipomatosis
- Lipomatosis of nerve
- Lipoblastoma/lipoblastomatosis
- Angiolipoma
- Myolipoma of soft tissue
- Chondroid lipoma
- Spindle cell/pleomorphic lipoma
- Hibernoma.

Superficial lipoma is far more common than deep lipoma. Microscopically, they are composed of mature fat cells (adipocytes) and are well vascularized. Occasionally they contain other mesenchymal elements such as fibrous connective tissue, mucoid substances, cartilaginous or osseous tissue, or smooth muscle. Although the etiology is uncertain, solitary lipomas are associated with rearrangements of chromosome 12 (Weiss, 1996).

Lipomas generally are slow-growing nodules with a firm, rubbery consistency (Luba et al., 2003) and typically present in middle age (fifth and sixth decades of life) (Bancroft, Kransdorf, Peterson, & O'Connor, 2006). Most lipomas are less than 5 cm in diameter, but some can be much larger (Rydholm & Berg, 1983). In general, they are asymptomatic unless they are compressing a nerve. They usually are solitary lesions that occur on the trunk, shoulders, posterior neck, and axillae (Luba et al.) and are unusual in the hand and foot (Bancroft et al.). Lipomas are diagnosed clinically by physical examination and radiologic evaluation. They are well characterized on both computed tomography and magnetic resonance imaging because they have an appearance similar to subcutaneous fat.

Treatment of benign fatty tumors is dependent on the degree of clinical symptoms related to the lesion, location and growth pattern of the tumor, and concern regarding a potential malignant histology. In general, lipomas are not removed unless there are cosmetic concerns or diagnostic uncertainty or they are causing symptoms (i.e., pain) from compression of local structures. Treatment includes surgical excision or liposuction depending on the size, anatomic location, and clinical characteristics of the lesion. These modalities are associated with the risk of scarring, seroma, and hematoma formation.

There is a paucity of information in the literature regarding how lipomas in patients with cancer respond to RT, chemotherapy, and immunotherapy. Confirmation that the lesion is benign and does not represent a malignancy is important. Nodules that are directly in the field of radiation may become inflamed and cause discomfort during the treatment period. However, no documentation exists describing their typical response to radiation.

Cherry Angiomas

Cherry angiomas (CAs), also known as *Campbell de Morgan spots* or *senile angiomas*, are the most common cutaneous vascular proliferation (Luba et al., 2003). CAs are acquired vascular lesions that rarely appear in early adult life and are most commonly seen with advancing age. CA lesions appear most often on the trunk and extremities and can be up to several millimeters in diameter. They are asymptomatic, round, bright to dark red, nonblanching vascular papules. They are composed of dilated capillaries and postcapillary venules. Despite their frequency, the etiology and pathogenesis for the appearance of CA lesions are unknown. The term *eruptive cherry angioma* (ECA) means the sudden and extensive appearance of multiple CAs. ECA is a rare variant of CA whose sudden onset has been associated with solid organ transplantation, chronic graft-versus-host disease, cyclosporine therapy, sulfur mustard gas, 2-butoxyethanol (glycol ether solvent), bromide exposure, and argon laser therapy. Some women develop CA lesions during pregnancy, and the lesions involute after delivery. These lesions primarily are treated for cosmetic reasons. Options include laser treatment, electrodessication of typical lesions, and excision of larger lesions. Cryotherapy is not effective (Luba et al.).

CA lesions do not usually affect treatment for cancer. During RT, CA lesions may darken or become irritated because of surrounding dry desquamation. Chemotherapy and immunotherapy should not have any direct impact on the presence of a CA lesion.

Keloids

Keloids are benign dermal fibroproliferative tumors unique to humans with no malignant potential. By definition, keloids are scars that continue to grow and extend beyond the confines of the original wound (Butler, Longaker, & Yang, 2008). In contrast to hypertrophic scars, which stay within the boundaries of the original wound and increase in size by pushing out the edge of the scar, keloids "invade" the skin beyond the perimeter of the original wound with a leading edge that is often erythematous and pruritic (Butler et al.). Classically, these scars are preceded by traumatic insult to the skin. They represent a form of pathologic wound healing affecting a substantial segment of the U.S. population. Keloids are more common among African Americans, Asian Americans, Latin Americans, and people of other darker-pigmented ethnicities (Butler et al.). They usually appear as firm, broad nodules, often erythematous and with a shiny surface, and sometimes with telangiectasias. The vast majority of keloids result in some minor cosmetic defect; however, some can grow large enough to become symptomatic by causing deformity, pain, and pruritus.

Histologically, keloids have a normal epidermal layer, abundant vasculature, increased mesenchymal density as manifested by a thickened dermis, and increased inflammatory cell infiltrate when compared with normal scar tissue (Butler et al., 2008). The diagnosis can be confirmed histologically after a biopsy. Unfortunately, a single effective therapeutic regimen has yet to be established for treatment of keloids. Although no single definitive treatment modality exists, numerous therapeutic regiments have been described, including occlusive dressings, compression therapy, intralesional steroid injections, cryosurgery, surgical excision, laser treatment, RT, interferon therapy, bleomycin, 5-fluorouracil, verapamil, imiquimod cream, transforming growth factor-beta 3, interleukin-10, and combinations of all of these (Butler et al.). Radiotherapy has been attempted as a monotherapy for keloids but remains controversial because of anecdotal reports of carcinogenesis occurring after treatment. More recently, radiotherapy after surgical excision of keloids has shown some promise with no evidence of increased risk of malignancy (Butler et al.).

In the oncology setting, keloids can present a challenge to the clinician and require careful planning and informed consent for treatment. Although chemotherapy and RT do not have a negative impact on keloids, their presence in a patient with cancer may impede therapy. In an individual who has a history of keloid formation, any trauma to the skin from an invasive procedure (e.g., surgery, central line placement) may result in keloid formation. Careful consideration is needed to avoid unnecessary procedures. The informed consent for surgery should include a discussion about the potential risk of keloid formation and techniques to reduce the risk. If chemotherapy is necessary for treatment, a vascular access device may be beneficial, but the placement of the incision should not be directly over the access port because of the potential for a keloid to form and block access. In addition, keloids near joints can reduce range of motion and impede positioning for radiology procedures or radiation treatments. Patients with a significant medical history may already have a number of keloids that prevent peripheral IV access or central line placement.

Dermatofibromas

Dermatofibromas are nodules derived from mesodermal and dermal cells. It is unclear whether they are true neoplasms or are fibrous reactions to minor trauma, insect bites, viral infections, ruptured cysts, or folliculitis (Pariser, 1998). The nodules may be found anywhere on the body but most commonly appear on the anterior surface of the lower legs (Luba et al., 2003). They usually are asymptomatic firm, raised papules, plaques, or nodules that vary in size from 3–10 mm in diameter and range in color from brown to purple, red, yellow, and pink (Luba et al.). Multiple lesions (more than 15) have been associated with autoimmune disorders such as systemic lupus erythematosus or immunosuppression. The diagnosis of dermatofibromas is based on physical appearance; however, they can be confused with melanoma. Histologic diagnosis should be obtained when the clinician is unsure of the presentation.

In general, oncologic treatment is not contraindicated in patients with a dermatofibroma. The lesions may respond to RT with local inflammation and acute discoloration. No documentation exists on the long-term effects of treatment.

Pigment Disorders

Hypomelanotic Skin Disorders

Hypomelanotic skin disorders are cutaneous pigment disorders characterized by reduced melanin content in the skin that results in a lightening of the skin. Hypomelanosis can be congenital or acquired, and the hypopigmented or depigmented lesions may appear in a localized form or a diffuse pattern. *Acquired localized hypomelanotic* skin disorders may include infectious entities such as pityriasis versicolor, postinflammatory disorders including pityriasis alba, chemical and physical agents, lupus erythematosus, or scleroderma. Other disease entities include lichen sclerosis, vitiligo, halo nevus, and melanoma-associated leukoderma. *Acquired diffuse hypomelanotic* skin disorders may include idiopathic guttate hypomelanosis, leukoderma punctata, or progressive macular hypomelanosis of the trunk (Mollet et al., 2007).

Establishing the correct diagnosis for hypomelanotic skin disorders requires a good history, a detailed physical examination, the use of special lighting techniques, such as a Wood's light (ultraviolet light), and possibly a biopsy of the abnormally pigmented skin and the normally pigmented skin (Mosher, Fitzpatrick, Ortunne, & Hori, 1999). This section will focus on the most common hypomelanotic skin disorders, vitiligo and albinism.

Vitiligo (generalized): Vitiligo is an acquired cutaneous disorder in which patches of depigmented skin, overlying hair, and oral mucosa result from progressive autoimmune loss of melanocytes from the involved areas. Perhaps the most common pigment disorder, vitiligo results from a complex interaction of environmental, genetic, and immunologic factors that contribute to melanocyte destruction resulting in the characteristic depigmented lesions (Spritz, 2008). Vitiligo usually begins in childhood or young adulthood and has an unpredictable but often progressive course, with phases of stability and spreading of lesions. It has four distinct clinical presentations (Passeron & Ortonne, 2005):

- Segmental vitiligo with a dermatomal pattern of the lesions
- Focal vitiligo characterized by a limited number of depigmented macules without segmental distribution
- Universal vitiligo, which involves complete or almost complete body surface area
- Generalized vitiligo, the most common type, characterized by a bilateral and symmetrical distribution of the lesions.

Several major hypotheses for the pathogenesis of vitiligo exist and are not exclusive of each other: autoimmune, autocytotoxic/metabolic, and neural dysfunctional. Recent data have supported an autoimmune pathogenesis of vitiligo (Passeron & Ortonne, 2005). The diagnosis of vitiligo is confirmed clinically with a biopsy of the skin. The current consensus on the histologic presentation in vitiligo is a complete absence of melanocytes in the amelanotic lesions (Passeron & Ortonne).

Various factors are suspected to affect the progression of vitiligo including emotional shock, sunburn, pregnancy, physical illness, and trauma. The latter is known as the *Koebner phenomenon*, which is defined as the development of macules at the site of trauma, such as a cut, burn, or abrasion. In the oncology setting, scarce data are available regarding the impact of chemotherapy or RT on vitiligo. The key is careful skin assessment and documentation prior to treatment, as well as during and after treatment, to assess for long-term damage. Further depigmentation has been described in association with irradiation (Levine & Ribeiro, 1994). The patient and family should receive a clear informed consent indicating the limited knowledge of the impact of treatment on the skin and the potential risks and benefits.

Albinism: Oculocutaneous albinism (OCA) is a group of four autosomal recessive disorders caused by either a complete lack or a reduction of melanin biosynthesis in the melanocytes resulting in hypopigmentation of the hair, skin, and eyes. The clinical spectrum of OCA varies, with OCA 1A being the most severe type, characterized by a complete lack of melanin production throughout life, whereas the milder forms OCA 1B, OCA 2, OCA 3, and OCA 4 show some pigment accumulation over time. The types of OCA are caused by mutations in different genes; however, the clinical phenotype is not always distinguishable (Gronskov, Ek, & Brondum-Nielsen, 2007). The diagnosis of OCA is based on clinical findings of hypopigmentation of the skin and hair, in addition to the characteristic ocular symptoms described below. Molecular diagnosis is necessary to establish the gene defect and, thus, the OCA subtype (Gronskov et al.).

Albinism can affect people of all ethnic backgrounds, with approximately 1 in 17,000 people having one of the types of albinism (Gronskov et al., 2007; Witkop, 1979). Prevalence of albinism varies considerably worldwide, partly explained by the different founder mutations in specific genes. Additionally, it can be difficult clinically to distinguish between the subtypes of albinism among the large normal spectrum of pigmentation (Gronskov et al.). OCA 2 is the most prevalent form worldwide.

The degree of skin and hair hypopigmentation varies with the type of albinism. In OCA 1A, the hair, eyelashes, and eyebrows are white, and the skin is white and does not tan. The iris of the eye is light blue to almost pink and is fully translucent. Pigment does not develop, and amelanotic nevi may be present. In OCA 1B, the hair and skin may develop some pigment with time (after one to three years), and the blue iris may change to a green/brown color. In OCA 2, the amount of cutaneous pigment may vary, and a newborn will nearly always have pigmented hair. Nevi and ephelides are common. The iris color varies, and the pink eyes seen in OCA 1A usually are absent. OCA 3 results in rufous or red OCA in African individuals, who present with red hair and reddish-brown skin (xanthism) (Gronskov et al., 2007).

Most people with albinism are highly susceptible to sun-induced damage to the skin. Studies have documented a high frequency of actinic keratoses and skin cancers in these patients (Lookingbill, Lookingbill, & Leppard, 1995). The frequency of these findings appears to be highest in populations living closest to the equator. Therefore, it is reasonable to expect poor tolerance to RT. It is crucial that the radiation oncology clinician participate in the initial treatment plan for a patient with albinism to determine if RT will be a safe and appropriate treatment. Large fields and high doses of treatment may result in significant skin breakdown and lead to treatment breaks or discontinuation. Careful skin assessments should be performed during RT to assess for tolerance and early identification of desquamation.

Xeroderma Pigmentosum

Xeroderma pigmentosum is a rare autosomal recessive disease characterized by clinical and cellular sensitivity to ultraviolet (UV) light (Arlett et al., 2006). Because of the rarity of the disease, very little has been published on the impact of oncologic therapy on these patients. However, it is generally acknowledged that these patients are clinically hypersensitive to ionizing radiation.

Inflammatory Disorders

Allergic Contact Dermatitis

Contact dermatitis can be either allergic or irritant in etiology. The diagnosis is not usually apparent from history or physical examination alone and may require a patch test to delineate the cause (Belsito, 2000). Although allergic contact dermatitis (ACD) can occur in any setting, many causes are related to exposures in the workplace. Despite all the clinical and scientific research, a thorough understanding of the disease remains elusive (Belsito).

The clinical manifestations of ACD vary depending on its location and duration. Acute eruptions typically are characterized by macular erythema and papules, vesicles, or bullae, depending on the intensity of the allergic response (Belsito, 2000). In contrast, chronic ACD of most cutaneous sites presents as a lichenified, scaling, or fissured dermatitis, with or without accompanying papulovesiculation. ACD initially involves the cutaneous site of the principal exposure and, as it evolves, may spread to distant sites either by inadvertent contact or, under certain circumstances, by autosensitization (Belsito).

The identification of the allergen is vital to treatment. Krasteva et al. (1999) identified the most frequently encountered causes of ACD in the major anatomic areas of the body. Careful clinical assessment of the patient is critical to this process. The assessment should include the size, type, extent, and anatomic location of the lesion. For example, a lesion on the face may be related to chemicals in personal cleansers (i.e., shampoo, body soap), components of facial cosmetics, grooming aids, makeup applicators, or airborne contaminants in the home or workplace. The only useful and reliable method for diagnosis is the patch test, but not all of the common allergens in the environment are represented in the test, thus leaving the clinician to rely heavily on the patient's history and accurate description of exposure. Patient education about avoiding the allergen and possible cross-reacting allergens is important. Treatment of symptoms may include the use of drying agents in the presence of weeping eruptions, as well as controlling pruritus with oral or topical agents.

In terms of oncologic treatment, patients with ACD should be treated aggressively so as to avoid development of a local cellulitis from scratching during periods of immunosuppression. Individuals with long-standing ACD and many potential allergens may require careful assessment of the treatment environment to avoid such allergens (e.g., providing their own linens). It may be difficult to assess the difference between ACD and other skin lesions such as early fungal infections in some patients. Documentation of skin rashes prior to treatment may help to alleviate this problem.

Atopic Dermatitis

Atopic dermatitis is an eczematous, highly pruritic, chronic, inflammatory skin disease (Simpson & Hanifin, 2006). It usually starts early in life and often occurs in people with a personal or family history of asthma and allergic rhinitis. The prevalence is high, especially in children, and has been rising in recent decades, in parallel with asthma prevalence (Simpson & Hanifin). The precise cause of atopic dermatitis is unknown. It is thought to be a combination of genetic and environmental factors, defects in the skin barrier, and cutaneous immune dysfunction (Munzenberger & Montejo, 2007).

The disease usually presents in infancy on the face and extensor extremities, moves to flexural areas during childhood, and often resolves before puberty. If it persists into adulthood, it most commonly manifests as *hand eczema*. In the acute setting, the rash may appear erythematous and have papules, excoriation, oozing, or crusting. In the chronic setting, the skin may appear dry and scaly with lichenification.

The treatment of atopic dermatitis is targeted at the combined causes. Along with good daily skin care to maintain an effective skin barrier and avoidance of known environmental triggers, several pharmacologic agents often are required for long-term management (Munzenberger & Montejo, 2007). Agents such as topical corticosteroids and topical calcineurin inhibitors (TCIs) reduce inflammation at the site of the atopic dermatitis by acting on the immune system. Recently, safety concerns have arisen over the use of the TCIs because of the potential risks associated with prolonged immunosuppression and theoretical risk of malignancy.

No reports exist on the impact of cancer therapies on atopic dermatitis. However, extensive reporting has been done on the use of UVA, UVB, and psoralen plus UVA phototherapy to control atopic dermatitis with some success (Meduri, Vandergriff, Rasmussen, & Jacobe, 2007). Patients with atopic dermatitis in need of chemotherapy and/or RT should have careful skin assessments before and during treatment. The atopic dermatitis may worsen as a result of the stress of the diagnosis and treatment and may require aggressive management to facilitate the oncology treatment.

Psoriasis

Psoriasis vulgaris is a genetic, T-cell mediated, systemic, inflammatory, chronic disorder affecting approximately 2% of the population (Menter et al., 2008). It may be associated with other inflammatory disorders such as psoriatic arthritis, autoimmune diseases such as inflammatory bowel disease, components of the metabolic syndrome such as diabetes, cardiovascular disease, and lymphoma. Psoriasis is a chronic disease that waxes and wanes during a patient's lifetime and often is modified by treatment. The major manifestation of psoriasis is chronic inflammation of the skin. It is characterized by disfiguring, scaling, and erythematous plaques that may be painful or often severely pruritic.

Plaque psoriasis is the most common form, affecting approximately 80%–90% of patients (Menter et al., 2008). Plaque psoriasis manifests as well-defined, sharply demarcated, erythematous plaques varying in size from 1 cm to several centimeters. Patients may have involvement ranging from only a few plaques to numerous lesions covering almost the entire body surface. The plaques are irregular, round to oval in shape, and most often located on the scalp, trunk, buttocks, and limbs, with a predilection for extensor surfaces such as the elbows and knees. Smaller plaques or papules may coalesce into larger lesions, especially on the legs and trunk. Painful fissuring within plaques can occur when lesions are present over joint lines or on the palms and soles. Approximately 80% of those affected with psoriasis have mild to moderate disease, with 20% having moderate to severe psoriasis affecting more than 5% of the body surface area or affecting crucial body areas such as the hands, feet, face, or genitals (Menter et al.). Other less common forms of psoriasis include inverse, erythrodermic, pustular, and guttate disease. Nail disease (psoriatic onychodystrophy) can occur in all psoriasis subtypes. Fingernails are involved in approximately 50% of all patients who are psoriatic, and toenails are involved in 35% of patients. The changes include pitting, onycholysis, and subungual hyperkeratosis (Menter et al.).

Traditional therapies for psoriasis include topical drugs, such as corticosteroids, retinoids, and vitamin D analogs; systemic drugs, such as methotrexate, cyclosporine, and retinoids; and phototherapy (Magliocco, 2005). These mainstays of treatment are efficacious for the treatment of severe disease; however, most are associated with toxicities or are inconvenient. Recent advances in biotechnology have produced new pharmaceuticals that interfere with immune responses thought to be involved in the pathogenesis of psoriasis and other inflammatory diseases. The *immunobiologics*, one new family of drugs, consist of T-cell inhibitors and tumor necrosis factor (TNF) inhibitors. Many have demonstrated efficacy in treating psoriasis. Some appear to offer safety benefits over traditional therapies, but further monitoring and surveillance of these agents are required to adequately establish safety profiles (Magliocco). The potential risk of lymphoma, melanoma, cutaneous T-cell lymphoma, and nonmelanoma skin cancer in patients treated with the TNF inhibitors has been raised recently in the literature (Magliocco).

In terms of oncologic treatment, psoriasis is a challenge for clinicians. Case reports in the literature have described episodes of exacerbation of psoriasis following radiotherapy, while others have reported the use of low-dose radiotherapy for the treatment of the disease (Charalambous, 2001; Schreiber, 1991). Some of the chemotherapy agents used to treat malignancy also are being used to treat psoriasis. Therefore, it is imperative that the oncology clinician work closely with the patient's dermatologist to plan oncologic treatment. Some patients with psoriasis who have received long courses of biologics or chemotherapy agents may be at risk for immunosuppression that might take longer to resolve. Other patients may experience exacerbations of their psoriasis that will take priority over treatment for their cancer. Communication and careful informed consent are crucial to a successful outcome.

Collagen Vascular Disease

Patients with collagen vascular diseases (CVDs) include those with rheumatoid arthritis, systemic lupus erythematosus, Raynaud phenomena, fibromyalgia, polymyositis, dermatomyositis, Sjögren syndrome, scleroderma, and polymyalgia rheumatica. CVD is believed to predispose patients to increased toxicity, and many clinicians believe that a diagnosis of CVD is a relative contraindication to RT. The finding that some commonly prescribed medications, many of which are used in patients with CVD, may alter the radiation toxicity profile is a further complication to treatment. Lin, Abu-Isa, Griffith, and Ben-Josef (2008) performed a large matched-control analysis of acute and late complications in 73 patients with CVDs receiving RT. They found that although a diagnosis of CVD appears to predispose patients to a greater risk of late RT toxicity, treatment generally is well tolerated, with a relatively low incidence of severe acute or late toxicity. Patients with CVD had a higher incidence of any late toxicity (29.1% versus 14%; p = 0.001) and a trend toward an increased rate of severe late toxicity (9.3% versus 3.7%; p = 0.079). RT delivered to the breast increased the risk of severe acute toxicity, whereas RT to the pelvis increased the risk of severe acute and late toxicity. RT administered in the setting of scleroderma carried a higher risk of any severe late toxicity (41.2% versus 19.1%) compared to controls, whereas RT to patients with systemic lupus erythematosus carried a higher risk of severe acute (29.4% versus 11.9%) and late toxicity (35.3% versus 4.8%).

Other factors can affect the risk of toxicity including the site of irradiation, the RT dose, and the use of concurrent chemotherapy. In patients who may be at particularly high risk because of a CVD subtype or RT site, careful attention to toxicity is required. Treatment modifications such as reduction of fraction size, twice-daily treatment, or reduction of total dose for these patients may be considered. These factors should be taken into consideration in the risk-benefit analysis at the time of consultation (Lin et al., 2008).

Conclusion

Skin disorders can have a significant negative impact on the treatment of cancer. Careful assessment, early diagnosis, and management are key to a successful outcome. Collaboration with other healthcare providers, including surgeons, wound care experts, and dermatologists, will provide patients who have a benign skin disorder with a multidisciplinary approach to manage and reduce the risk of significant complications.

References

Arlett, C.F., Plowman, P.N., Rogers, P.B., Parris, C.N., Abbaszadeh, F., Green, M.H.L., et al. (2006). Clinical and cellular ionizing radiation sensitivity in a patient with xeroderma pigmentosum. *British Journal of Radiology, 79*(942), 510–517.

Bancroft, L.W., Kransdorf, M.J., Peterson, J.J., & O'Connor, M.I. (2006). Benign fatty tumors: Classification, clinical course, imaging appearance, and treatment. *Skeletal Radiology, 35*(10), 719–733.

Belsito, D.V. (2000). The diagnostic evaluation, treatment and prevention of allergic contact dermatitis in the new millennium. *Journal of Allergy and Clinical Immunology, 105*(3), 409–420.

Butler, P.D., Longaker, M.T., & Yang, G.P. (2008). Current progress in keloid research and treatment. *Journal of the American College of Surgeons, 206*(4), 731–741.

Charalambous, H., & Bloomfield, D. (2000). Psoriasis and radiotherapy: Exacerbation of psoriasis following radiotherapy for carcinoma of the breast (the Koebner phenomenon). *Clinical Oncology, 12*(3), 192–193.

Fletcher, C.D.M., Unni, K.K., & Mertens, F. (Eds.). (2002). *Pathology and genetics: Tumours of soft tissue and bone.* Lyon, France: IARC.

Gorwitz, R.J., Jernigan, D.B., Powers, J.H., & Jernigan, J.A. (2006, March). *Strategies for clinical management of MRSA in the community: Summary of an experts' meeting convened by the Centers for Disease Control and Prevention.* Retrieved June 15, 2008, from http://www.cdc.gov/ncidod/dhqp/pdf/ar/CAMRSA_ExpMtgStrategies.pdf

Gronskov, K., Ek, J., & Brondum-Nielsen, K. (2007, November). Oculocutaneous albinism. *Orphanet Journal of Rare Diseases, 2*(2), 43.

Kazandjieva, J., & Tsankov, N. (2007). Tattoos: Dermatological complications. *Clinics in Dermatology, 25*(4), 375–382.

Krasteva, M., Kehren, J., Sayag, M., Ducluzeau, M.T., Dupuis, M., Kanitakis, J., et al. (1999). Contact dermatitis II. Clinical aspects and diagnosis. *European Journal of Dermatology, 9*(2), 144–159.

Lebwohl, M., Clark, L., & Levitt, J. (2007). Therapy for head lice based on life cycle, resistance, and safety considerations. *Pediatrics, 119*(5), 965–974.

Levine, E.L., & Ribeiro, G.G. (1994). Vitiligo and radiotherapy: The Koebner phenomenon demonstrated in patients with vitiligo undergoing radiotherapy for carcinoma of the breast. *Clinical Oncology, 6*(2), 133–134.

Lin, A., Abu-Isa, E., Griffith, K.A., & Ben-Josef, E. (2008). Toxicity of radiotherapy in patients with collagen vascular disease. *Cancer, 113*(3), 648–653.

Lookingbill, D.P., Lookingbill, G.L., & Leppard, D.M. (1995). Actinic damage and skin cancer in albinos in northern Tanzania: Findings in 164 patients enrolled in an outreach skin care program. *Journal of the American Academy of Dermatology, 32*(4), 653–658.

Luba, M.C., Bangs, S.A., Mohler, A.M., & Stulberg, D.L. (2003). Common benign skin tumors. *American Family Physician, 67*(4), 729–738.

Magliocco, M.A. (2005). Emerging drugs for moderate-to-severe psoriasis. *Expert Opinion on Emerging Drugs, 10*(1), 35–52.

Mays, S.R., & Cohen, P.R. (2006). Emerging dermatologic issues in the oncology patient. *Seminars in Cutaneous Medicine and Surgery, 25*(4), 179–189.

Meduri, N.B., Vandergriff, T., Rasmussen, H., & Jacobe, H. (2007). Phototherapy in the management of atopic dermatitis: A systematic review. *Photodermatology, Photoimmunology, and Photomedicine, 23*(4), 106–112.

Menter, A., Gottlieb, A., Feldman, S., Van Voorhees, A.S., Leonardi, C.L., Gordon, K.B., et al. (2008). Guidelines of care for the management of psoriasis and psoriatic arthritis: Section 1. Overview of psoriasis and guidelines of care for the treatment of psoriasis with biologics. *Journal of the American Academy of Dermatology, 58*(5), 826–850.

Mollet, I., Ongenae, K., & Naeyaert, J.M. (2007). Origin, clinical presentation, and diagnosis of hypomelanotic skin disorders. *Dermatologic Clinics, 25*(3), 363–371, ix.

Mosher, D.B., Fitzpatrick, T.B., Ortonne, J.P., & Hori, Y. (1999). Normal skin color and general considerations of pigmentary disorders. In I.M. Freedberg, A.Z. Eisen, K. Wolff, K.F. Austen, L.A. Goldsmith, S.I. Katz, et al. (Eds.), *Fitzpatrick's dermatology in general medicine* (5th ed., pp. 936–944). New York: McGraw-Hill.

Munzenberger, P.J., & Montejo, J.M. (2007). Safety of topical calcineurin inhibitors for the treatment of atopic dermatitis. *Pharmacotherapy, 27*(7), 1020–1028.

Pallin, D.J., Egan, D.J., Pelletier, A.J., Espinola, J.A., Hooper, D.C., & Camargo, C.A., Jr. (2008). Increased US emergency department visits for skin and soft tissue infections, and changes in antibiotic choices, during the emergence of community-associated methicillin-resistant Staphylococcus aureus. *Annals of Emergency Medicine, 51*(3), 291–298.

Panconesi, E. (2007). Body piercing: Psychosocial and dermatologic aspects. *Clinics in Dermatology, 25*(4), 412–416.

Pariser, R.J. (1998). Benign neoplasms of the skin. *Medical Clinics of North America, 82*(6), 1285–1307.

Passeron, T., & Ortonne, J.-P. (2005). Physiopathology and genetics of vitiligo. *Journal of Autoimmunity, 25*(Suppl. 1), 63–68.

Quatresooz, P., Pierard-Franchimont, C., Arrese, J.E., & Pierard, G.E. (2008). Clinicopathologic presentations of dermatomycoses in cancer patients. *Journal of the European Academy of Dermatology and Venereology, 22*(8), 907–917.

Rydholm, A., & Berg, N.O. (1983). Size, site and clinical incidence of lipoma. Factors in the differential diagnosis of lipoma and sarcoma. *Acta Orthopedica Scandinavica, 54*(6), 929–934.

Schreiber, G.J., & Muller-Runkel, R. (1991). Exacerbation of psoriasis after megavoltage irradiation. The Koebner phenomenon. *Cancer, 67*(3), 588–589.

Simpson, E.L., & Hanifin, J.M. (2006). Atopic dermatitis. *Medical Clinics of North America, 90*(1), 149–167.

Spritz, R.A. (2008). The genetics of generalized vitiligo. *Current Directions in Autoimmunity, 10*, 244–257.

Swygert, K., Parrish, C.A., Cashman, R.E., Lin, R., & Cockerell, C.J. (2007). Melanoma in situ involving an epidermal inclusion (infundibular) cyst. *American Journal of Dermatopathology, 29*(6), 564–565.

Vicente, J., & Vazquez-Doval, F.J. (1998). Proliferations of the epidermoid cyst wall. *International Journal of Dermatology, 37*(3), 181–185.

Weiss, S.W. (1996). Lipomatous tumors. *Monographs in Pathology, 38,* 207–239.

Witkop, C.J. (1979). Albinism: Hematologic-storage disease, susceptibility to skin cancer, and optic neuronal defects shared in all types of oculocutaneous and ocular albinism. *Alabama Journal of Medical Sciences, 16*(4), 327–330.

CHAPTER 4

Malignant Cutaneous Diseases

Sandra Cochran, RN, BSN, CWOCN, and Pamela R. Jakubek, MSN, RN, CWOCN

Introduction

Malignant cutaneous diseases are a true challenge to healthcare professionals. *Malignant cutaneous disease,* also referred to as *malignant fungating wounds,* is defined according to the British Columbia Cancer Agency (2001) as

> A cancerous lesion involving the skin, which is open and may be draining. The lesion may be a result of a primary cancer, or a metastasis to the skin from a local tumor or from a tumor in a distant site. It may take the form of a cavity, an open area on the surface of the skin, skin nodules, or a nodular growth extending from the surface of the skin.

Thus, the cutaneous tumor can be a result of metastatic, recurrent, or locally advanced malignancies (Grocott & Cowley, 2001).

Fungating malignant wounds present as skin lesions caused by the abnormal cells penetrating the surrounding lymph and blood circulation, which may result in capillary enlargement and possible rupture leading to the formation of necrotic tissue (Collier, 1997; Foltz, 1980; Grocott, 1999; Hallett, 1995). An initial wound may appear as a series of multiple nontender, generally painless nodules with possible skin discoloration (Manning, 1998). Lesions are considered "fungating" once the cancerous tumor penetrates the skin through the processes of ulceration and proliferation, and the lesions may become very painful (Mortimer, 1998). The potential for extensive impaired skin integrity can occur when use of single or combination anticancer treatments is unsuccessful. This transpires through a combination of tumor growth, loss of local blood supply, and consequent loss of tissue viability. The malodor and exudate common with these wounds comes from this loss of tissue viability, arising from tissue hypoxia and the presence of anaerobic bacteria in the large amount of necrotic tissue (Bauer, Gerlach, & Doughty 2000; Hampson, 1996; Thomas & Hay, 1991).

Although rare, an estimated 5%–10% of patients with cancer will develop such a wound (Seaman, 2006). Fungating wounds primarily occur in patients aged 60 and older, usually developing near the end of life (Haisfield-Wolfe & Rund, 1997; Ivetic & Lyne, 1990). Lesions may be a metastasis from a primary site, such as breast carcinoma, or may arise from any other type of cancer, including head and neck, kidney, lung, ovarian, colon, penile, skin, and bladder cancers (Gallagher, 1995). Metastatic skin lesions also may occur with melanoma, leukemia, and lymphoma, albeit not as commonly (Goldberg & McGinn-Byer, 2007).

Although these wounds are identified with a poor treatment outcome, some degree of healing is achievable with good topical care in conjunction with combination chemotherapy and/or radiation therapy. If healing is part of the care plan for management, it should be recognized that healing of metastatic wounds differs from that of normal wound healing. Platelets, normally present in acute wounds, are absent from the stroma in metastatic lesions. Their role is taken over by tumor cells, leading to a reduced number of leukocytes in the wound bed and increasing the amount of bleeding. Furthermore, tumor cells produce clotting and growth factors that are specific to the tumor cells and may damage healthy tissue (Bauer et al., 2000). Lesions caused by tumors lack the ability to contract; "therefore, as wound healing occurs, a larger deficit occurs as compared with other wounds in which contraction is present" (Bauer et al., p. 248).

This chapter will provide a summary of the unique nature of skin neoplasms and an overview of the care of malignant fungating wounds. With a greater understanding of the complexity of these difficult wounds, healthcare professionals can provide quality, meaningful care for their patients.

Common Primary Skin Malignancies

With more than one million cases of nonmelanoma skin cancers diagnosed each year in the United States, *basal cell carcinoma* (BCC) and *squamous cell carcinoma* (SCC) together are the most common forms of skin cancer that, if left untreated, can create very complex wounds (Alam & Ratner, 2001). Sun exposure is a common risk factor for nonmelanoma skin cancer, which explains the high incidence of occurrence in sun-exposed areas such as the central face, postauricular region, forehead, scalp, lips, and hands (Christenson et al., 2005; Wong, Strange, & Lear, 2003).

The most characteristic presentation of BCC is an asymptomatic, nodular, ulcerative lesion that is elevated from surrounding skin with a pearl-like quality that may also contain telangiectatic vessels (Christenson et al., 2005). When BCC becomes advanced, it often presents as an ulcerative, bleeding lesion.

SCC can be an isolated lesion or present as multiple lesions. The presentation of invasive cutaneous SCC can vary depending on whether it is a well or poorly differentiated lesion. Well-differentiated cutaneous SCC usually appears as an indurated or firm papule, plaque, or nodule with hyperkeratosis or ulceration. The lesions usually are asymptomatic, but occasionally patients report that the area itches and bleeds easily. Poorly differentiated SCC lesions are typically fleshy, soft, granulomatous papules or nodules that sometimes present as hemorrhaging ulcerations or with deep necrosis (Alam & Ratner, 2001).

Advanced stages of BCC and SCC are relatively rare (Rowe, Carroll, & Day, 1989 ; Wagner & Casciato, 2000), mostly because of medical advances in treating these skin cancers. Large ulcerative lesions are usually lesions that the patient has neglected or left untreated. As with any ulcerative lesion, the problems of odor, drainage, and discomfort are the most difficult aspects of the care of these sites. Wound management and supportive care are discussed later in this chapter.

Sun exposure is a contributing factor for malignant melanoma (MM), along with other risk factors such as family history, presence of pigmented lesions, and atypical moles, or dysplastic nevi (Rigel et al., 1989). MM occurs more than 50% of the time in areas of sun exposure; however, it can occur in nonexposed body structures (Desmond & Soong, 2003). The classic presentation of MM can be summarized with the ABCDE acronym (American Academy of Dermatology, 2009) as follows:

- **A**symmetry of the mole
- **B**order irregularity
- **C**olor variegation
- **D**iameter greater than 6 mm
- **E**volving in size, shape, or color.

MM is well recognized for its ability to spread locally and its ability to metastasize to other areas of the body, creating ulcerative, draining wounds that defy standard wound care treatments. Locally advanced MM can present as a simple full-thickness, dry wound, or as a fungating, draining, and necrotic wound.

Uncommon Primary Skin Malignancies

Merkel cell carcinoma (MCC) is a relatively rare skin malignancy found in sun-exposed skin, with the highest incidence in Caucasian men (Jabbour et al., 2007). MCC is aggressive and is similar to MM when comparing the rates of recurrence, metastatic spread, and mortality. With MCC, a simple lesion is the presenting symptom (Dinh, Feun, Elgart, & Savaraj, 2007). This lesion typically is described as a rapidly growing, solitary, firm, cutaneous, nontender nodule with a red or bluish color; as a dome-shaped nodule; or as an indurated plaque measuring up to several centimeters in diameter (Dinh et al.; Gollard et al., 2000).

MCC is treatable but with an unpredictable response to treatment (Allen et al., 2005). Wide excision surgery often is used along with adjuvant radiation therapy (Garneski & Nghiem, 2007). Overall survival benefits of chemotherapy have not been demonstrated in controlled studies of patients with MCC. Recurrence is frequent (mean time of 18 months), and distant metastasis also can occur (Dinh et al., 2007). If left untreated, MCC has a tendency to increase rapidly in size over the course of a few weeks or months. The aggressive speed of this disease can lead to deep tissue injury with a wound that has limited ability to heal. Wound necrosis, drainage, and pain are the biggest patient care challenges.

Kaposi sarcoma (KS) is a soft-tissue sarcoma that affects the skin, oral cavity, esophagus, and anal canal (Levine & Tulpule, 2001). It is the most common form of neoplasm associated with HIV infection (Lim, Tupule, Espina, & Levine, 2005). However, KS was not always known as an AIDS-related cutaneous neoplasm but rather a rare cancer. *Classic KS* is the term used for the rare form, and it commonly runs a benign, indolent course for 10–15 years or more, with slow enlargement of the original tumors and the gradual development of additional lesions. The immunologic deficiency in AIDS creates a predisposition to opportunistic infections and unusual neoplasms, including KS; this type of KS is referred to as *epidemic KS*. Epidemic KS usually remains localized to the skin; however, widespread cutaneous, mucocutaneous, or visceral organ involvement is common in severely immunosuppressed patients (Safai, 1997).

Epidemic KS can be diagnosed at any stage of HIV infection, and the presentation is variable, ranging from minimum disease to explosive growth, contributing to significant morbidity and mortality (Di Lorenzo et al., 2007). The lesions that develop in the skin appear on the lower extremities and face, especially on the nose. The lesions can be described as elliptical papules and may be found in a linear formation, along skin tension lines. Lesions can vary in color ranging from pink, red, and purple to brown. The degree of vascularity will affect the color; deeper colors usually will have more vasculature within them. A yellow halo also may be present around the perimeter of the lesion. The lesions often are reported as painless and nonpruritic. Most early lesions do not extend into the underlying structures below the skin surface and can easily be mistaken for purpura, hematomas, angiomas, dermatofibromas, or nevi. Advanced cutaneous KS lesions progress to form thick plaques that eventually form into nodular, tumor-like lesions. These tumors ulcerate and become deeply invasive, resulting in lesions that are disfiguring and painful (Vanni et al., 2006).

Cutaneous T-cell lymphomas (CTCL) are a rare group of disorders that are characterized by the localization of malignant lymphocytes to the skin. Approximately 1,500 new cases of CTCL are diagnosed each year (Willemze et al., 2005). The most common form of CTCL is *mycosis fungoides*, which accounts for approximately 60% of all new cases. *Sezary syndrome* is less common and accounts for approximately 5% of all new cases of CTCL (Trautinger et al., 2006).

Mycosis fungoides commonly presents as a scaly, red rash in areas of the body that usually are not exposed to the sun. The rash generally does not cause symptoms and may last for months or years. During this phase, it is hard to diagnose the rash as mycosis fungoides. Eventually, the rash will develop into a patch and then plaque, followed by a tumor phase (Siegel, Pandolfino, Guitart, Rosen, & Kuzel, 2000). Mycosis fungoides patches can be described as a thin, reddened, eczema-like rash on the skin surface. Plaques are thickened red patches or reddened skin. The tumor phase occurs when a tumor-like growth presents on the surface of the skin. These tumors may develop into deep, painful ulcerations, which can become infected and involve the surrounding skin. In Sezary syndrome, which is the more advanced form of mycosis fungoides, the skin all over the body is reddened, pruritic, and painful and has dry desquamation. Patches, plaques, and tumors also are typically present (Siegel et al.).

Treatment for CTCL lesions involves chemotherapy. It is a palliative treatment to slow the progress of the disease; therefore, the skin lesions can persist and become a wound care challenge even during active treatment. The painful lesions associated with mycosis fungoides and Sezary syndrome are difficult to manage and require patient, meticulous nursing care. Wound management and supportive care are discussed later in this chapter.

Primary cutaneous B-cell lymphomas may involve the skin either as a primary tumor or as cutaneous spread from systemic disease. Approximately 6%–10% of patients with systemic primary B-cell lymphoma will develop cutaneous disease during their illness (Sterry, Kruger, & Steigleder, 1984). The cutaneous lesions may present as a single or multiple erythematous, painless, nonpruritic papules, nodules, or plaques on the head, neck, and trunk. These lesions are painless, smooth, and nonulcerating and can have superficial scaling. General care is discussed in the next section.

General Care

The management of a fungating wound is complex; it often involves a multidisciplinary approach that changes as the disease progresses and/or the wound evolves. Fungating wounds rarely heal (Goldberg & McGinn-Byer, 2007), so the treatment is based on palliation and symptom management, with a goal of improving the patient's overall quality of life.

Palliative care with symptom and local wound management are the mainstay treatment for fungating malignant wounds (Dowsett, 2002; West, 2007; Wilson, 2005). The World Health Organization (n.d.) defined *palliative care* as "an approach that improves the quality of life of patients and their families facing the problem associated with life-threatening illness, through the prevention and relief of suffering by means of early identification and impeccable assessment and treatment of pain and other problems, physical, psychosocial and spiritual." Further, as defined by WHO, palliative care
- Provides relief from pain and other distressing symptoms;
- Affirms life and regards dying as a normal process;
- Intends neither to hasten or postpone death;

- Integrates the psychological and spiritual aspects of patient care;
- Offers a support system to help patients live as actively as possible until death;
- Offers a support system to help the family cope during the patients illness and in their own bereavement;
- Uses a team approach to address the needs of patients and their families, including bereavement counseling, if indicated;
- Will enhance quality of life, and may also positively influence the course of illness;
- Is applicable early in the course of illness, in conjunction with other therapies that are intended to prolong life, such as chemotherapy or radiation therapy, and includes those investigations needed to better understand and manage distressing clinical complications. (www.who.int/cancer/palliative/definition/en/print.html)

Wound bed preparation is essential for any wound care (Vowden & Vowden, 2002). The proposed wound bed preparation in palliative care for fungating wounds consists of (Grocott, 2007)

- Clearance of dead tissue
- Management of bacterial overload
- Symptom control of odor
- Management of exudate
- Minimization of damage to periwound skin
- Management of soiling.

If the patient is actively receiving local treatment (i.e., radiation), the wound may get worse before it gets better, and the skin surrounding the wound may experience desquamation depending on the total dose and size of the treatment area.

An extensive literature review was performed to search for evidence-based practice for the care of fungating wounds. The results revealed a paucity of scientific evidence. However, expert and anecdotal reports on successful treatment of these challenging wounds can prove helpful for practitioners and nurses because the care of these wounds is often based on anecdotal experience or institution protocol. With that in mind, the following sections are designed as a reference in assessing, understanding, and caring for these complex and distressing rare wounds that present in patients with cancer.

Assessment

Understanding the disease process is an important first step in the assessment of a patient with a malignant cutaneous wound. The primary site and stage of the disease can give an indication of the probable progression of the cancer (Hallett, 1995). A thorough history and physical, including past and present treatment regimens, is essential when developing a plan of care (Bradley, 2004; Collier, 1997). A commonly cited key component in obtaining a history and physical is the nurse's ability to establish a personal relationship with the patient, engendering trust and empathy. This requires time and devotion (Wilson, 2005). It is critical that nurses assess patients holistically in order to address all issues related to the wound.

The assessment of malignant cutaneous wounds lacks a widely accepted classification system; thus, detailed documentation is the most reliable form of describing these wounds. Haisfield-Wolfe and Baxendale-Cox (1999) conducted a pilot study using the Hopkins Wound Assessment Tool (Baxendale-Cox, 1995) and careful examination of digital photographs. They proposed a wound classification system that described four stages of malignant wounds based on the parameters of wound color, the patient's hydration status, the absence or presence of nodules, drainage, pain, odor, and tunneling. However, further research is needed to validate this pilot study.

Key factors in the assessment process should include the following.

- Location and etiology: Crucial for determining the type of dressing choice, which will ultimately affect the outcome
- Appearance: Is the wound fungating or ulcerative? Does it have adherent or nonadherent tissue? Are necrosis or slough present? What is the color (gray/brown/black, green/yellow)? Is the tissue friable or bleeding? Is there evidence of a fistula or sinus formation?
- Signs of infection: Increased odor, erythema, warmth, induration, presence of fever, and leukocytosis. Many wounds can be colonized but not necessarily infected (Landis, 2008).
- Size: Length, width, depth (i.e., superficial or deep layers of skin involved), and assessment for tunneling or undermining
- Exudate: Amount, type, color, and odor of exudate
- Periwound skin: Erythematous, fragile or denuded, macerated, nodular, signs of infection, such as erythema, warmth, induration, and fever
- Description of pain: Intensity, aching, burning, or pruritic quality
- Other symptoms: Investigate any other symptoms or potential complications of the wound that need to be assessed, such as the new appearance of necrotic tissue, and document prior to initiating or altering therapy (Seaman, 2006; Wilson, 2005).
- Psychosocial issues: How the wound affects the patient's self-image and what concerns the patient most about the wound should be included in the assessment (Grocott, 1995). The patient's primary concern may not always be related to the treatment but may involve another issue (e.g., financial concerns, feelings of isolation).

Upon completion of a preliminary wound assessment, specific issues should be acknowledged to ensure that a comprehensive, evidence-based care plan is initiated (Wilson, 2005). According to Collier (2000), the results obtained from a thorough assessment should be able to provide answers to the following questions.

1. What is the location and etiology of the wound?
2. Using an objective grading tool, how should the wound be graded?
3. What is the primary treatment objective for this wound?
4. What treatment regimen is vital to achieve the recognized treatment objective?

Management

In general, the four main problems associated with malignant wounds that require symptom management are odor, exudate, bleeding, and pain. However, protecting the periwound skin, controlling infection, and optimizing the emotional well-being of patients and caregivers remain key for optimal management. Although symptom management is the primary goal, ongoing treatment aimed at reducing the fungating tumor, such as chemotherapy, hormone therapy, and radiotherapy, may continue to be incorporated (Haisfield-Wolfe & Rund, 1997; Hallett, 1995). If treatment is effective, the wound may show improvement; it may worsen if the tumor does not respond to therapy. However, it is certain that if the majority of management is palliative, healing is an unrealistic expectation (Bird, 2000).

Odor Control

It is well documented that the effects of uncontrolled foul odor can have a devastating impact on patients' quality of life, leading to psychological stress and social withdrawal (Adderley & Smith, 2007; Bale, Tebbie, & Price, 2004; Clark, 2002; Seaman, 2006). Strong, foul wound odors can lead to involuntary gagging, vomiting, and the decrease of one's sense of taste and appetite, eventually affecting the patient's nutrition status (Hack, 2003).

Odor can be difficult to assess objectively, and without a standard measure, the practitioner is left to assess the presence and severity of odor subjectively, depending on several variables. Assessment of the "level" of odor is minimally addressed or documented in the literature; however, one scoring tool was created in 1995 but has not been widely used (Haughton & Young, 1995). The patient's subjective opinion usually is the best indicator in creating a plan of action (Clark, 2002).

Several theories exist as to why fungating tumors produce an odor.
- The breakdown of proteins in the necrotic tissue by anaerobic bacteria produce a chemical compound and fatty acids, which will emit extremely foul-smelling odor (Thomas, Fisher, Fram, & Waring, 1998).
- Aerobic bacteria (often isolated in these wounds) have odor characteristics of their own, which tend to be less strong (Thomas et al., 1998).
- Presence of clinical infection (Schiech, 2002)
- Presence of necrotic and/or slough tissue
- Stagnant exudate, especially within a saturated dressing (Collier, 1994)

The three anecdotal approaches commonly reported for malodor management are systemic antibiotic treatment, topical antimicrobials, and dressings such as charcoal and silver (Grocott & Cowley, 2001). In addition, sugar paste, honey, natural live yogurt, occlusive dressings, deodorizers, and pouching or bagging the wound area have been reported, but further research is warranted (Schiech, 2002). Debridement may be beneficial but is best performed using autolytic and/or a gentle mechanical method to prevent further bleeding, which can be difficult to manage if excessive. Surgical debridement can be performed when extensive necrotic tissue is present to prevent possible infection and its potential for odor; however, pain and bleeding are a concern (Grocott & Cowley).

Because fungating wounds are chronic in nature, assessment for signs and symptoms of infection should be ongoing. Exudate increases significantly when infection is present. A culture of the wound can confirm the presence or absence of infection and will isolate the main organism or organisms (Draper, 2005). Systemic antibiotics should be prescribed along with topical antimicrobials that act by decreasing the bacterial load, thus decreasing the exudate production (Sarvis, 2006). However, with the increasing rise of MRSA and antibiotic resistance, caution with abundant use is suggested. Some doubt exists that therapeutic drug levels can be obtained because of the lack of blood supply to the necrotic tissue (Grocott, 1999; Naylor, 2002; Thomas et al., 1998). Systemic antibiotics such as metronidazole have been suggested as useful in the treatment of clinical wound infection only (Collier, 2000). Side effects may include nausea, vomiting, and peripheral neuropathy. Little evidence exists to suggest appropriate doses and should be individualized because in these cases it is considered off-label use.

Cleansing

Cleansing of the wound can reduce odor by removing necrotic debris and decreasing the bacterial count. Several different cleansing techniques have been reported. Ambulatory patients should use the shower, as this method provides local cleansing along with the added psychological benefit of helping the patient to feel clean. The shower head or force of the water should be directed to spray above the lesion and allowed to run over it (Draper, 2005; Seaman, 2006).

Many wounds may not be amenable to showering, especially those wounds that are friable or for patients who are unable to tolerate or participate in a shower. Gentle irrigation with warmed normal saline or a pH-balanced commercial skin cleanser can decrease the bacterial load on the wound's surface. If pain becomes an issue with the use of wound cleansers directly on the wound surface, the cleansers should only be used on the surrounding skin.

The use of topical antiseptics remains controversial. Antiseptic solutions may be toxic to healthy tissue, may result in a local reaction to the solution, or may result in wound desiccation causing increased pain and bleeding (Goldberg & McGinn-Byer, 2007; Holloway, 2004; Naylor, 2002). Individual patient assessment of the potential advantages may outweigh the disadvantages of the use of topical antiseptic solutions (Watret, 2002). In general, the consensus is that whatever technique is chosen, gentle care of the fungating tumor will help to prevent damage, pain, and bleeding.

Topical Treatment: Metronidazole

Researchers have agreed that oral metronidazole should be limited to the treatment of a clinically documented wound infection and should not be used for local bacterial colonization. The literature also argues that oral preparations should not be an alternative because of the high incidence of associated side effects, such as gastrointestinal distress, metallic taste in mouth, pruritus, anemia, and central nervous system disturbances (Moody, 1998). These side effects usually accompany high doses of the drug; lowering the doses may avoid the unwanted side effects while still providing a therapeutic effect (Twycross, Wilcock, Charlesworth, & Dickman, 2002).

Evidence does support the use of metronidazole 0.75% gel for the reduction or elimination of odor in the presence of anaerobic and aerobic organisms (Thomas & Hay, 1991). The effectiveness of this synthetic drug on reducing the bacterial burden in the wound works by preventing bacterial replication through binding to their DNA (Hampson, 1996). Although more expensive than oral metronidazole, its reported side effects are minimal, if any. The use of gel should be reconsidered for deep wounds where insufficient tissue penetration may decrease its effect. The use of gel also has been debated in wounds that are heavily exudating, as the gel may become ineffective when diluted by the wound drainage (Grocott, 2000).

After proper cleansing of the wound with warmed normal saline, it is recommended the gel be applied liberally and topped with a secondary dressing that is nonadhesive, such as foam or alginate. This procedure can be done once or twice daily. Research has shown that this procedure is safe and effective for controlling odor within two to three days (Bale et al., 2004; Bower et al., 1992; Finlay, Bowszyc, Ramlau, & Gwiezdzinski, 1996; Moody, 1998). It also has been reported that metronidazole gel played a significant role in the reduction of pain, exudate, and cellulitis. The use of metronidazole gel in combination with other gels, such as hydrogels, may cause a potential interaction between the products and is not recommended.

As a less expensive alternative to the gel form, oral tablets of metronidazole can be crushed and applied to the surface of a malignant fungating wound. To assist with controlling wound malodor, 250 mg or 500 mg metronidazole tablets crushed to a powder-like consistency can be applied in an even layer over the wound surface (Bauer et al., 2000). There have been no studies with regard to odor management comparing the 250 mg tablets to the 500 mg tablets used in this technique. According to Bauer et al., some clinicians have not noticed a difference in odor reduction when comparing the two strengths of the medication when crushed. It is recommended that if using crushed metronidazole, start with the lower dose because absorption of topical metronidazole has not been studied and remains an off-label use.

Without significant supporting evidence, the question still remains: How much application of the topical metronidazole is warranted to reduce the effects of the bacterial load, adequately deodorize, and decrease pain and exudate? Although side effects from topical metronidazole have not been reported, the expense of this product should be considered, and more evidence is needed to describe its exact role. It is important to remember that although use of this agent may reduce wound odor, adequate wound cleansing, exudate management, use of airtight dressings, and immediate disposal of soiled dressings will add to the management of odor control as well (Woodward & Haisfield-Wolfe, 2003).

Topical Treatment: Dakin's Solution

Dakin's solution (sodium hypochlorite) comes in a variety of solution strengths, most frequently found in strengths of 0.25% or 0.025% for wound care. Dakin's can be a powerful defense against aerobic and anaerobic organisms (Heggers et al., 1991). Clinicians find it a very effective deodorizer (Schiech, 2002) in malignant fungating wounds, most likely because of its negative effect on microorganisms. Dakin's solution is not intended to be used long term in the treatment of a fungating wound (Laverty, Taylor, & Soady, 2001); however, it will significantly reduce offensive odors so that maintenance care of the wound can be initiated. Dakin's can be used as a cleanser, or the solution may be applied to gauze, placed on the wound, and changed twice a day. The surrounding skin must be protected from the solution because it can irritate intact skin (Bauer et al., 2000).

As with many suggestions on odor reduction, studies have not been completed on the use of Dakin's solution for effectively reducing the odor of a malignant wound; recommendations for appropriate strength of the solution; how often dressings should be changed; comparison of use of Dakin's as a wound cleanser versus topical treatment; and whether the solution can be absorbed through the wound bed and at what levels it may be dangerous. Further studies are warranted on this effective chemical.

Specialty Dressings

A number of silver-impregnated dressings are available for wound care. Research has shown that silver acts as an antimicrobial and when in use may inhibit bacterial growth (Lansdown, 2002). These dressings may be useful in fighting infection or preventing significant colonization in fungating wounds (Thomas & McCubbin, 2003). Unfortunately, these dressings are expensive, and with the possibility of frequent dressing changes, one needs to justify the benefit to outweigh the added expense.

Charcoal dressings, which contain activated charcoal, are effective in reducing odor by acting as a filter to absorb volatile chemicals from the wound before they pass into the air (Thomas et al., 1998). Two issues arise with their use. First, they become ineffective once they are wet, resulting in frequent dressing changes (Collier, 2000). Second, they must be applied as a sealed unit, making it difficult to fit awkwardly shaped wounds (Grocott, 1999). Charcoal dressings can be applied as either primary or secondary dressings; however, the effectiveness of activated charcoal is only maintained if it remains dry, so it may be used best as a secondary dressing (Thomas et al.). In practice, unless the dressings can maintain a tight seal, they remain ineffective because volatile malodorous chemicals simply escape into the air (Grocott, 1998; Thomas et al.). Care should be taken during application to follow the manufacturer's instructions for use. Caution also should be taken to avoid contamination of the wound if the charcoal dressing is cut to fit a wound (Benbow, 1999).

Activated charcoal dressings come in different forms, including dressings that also contain silver. However, no studies have compared the different dressings on different types of fungating wounds. Thomas et al. (1998), in an in vitro study, tested different dressings and their effectiveness in the prevention of the passage of volatile compounds. Two factors determined the ability of a dressing to contain odor: physical absorbency and the activity of the charcoal itself. This study supported the use of multilayered dressings (such as foam) as most efficient; however, more research is recommended to provide strong evidence supporting the choice of any one particular dressing.

Alternatives

A number of alternative products and procedures have been described in the literature for odor control. Pouching or bagging a fungating wound to control odor may be effective, yet is difficult to achieve with a more challenging fungating wound site. Room deodorizers may help to camouflage the odor but offer no aid in resolution of the problem (Young, 1997).

Honey, a form of autolytic debridement, has been used to debride and deodorize fungating tumors with positive results (Dunford, Cooper, Molan, & White, 2000; Kingsley, 2001; Molan, 2006; White, 2005). Certain types of honey contain hydrogen peroxide at levels lethal to bacteria yet harmless to healthy tissue (Booth, 2004). Sterilized honey is the preferred product because unsterilized products could cause botulism or may even be toxic (Topman, 1994). Manuka honey contains large levels of plant-derived substances (Allen, Molan, & Reid, 1991) and can be purchased with standardized levels of antibacterial activity (Dunford et al., 2000). Despite this, difficulties arise with the application of honey. Honey becomes liquid at higher temperatures, and management of the additional exudate requires dressings with sufficient absorbent qualities; otherwise, odor may become an even bigger dilemma (Cooper & Molan, 1999). Booth (2004) suggested that very little evidence exists to support the use of honey and recommended more research.

The use of natural live yogurt has been suggested but remains controversial, as live *Lactobacillus* spp. can cause an infection in the wound (Haughton & Young, 1995). It is speculated that yogurt lowers the pH of the wound environment and thus prevents the growth of bacteria. This procedure, although unconventional, has been found by some clinicians to be useful in the management of malodor (Schulte, 1993).

Debridement generally is not an option because of the potential result of excessive, uncontrolled bleeding (Dowsett, 2002; Goode, 2004). If warranted, autolytic and/or gentle mechanical methods, such as lightly scrubbing the necrotic tissue with gauze saturated with normal saline, are recommended. Management of malodor with this type of procedure is preferred over sharp debridement, which may cause significant bleeding. Surgical debridement may be indicated if an excess of tumor tissue is present to aid in the prevention of infection, odor control, and management of exudate but should be performed with caution (Seaman, 2006). Hydrogels can be used to soften hard eschar, promoting autolytic debridement (Dowsett); however, steps must be taken to contain and manage the increased volume of exudate that may occur with the use of such products (Vuolo, 2004). Larval (maggot) therapy has been effective for debriding necrotic tissue, but patients may be repelled by the thought of its use, and no studies have been done in this patient population to support this approach (Thomas et al., 1998).

Exudate Management

Next to odor, exudate is probably the most common problem associated with these wounds. Exudate is a result of the increased capillary permeability within the wound, caused by the disorganized tumor vasculature (Naylor, 2002). Another contributing factor of increased exudate levels is the autolysis of necrotic tissue by bacterial proteases (Collier, 1997). A slight amount of exudate is beneficial to most wounds in that it maintains the necessary moist environment to promote healing. Too much exudate can cause maceration of the skin, along with the challenge of containing the fluids. Because inflammation and edema are present in fungating lesions, the drainage tends to be significant, and a great deal of patient embarrassment is accompanied by the fear of leakage. If not managed appropriately, exudate and its related problems can spiral out of control (Grocott, 1999).

Dressings should be aesthetically, emotionally, and physically comfortable, with the choice of treatment options given to the patient (Hallett, 1995). Similar to the recommendations for odor control, pouching for the management of exudate is an option, particularly for smaller fungating ulcers that have an existing pouchable plane. Pouching may be considered when dressings require changing more than two to three times daily or have an exudate of greater than 150 ml in eight hours. Pouching is also effective for rapid removal of exudate or if measurement of the amount of drainage is necessary (Sarvis, 2006).

The use of negative pressure wound therapy or a vacuum-assisted closure system is contraindicated. One of the major concerns with fungating wounds is bleeding, and these systems may increase the risk of profuse bleeding and possible malignant growth exacerbation (KCI, 2007). In addition, wet-to-dry dressings with normal saline are not recommended because they can increase the risk of periwound maceration and result in excessive bleeding when removed (Baranoski & Ayello, 2004).

Current wound care practice of nonfungating wounds is substantially based on Winter's (1962, 1965) theory of moist wound healing. Moist wound healing defines the benefits of a moist wound environment for the purposes of epithelialization. However, Winter's theory may not be transferrable to fungating wounds because moisture-conserving dressings allow exudate to accumulate, giving rise to problems such as maceration and leakage (Grocott, 1998, 2000). In addition, the focus of care is not on "healing" but rather on palliative care of the wound.

The choice of dressing depends on the amount of exudate while facilitating a moist wound environment to minimize the risk of pain and bleeding at dressing change. Hydrogels and hydrocolloids are useful for low exudating wounds and help with preservation of the surrounding skin (Collier, 2000; Naylor, 2002). Dressings such as foams, alginates, and hydrofibers are recommended to absorb excessive drainage and are less bulky and more acceptable to patients (Young, 2000).

The protection of the periwound skin remains extremely important to aid against maceration. This can be accomplished with the use of an alcohol-free barrier film or skin protectant. The use of hydrocolloid strips, "window framing" a taping surface while minimizing the use of tape, is recommended. Using netting, gauze, nonadherent dressings, and clothing to secure the dressings should be considered (Young, 2000).

Little evidence exists to support the use of any individual brand of dressing, but an extensive research project performed by Grocott (2000) determined two systems that performed best. The first was a nonadherent wound contact layer, which allowed the exudate to pass into a second layer, and consisted of an absorbent pad from which moisture can evaporate. The second was an absorbent contact layer on the wound such as an alginate or hydrofiber, with a secondary retention layer of foam followed by two-layer controlled permeability. Although neither system is without faults, Grocott's important study provided the best evidence to guide dressing choice. It remains important that no matter what dressing is chosen for management, it should be changed as frequently as needed to control exudate and odor.

Management of Bleeding

A malignant cutaneous wound may bleed easily because of its fragile vasculature and erosion of capillaries by the tumor (Goldberg & McGinn-

Byer, 2007). In addition, patients with cancer may experience coagulation defects related to their disease process or treatments that contribute to their risk of bleeding (Gagnon, Mancini, Pereira, & Bruera, 1998). If not addressed, bleeding can cause acute and chronic anemia. Bleeding also can be distressing for patients and families and, if it occurs spontaneous or profusely, may become life threatening (Sarvis, 2006). Patient education is crucial for the prevention and management of bleeding. Patients and their families should be informed of when it is critical to seek medical attention. If a large amount of bleeding does occur, a blood hemoglobin level should be considered to assess the need for transfusions (Dowsett, 2002). The most significant way to deal with bleeding is prevention. Methods to reduce the incidence of bleeding include (Dowsett, 2002; Schiech, 2002; Seaman, 2006)

- Mild cleansing of the wound
- Gentle application and removal of the dressing
- Using a delicate nonadherent contact layer dressing
- Maintaining a moist wound bed
- Avoiding unnecessary dressing changes
- Avoiding or using caution with debridement.

When a dressing adheres to the wound bed, it should be soaked with normal saline before its removal to lessen the trauma (Schiech, 2002; Seaman, 2006). This also may be accomplished in the shower with warm water. Patients should be taught when to seek help if a dressing adheres and be given instructions on how to manage bleeding when it does occur. There are several key approaches to controlling bleeding in a wound. They include

- Application of direct pressure for 10–15 minutes
- Application of ice packs to the wound
- Use of coagulant topical or hemostatic agents/sponges (Adderley & Smith, 2007; Seaman, 2006)
- Use of oral antifibrinolytics to help to control severe bleeding
- Application of topical sucralfate (Carafate®, Axcan Pharma) suspension, used to coat the surface of friable blood vessels to aid in the prevention of trauma-induced bleeding and enhance clotting (Cooper & Cooper, 1993; Sarvis, 2006)
- Application of silver nitrate sticks, especially in small areas of bleeding
- Surgical intervention such as cauterization if a tumor has eroded into a major vessel (McMurray, 2003)
- For extreme, severe bleeding, a short course of radiation may be given until the bleeding discontinues.
- Chemotherapy, initiated to reduce the size of the wound (Sarvis, 2006).
- Use of topical epinephrine 1:1,000 (in the form of a soak), another agent for profuse bleeding (Sarvis, 2006). (It is recommended in the literature that only knowledgeable practitioners should apply this therapy, as critical ischemia can occur from extreme local vasoconstriction.)

Managing Pain and Itching

Multiple factors contribute toward pain, and 55%–95% of patients with malignant wounds experience pain (Downing, 1999). A careful and thorough assessment is required to accurately control a patient's discomfort. Assessment of pain should include the site, nature, duration, onset, frequency, and severity, as well as the impact on the patient's daily activities. In addition, aggravating and alleviating factors, the patient's current pain regimen, and the effects of the current treatment should be considered (Naylor, 2001). A reliable assessment tool is recommended to enhance an assessment (Dowsett, 2002). Several are available, but the most frequently used are a visual analog scale and descriptive scales (Naylor).

Assessment of pain is critical when developing a care plan. This should include specific pain at the wound site noted by the patient as well as pain with dressing changes or other activities of daily living (e.g., showering). The initial assessment should include the location, duration, nature, severity, onset, frequency, and how pain affects activities and sleep. Aggravating factors, type of analgesia, and effects of treatment for pain are useful details to obtain when tailoring the treatment plan (Dowsett, 2002). It is important to distinguish between pain caused by stimulation of nerve endings (nociceptive pain) and pain resulting from nerve dysfunction (neuropathic pain), because different treatments are suggested (Dowsett; Seaman, 2006; Wilson, 2005). Several causes of pain in malignant wounds have been documented, including pressure from the tumor on the nerves and blood vessels, exposure and drying of the dermis (Manning, 1998), and inappropriate dressing procedures (Jones, Davey, & Champion, 1998).

Just as bleeding is best managed with prevention, so is pain. Management may include several approaches, including administering medications (sometimes in combination), monitoring pain levels, providing emotional support, and determining when changes are necessary (Grocott, 2007). The same principles for the management of bleeding apply with pain management: nonadherent dressings, gentle cleansing, and maintaining a moist wound environment. A helpful reference to guide pain management is the World Health Organization's analgesic ladder.

Application of a local and topical anesthetic (e.g., lidocaine gel) directly to the wound surface has been reported to be effective. Such agents act by blocking the action potential (Laverty et al., 2001). The gel should be applied 10–15 minutes before any procedure such as removal of an adhering dressing and may decrease the patient's level of discomfort. Prior to dressing changes, administering an analgesic and/or local anesthetics may be helpful in reducing pain (Sarvis, 2006). The use of opioids topically, such as morphine, is noted to bind to peripheral opioid receptors. When mixed with a carrier gel or hydrogel, the solution can be applied directly on the wound surface, causing immediate local analgesia and decreasing the inflammation process. Several case studies have demonstrated a positive effect when topical opioids were used (Dowsett, 2002); however, this remains an off-label use.

The use of a systemic analgesic remains the gold standard for pain management, and short-acting analgesics should be administered prior to dressing changes (Seaman, 2006). Nonsteroidal anti-inflammatory medications may be helpful if the pain is associated with skin surface pain or local inflammation (Laverty et al., 2001; Sarvis, 2006). Evans (2003) assessed the effectiveness of nitrous oxide and oxygen (sometimes referred to as entonox) prior to dressing changes in several case studies; however, there is no research evidence to support its use (Laverty et al.). Adjuvant analgesia, such as antidepressants and anticonvulsants, has been studied for their use in neuropathic pain with successful outcomes (Naylor, 2001).

Palliative care may include radiation and/or chemotherapy to reduce the tumor volume and promote pain control. Obtaining a cure from these treatments is not the objective, yet it may prolong life and ease pain and bleeding, thus improving the quality of life (Seaman, 2006). The potential side effects of the therapy must be considered and balanced with the potential benefit.

Along with pain, pruritus of the adjacent skin often is a chronic problem during the beginning phases of tumor development. It is the result of the stretching skin irritating the nerve endings, which causes a biochemical reaction leading to local inflammation. Patients often describe it as a "creeping" intense itching sensation (Sarvis, 2006). Although pruritus is a challenge to treat, recommendations have been developed to manage the intense itching. Chilled hydrogel sheets are soothing and cooling on contact and may offer relief. The application of menthol creams, showering in cool water, using low pH-balanced cleansers, avoiding alcohol-containing products, and wearing lightweight, nonbinding clothing have all been suggested (Sarvis). Significant reduction in itching has been reported with the use of transcutaneous electrical nerve stimulation (Grocott, 2000). Limited research exists, and further study is warranted (Grocott, 2007). Antihistamines generally are ineffective in management of pruritus associated with malignant wounds (Sarvis).

Patient Education

Effective communication between healthcare providers and patients and families is paramount for the successful management of malignant cutaneous wounds. Involving patients and their caregivers in the plan of care early in the process is central to this practice. Dressing selection should include considerations other than efficacy; concerns such as cost, reimbursement, availability, number of dressing changes required, complexity of the procedure, extent of education necessary, and presence of a caregiver all require careful consideration (Goldberg & McGinn-Byer, 2007).

With the trend toward home care, achieving a realistic plan of care with measurable goals is the cornerstone of successful management. Treating patients and family members with respect and compassion will help to build the trust required to maintain open communication. Sensitive issues regarding these types of wounds are extremely personal and need to be addressed in an empathetic manner.

Education on basic wound care, such as hand washing and dressing change procedures, also applies to the care of these wounds and should be part of the educational process (Seaman, 2006). It has been confirmed throughout the literature that no one dressing is the ultimate answer to the management needs of patients experiencing this type of wound (Grocott, 2000). Because wound healing is often not achievable, educating patients and caregivers on management of odor and bleeding, containment of exudate, alleviation of pain, and protection of the periwound skin should remain the focus of education. The dressing selection should be continually assessed for effectiveness and appropriate changes made where necessary.

Patients and caregivers should be involved with the choice of options and informed on conditions that require the notification of a practitioner. Patients and caregivers need to know the importance of reporting an increase in exudate, pain, and bleeding. The inability of the patient or caregiver to obtain wound care products or manage the wound regimen is significant to report to the practitioner. Issues such as the development of a fever, unusual changes in the wound, or the onset of severe emotional distress should be included when educating patients and caregivers on when to notify the practitioner. Documentation remains critical for overall success in the management of these wounds and should include

- Wound presentation
- All interventions and plan of care
- Patient and family instruction
- Evaluation of interventions
- Rationale for any changes in plan of care
- Emotional impact on patients and caregivers
- Patients' psychosocial state.

A critical area to be addressed when caring for this patient population is their psychosocial welfare. Although the literature identifies the devastating psychosocial issues associated with malignant wounds, it does not provide researched strategies to meet the needs of patients and families (Lazelle-Ali, 2007). The National Comprehensive Cancer Network (NCCN, 2008) guidelines for distress management outline the standards and assessment and treatment processes to help practitioners to guide patients with cancer as they experience a wide variety of psychological stressors. Some of the factors that may relate to the distress felt by patients with a fungating wound include the following (NCCN) (see Chapter 12 for additional information).

- Vulnerability
- Sadness
- Fear
- Depression
- Anxiety
- Panic

- Social isolation
- Existential and spiritual crisis

Keeping in mind these potential issues surrounding the complications of people with fungating wounds will give way to a holistic and sympathetic plan of care (Sarvis, 2006).

Common psychosocial aspects that accompany fungating wounds include experiencing grief, anxiety, embarrassment, and withdrawal from social situations. Malodorous and exudating fungating wounds have such a significant impact on the patient's body image and self-worth that social isolation becomes an increasing problem. More visible malignant wounds play a major role in a patient's social isolation compared to wounds on the breast, which may cause concerns such as with sexuality (Dowsett, 2002). Physical symptoms, such as malodor and exudate, contribute to patient embarrassment and withdrawal from family and friends, leading to social isolation. Losing one's social support can ultimately be a causative factor in the development of depression when this important coping mechanism has been severed (Sarvis, 2006).

Patients may be reluctant to seek medical attention and can present with lesions in advanced stages. These wounds can have a significant impact on body image, as well as other psychosocial concerns, including a loss of dignity and independence. During the initial assessment, it is imperative to determine the wound's effect on a patient's activities of daily living and self-image (Grocott, 1995). The assessment should include what concerns the patient most about the wound (Grocott, 1995), as the patient's primary concern may not always be treatment related but may involve another issue (e.g., financial or feelings of isolation).

Experiencing poor body image is not uncommon, especially when the wound is visible and difficult to conceal. Location of the wound is significant to the patient's body image and dressing application. Interventions such as creative dressing techniques; low-profile dressings; and filling cavities to create symmetry all may help to improve cosmetic appearance and overall body image (Haisfield-Wolfe & Rund, 1997).

Intimacy and relationships may be challenged if the wounds are located within the genitals or breasts and produce malodor or exudate (Sarvis, 2006). Addressing patients' issues regarding sexual activity is necessary, as is finding a resolution to the patient's specific concerns.

Effective communication and listening are essential when exploring not only the physical but also the psychological aspects of dealing with a chronic wound. Counseling with instruction on the use of coping mechanisms is helpful when patients and families are adjusting to the presence of a complex wound (Laverty et al., 2001). Tapping into the interdisciplinary team, such as a social worker and/or family support, offers assistance with patients' care. Specially trained colleagues may contribute to an extended care plan when offering specific skills and knowledge (Grocott, 2007). Obtaining a psychiatric or psychological counseling consult or suggesting attending a support group also may be beneficial (Schiech, 2002).

Providing ongoing education and reevaluation of the effectiveness of the present care plan will, in the end, allow patients and significant others to live their lives to their fullest. Continual and effective communication with patients and caregivers is vital in this ever-challenging field of wound care. Ultimately, evaluating the outcomes from a psychosocial perspective should answer the question of whether the symptom management, communication skills, and overall advice from the practitioner have improved the patient's quality of life (Laverty et al., 2001).

Conclusion

No matter what the primary disease is, fungating tumors have this in common: They are very difficult to treat, remaining a major management challenge for oncology nurses and healthcare practitioners. Wound healing is slow during most chemotherapy regimens, and proper wound care is essential to prevent infection and promote healing. Complete resolution is rare, and supportive care becomes the primary goal of treatment. These wounds present both physical and emotional challenges to patients and families. They are often disfiguring and malodorous and can have heavy exudate accompanied by bleeding and pain. To maintain a framework for the consistent care of fungating wounds, further research is warranted.

References

Adderley, U.J., & Smith, R. (2007). Topical agents and dressings for fungating wounds. *Cochrane Database of Systematic Reviews* 2007, Issue 2. Art. No.: CD003948. DOI: 10.1002/14651858.CD003948.pub2.

Alam, M., & Ratner, D. (2001). Cutaneous squamous cell carcinoma. *New England Journal of Medicine, 344*(13), 975–983.

Allen, K.L., Molan, P.C., & Reid, G.M. (1991). A survey of the antibacterial activity of some New Zealand honeys. *Journal of Pharmacy and Pharmacology, 43*(12), 817–822.

Allen, P.J., Bowne, W.B., Jaques, D.P., Brennan, M.F., Busam, K., & Coit, D.G. (2005). Merkel cell carcinoma: Prognosis and treatment of patients from a single institution. *Journal of Clinical Oncology, 23*(10), 2300–2309.

American Academy of Dermatology. (2009). *Malignant melanoma.* Retrieved February 5, 2009, from http://www.aad.org/public/publications/pamphlets/sun_malignant.html

Bale, S., Tebbie, N., & Price, P. (2004). A topical metronidazole gel used to treat malodorous wounds. *British Journal of Nursing, 13*(11), S4–S11.

Baranoski, S., & Ayello, E.A. (2004). *Wound care essentials: Practice principles.* Philadelphia: Lippincott Williams & Wilkins.

Bauer, C., Gerlach, M.A., & Doughty, D. (2000). Care of metastatic skin lesions. *Journal of Wound, Ostomy, and Continence Nursing, 27*(4), 247–251.

Baxendale-Cox, L. (1995). [Quantification of wound status]. Johns Hopkins University, School of Nursing, Department of Radiology, Surgery, and Biomedical Engineering Applied Physics Lab. Unpublished raw data.

Benbow, M. (1999). Malodorous wounds: How to improve quality of life. *Community Nurse, 5*(1), 43–46.

Bird, C. (2000). Supporting patients with fungating breast wounds. *Professional Nurse,* *15*(10), 649–652.

Booth, S. (2004). Are honey and sugar paste alternatives to topical antiseptics? *Journal of Wound Care, 13*(1), 31–33.

Bower, M., Stein, R., Evans, T.R., Hedley, A., Pert, P., & Coombes, R.C. (1992). A double-blind study of the efficacy of metronidazole gel in the treatment of malodorous fungating tumours. *European Journal of Cancer, 28A*(4–5), 888–889.

Bradley, M. (2004). When healing is not an option. Palliative care as a primary treatment goal. *Advance for Nurse Practitioners, 12*(7), 50–52, 57.

British Columbia Cancer Agency. (2001, January). *Chronic ulcerating malignant skin lesions.* Retrieved February 5, 2009, from http://www.bccancer.bc.ca/HPI/Nursing/References/SupportiveCare/Chronic/default.htm

Christenson, L.J., Borrowman, T.A., Vachon, C.M., Tollefson, M.M., Otley, C.C., Weaver, A.L., et al. (2005). Incidence of basal cell and squamous cell carcinomas in a population younger than 40 years. *JAMA, 294*(6), 681–690.

Clark, J. (2002). Metronidazole gel in managing malodorous fungating wounds. *British Journal of Nursing, 11*(Supp. 6), S54–S60.

Collier, M. (1994). Assessing a wound. *Nursing Standard, 8*(49), 3–8.

Collier, M. (1997). The assessment of patients with malignant fungating wounds—A holistic approach: Part 1. *Nursing Times, 93*(44), Suppl. 1–4.

Collier, M. (2000). Management of patients with fungating wounds. *Nursing Standard, 15*(11), 46–52.

Cooper, D., & Cooper, J. (1993). Managing malignant ulcers effectively. *Nursing Standard, 8*(2), 25–28.

Cooper, R., & Molan, P. (1999). The use of honey as an antiseptic in managing Pseudomonas infection. *Journal of Wound Care, 8*(4), 161–164.

Desmond, R.A., & Soong, S.J. (2003). Epidemiology of malignant melanoma. *Surgical Clinics of North America, 83*(1), 1–29.

Di Lorenzo, G., Konstantinopoulos, P.A., Pantanowitz, L., Di Trolio, R., De Placido, S., & Dezube, B.J. (2007). Management of AIDS-related Kaposi's sarcoma. *Lancet Oncology, 8*(2), 167–176.

Dinh, V., Feun, L., Elgart, G., & Savaraj, N. (2007). Merkel cell carcinomas. *Hematology/Oncology Clinics of North America, 21*(3), 527–544.

Downing, J. (1999). *Pain in the patient with cancer.* London: Nursing Times Books.

Dowsett, C. (2002). Malignant fungating wounds: Assessment and management. *British Journal of Community Nursing, 7*(8), 394–400.

Draper, C. (2005). The management of malodour and exudate in fungating wounds. *British Journal of Nursing, 14*(11), S4–S12.

Dunford, C., Cooper, R., Molan, P., & White, R. (2000). The use of honey in wound management. *Nursing Standard, 15*(11), 63–68.

Evans, A. (2003). Use of Entonox in the community for control of procedural pain. *British Journal of Community Nursing, 8*(11), 488–494.

Finlay, I.G., Bowszyc, J., Ramlau, C., & Gwiezdzinski, Z. (1996). The effect of topical 0.75% metronidazole gel on malodorous cutaneous ulcers. *Journal of Pain and Symptom Management, 11*(3), 158–162.

Foltz, A.T. (1980). Nursing care of ulcerating metastatic lesions. *Oncology Nursing Forum, 7*(2), 8–13.

Gagnon, B., Mancini, I., Pereira, J., & Bruera, E. (1998). Palliative management of bleeding events in advanced cancer patients. *Journal of Palliative Care, 14*(4), 50–54.

Gallagher, J. (1995). Management of cutaneous symptoms. *Seminars in Oncology Nursing, 11*(4), 239–247.

Garneski, K.M., & Nghiem, P. (2007). Merkel cell carcinoma adjuvant therapy: Current data support radiation but not chemotherapy. *Journal of the American Academy of Dermatology, 57*(1), 166–169.

Goldberg, M.T., & McGinn-Byer, M. (2007). Oncology-related skin damage. In R.A. Bryant & D.P. Nix (Eds.), *Acute and chronic wounds: Current management concepts* (3rd ed., pp. 471–489). St. Louis, MO: Elsevier Mosby.

Gollard, R., Weber, R., Kosty, M.P., Greenway, H.T., Massullo, V., & Humberson, C. (2000). Merkel cell carcinoma: Review of 22 cases with surgical, pathologic, and therapeutic considerations. *Cancer, 88*(8), 1842–1851.

Goode, M.L. (2004). Psychological needs of patients when dressing a fungating wound: A literature review. *Journal of Wound Care, 13*(9), 380–382.

Grocott, P. (1995). Assessment of fungating malignant wounds. *Journal of Wound Care, 4*(7), 333–336.

Grocott, P. (1998). Exudate management in fungating wounds. *Journal of Wound Care, 7*(9), 445–448.

Grocott, P. (1999). The management of fungating wounds. *Journal of Wound Care, 8*(5), 232–234.

Grocott, P. (2000). The palliative management of fungating malignant wounds. *Journal of Wound Care, 9*(1), 4–9.

Grocott, P. (2007). Care of patients with fungating malignant wounds. *Nursing Standard, 21*(24), 57–62.

Grocott, P., & Cowley, S. (2001). The palliative management of fungating malignant wounds—Generalising from multiple-case study data using a system of reasoning. *International Journal of Nursing Studies, 38*(5), 533–545.

Hack, A. (2003). Malodorous wounds—Taking the patient's perspective into account. *Journal of Wound Care, 12*(8), 319–321.

Haisfield-Wolfe, M.E., & Baxendale-Cox, L.M. (1999). Staging of malignant cutaneous wounds: A pilot study. *Oncology Nursing Forum, 26*(6), 1055–1064.

Haisfield-Wolfe, M.E., & Rund, C. (1997). Malignant cutaneous wounds: A management protocol. *Ostomy/Wound Management, 43*(1), 56–66.

Hallett, A. (1995). Fungating wounds. *Nursing Times, 91*(47), 78.

Hampson, J.P. (1996). The use of metronidazole in the treatment of malodorous wounds. *Journal of Wound Care, 5*(9), 421–425.

Haughton, W., & Young, T. (1995). Common problems in wound care: Malodorous wounds. *British Journal of Nursing, 4*(16), 959–963.

Heggers, J.P., Sazy, J.A., Stenberg, B.D., Strock, L.L., McCauley, R.L., Herndon, D.N., et al. (1991). Bactericidal and wound-healing properties of sodium hypochlorite solutions: The 1991 Lindberg Award. *Journal of Burn Care and Rehabilitation, 12*(5), 420–434.

Holloway, S. (2004). Recognising and treating the causes of chronic malodorous wounds. *Professional Nurse, 19*(7), 380–384.

Ivetic, O., & Lyne, P.A. (1990). Fungating and ulcerating malignant lesions: A review of the literature. *Journal of Advanced Nursing, 15*(1), 83–88.

Jabbour, J., Cumming, R., Scolyer, R.A., Hruby, G., Thompson, J.F., & Lee, S. (2007). Merkel cell carcinoma: Assessing the effect of wide local excision, lymph node dissection, and radiotherapy on recurrence and survival in early-stage disease—Results from a review of 82 consecutive cases diagnosed between 1992 and 2004. *Annals of Surgical Oncology, 14*(6), 1943–1952.

Jones, M., Davey, J., & Champion, M. (1998). Dressing wounds. *Nursing Standard, 12*(39), 47–56.

KCI. (2007, July). *V.A.C. therapy clinical guidelines: A reference source for clinicians.* San Antonio, TX: Author. Retrieved February 5, 2009, from http://www.kci1.com/Clinical_Guidelines_VAC.pdf

Kingsley, A. (2001). The use of honey in the treatment of infected wounds: Case studies. *British Journal of Nursing, 10*(Suppl. 22), S13–S16, S18, S20.

Landis, S. (2008). Chronic wound infection and antimicrobial use. *Advances in Skin and Wound Care, 21*(11), 531–540.

Lansdown, A.B. (2002). Silver. I: Its antibacterial properties and mechanism of action. *Journal of Wound Care, 11*(4), 125–130.

Laverty, D., Naylor, W., & Soady, C. (2001). Management of wounds related to cancer and cancer therapies. In W. Naylor, D. Laverty, & J. Mallett (Eds.), *The Royal Marsden Hospital handbook of wound management in cancer care* (pp. 73–122). London: Blackwell Science.

Lazelle-Ali, C. (2007). Psychological and physical care of malodorous fungating wounds. *British Journal of Nursing, 16*(15), S16–S24.

Levine, A.M., & Tulpule, A. (2001). Clinical aspects and management of AIDS-related Kaposi's sarcoma. *European Journal of Cancer, 37*(10), 1288–1295.

Lim, S.T., Tupule, A., Espina, B.M., & Levine, A.M. (2005). Weekly docetaxel is safe and effective in the treatment of advanced-stage acquired immunodeficiency syndrome-related Kaposi sarcoma. *Cancer, 103*(2), 417–421.

Manning, M.P. (1998). Metastasis to skin. *Seminars in Oncology Nursing, 14*(3), 240–243.

McMurray, V. (2003). Managing patients with fungating malignant wounds. *Nursing Times, 99*(13), 55–57.

Molan, P.C. (2006). The evidence supporting the use of honey as a wound dressing. *International Journal of Lower Extremity Wounds, 5*(1), 40–54.

Moody, M. (1998). Metrotop: A topical antimicrobial agent for malodorous wounds. *British Journal of Nursing, 7*(5), 286–289.

Mortimer, P.S. (1998). Management of skin problems. In D. Doyle, G.W.C. Hanks, & N. MacDonald (Eds.), *Oxford textbook of palliative medicine* (2nd ed., pp. 617–626). New York: Oxford University Press.

National Comprehensive Cancer Network. (2008). *NCCN Clinical Practice Guidelines in Oncology™: Distress management* [v.1.2008]. Retrieved December 10, 2008, from http://www.nccn.org/professionals/physician_gls/PDF/distress.pdf

Naylor, W. (2001). Assessment and management of pain in fungating wounds. *British Journal of Nursing, 10,* S33–S40.

Naylor, W. (2002). Malignant wounds: Aetiology and principles of management. *Nursing Standard, 16*(52), 45–53.

Rigel, D.S., Rivers, J.K., Kopf, A.W., Friedman, R.J., Vinokur, A.F., Heilman, E.R., et al. (1989). Dysplastic nevi. Markers for increased risk for melanoma. *Cancer, 63*(2), 386–389.

Rowe, D.E., Carroll, R.J., & Day, C.L. (1989). Long-term recurrence rates in previously untreated (primary) basal cell carcinoma: Implications for patient follow-up. *Journal of Dermatologic Surgery and Oncology, 15*(3), 315–328.

Safai, B. (1997). Kaposi's sarcoma and acquired immunodeficiency syndrome. In V.T. DeVita Jr., S. Hellman, & S.A. Rosenberg (Eds.), *AIDS: Etiology, diagnosis, treatment, and prevention* (4th ed., pp. 295–318). Philadelphia: Lippincott-Raven.

Sarvis, C. (2006). Providing relief for patients with malignant wounds. *Nursing Spectrum, Oncology Specialty Guide,* pp. 42–47.

Schiech, L. (2002). Malignant cutaneous wounds. *Clinical Journal of Oncology Nursing, 6*(5), 305–309.

Schulte, M.J. (1993). Yogurt helps to control wound odor. *Oncology Nursing Forum, 20*(8), 1262.

Seaman, S. (2006). Management of malignant fungating wounds in advanced cancer. *Seminars in Oncology Nursing, 22*(3), 185–193.

Siegel, R., Pandolfino, S.T., Guitart, J., Rosen, S., & Kuzel, T.M. (2000). Primary cutaneous T-cell lymphoma: Review and current concepts. *Journal of Clinical Oncology, 18*(15), 2908–2925.

Sterry, W., Kruger, G.R., & Steigleder, G.K. (1984). Skin involvement of malignant B-cell lymphomas. *Journal of Dermatologic Surgery and Oncology, 10*(4), 276–277.

Thomas, S., & Hay, N.P. (1991). The antimicrobial properties of two metronidazole-medicated dressings used to treat malodorous wounds. *Pharmaceutical Journal, 246,* 264–266.

Thomas, S., Fisher, B., Fram, P.J., & Waring, M.J. (1998). Odour-absorbing dressings. *Journal of Wound Care, 7*(5), 246–250.

Thomas, S., & McCubbin, P. (2003). An in vitro analysis of the antimicrobial properties of 10 silver-containing dressings. *Journal of Wound Care, 12*(8), 305–308.

Topman, J. (1994). What's new in wound treatment? Not a lot. *Journal of Tissue Viability, 4*(3), 86–89.

Trautinger, F., Knobler, R., Willemze, R., Peris, K., Stadler, R., Laroche, L., et al. (2006). EORTC consensus recommendations for the treatment of mycosis fungoides/Sezary syndrome. *European Journal of Cancer, 42*(8), 1014–1030.

Twycross, R., Wilcock, A., Charlesworth, S., & Dickman, A. (2002). *Palliative care formulary* (2nd ed.). Oxford, UK: Radcliffe Medical Press.

Vanni, T., Sprinz, E., Machado, M.W., Santana, R.C., Fonseca, B.A.L., & Schwartsmann, G. (2006). Systemic treatment of AIDS-related Kaposi sarcoma: Current status and perspectives. *Cancer Treatment Reviews, 32*(6), 445–455.

Vowden, K., & Vowden, P. (2002). *Wound bed preparation.* Retrieved January 10, 2007, from http://www.worldwidewounds.com/2002/april/Vowden/Wound-Bed-Preparation.html

Vuolo, J. (2004). Current options for managing the problem of excess wound exudate. *Professional Nurse, 19*(9), 487–491.

Wagner, R.F., & Casciato, D.C. (2000). Skin cancers. In D.A. Casciato & B.B. Lowitz (Eds.), *Manual of clinical oncology* (pp. 336–373). Philadelphia: Lippincott Williams & Wilkins.

Watret, L., & Armitage, M. (2002). Making sense of wound cleansing. *Journal of Community Nursing, 16*(4), 27–34.

West, D. (2007). A palliative approach to the management of malodour from malignant fungating tumours. *International Journal of Palliative Nursing, 13*(3), 137–142.

White, R. (2005). The benefits of honey in wound management. *Nursing Standard, 20*(10), 57–66.

Willemze, R., Jaffe, E.S., Burg, G., Cerroni, L., Berti, E., Swerdlow, S.H., et al. (2005). WHO-EORTC classification for cutaneous lymphomas. *Blood, 105*(10), 3768–3785.

Wilson, V. (2005). Assessment and management of fungating wounds: A review. *British Journal of Community Nursing, 10*(3), S28–S34.

Winter, G.D. (1962). Formation of the scab and the rate of epithelialisation of superficial wounds in the skin of the young domestic pig. *Nature, 193*(4812), 293–294.

Winter, G.D. (1965). A note on wound healing under dressings with special reference to perforated-film dressings. *Journal of Investigative Dermatology, 45*(4), 299–302.

Wong, C.S., Strange, R.C., & Lear, J.T. (2003). Basal cell carcinoma. *BMJ, 327*(7418), 794–798.

Woodward, L., & Haisfield-Wolfe, M.E. (2003). Management of a patient with a malignant cutaneous tumor. *Journal of Wound, Ostomy, and Continence Nurses Society, 30*(4), 231–236.

World Health Organization. (n.d.). *WHO definition of palliative care.* Retrieved February 5, 2009, from http://www.who.int/cancer/palliative/definition/en/print.html

Young, T. (1997). The challenge of managing fungating wounds. *Community Nurse, 3*(9), 41–44.

Young, T. (2000). *Managing wound exudate. Essential wound healing, Part 6.* London: Emap Healthcare.

CHAPTER 5

Wound Care Products and Treatments

Elizabeth A. Ayello, PhD, RN, ACNS-BC, ETN, FAPWCA, FAAN, and
Sharon Baranoski, RN, MSN, CWOCN, APN, DAPWCA, FAAN

Introduction

People with cancer may have wounds. The wounds can include surgical incisions, fistulas, skin tears from fragile skin, pressure ulcers from prolonged immobility, friction or shear, or even *malignant cutaneous wounds* (MCWs), sometimes called *fungating wounds*, from tumors that erupt on the skin. Wound care experts use the principles of wound bed preparation that include removal of nonviable tissue by debridement; infection and inflammation control; moisture balance correction by use of modern dressings; and epidermal edge closure (Schultz et al., 2003) to plan and implement wound healing protocols.

Surgical incisions usually are expected to heal. Sometimes, these wounds can dehisce and will require additional treatments, including debridement and appropriate dressings, and thus take longer to heal. Figures 5-1 through 5-6 illustrate a case example of a patient with breast cancer with wound dehiscence. This wound was able to be closed after four months using a combination of surgical debridement and appropriate modern advanced therapies.

For other patients, wound outcomes may be different. Sometimes the goal in wound healing may be to maintain the wound, whereas for others with a nonhealable wound, preventing complications and addressing patient-centered concerns such as pain, odor, and drainage may be paramount (Kirshen, Woo, Ayello, & Sibbald, 2006). Goals may change over the course of the person's cancer.

Palliative wound care is understudied. *Palliative wound care* uses strategies that focus on relief of suffering rather than wound closure (Ferris et al., 2007). Palliative wound care does not mean abandoning the patient but rather addressing quality-of-life issues for an individual with a chronic wound (Ferris et al.; Hughes & Van Onselen, 2001). An effective way to approach palliative

Figure 5-1. Wound Dehiscence

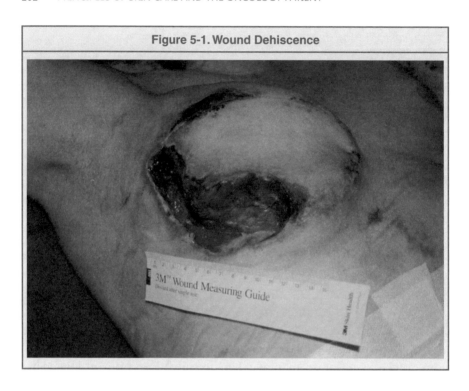

Figure 5-2. Surgical Debridement

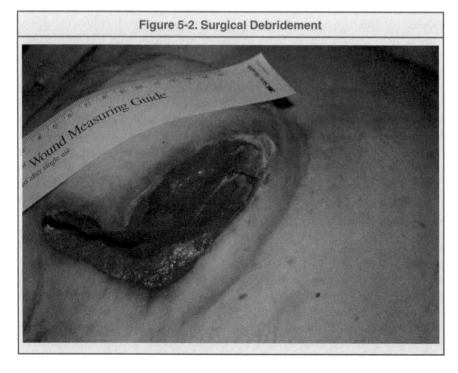

Figure 5-3. Granular Wound Bed

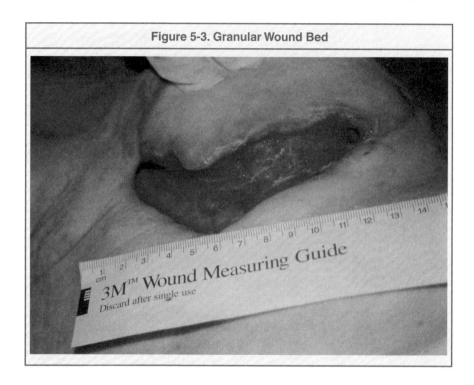

Figure 5-4. Granular Wound Bed With Good Closure Occurring

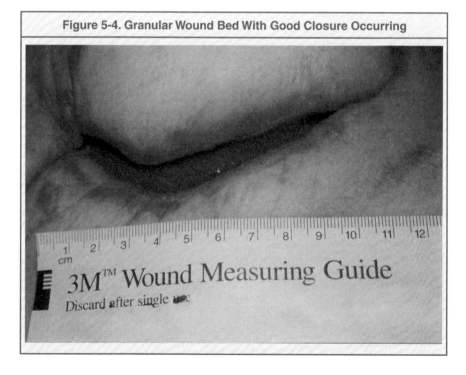

Figure 5-5. Healing After Two Months

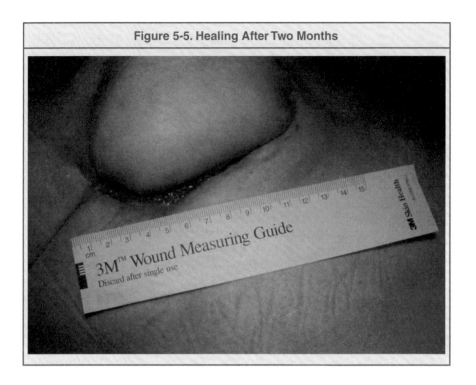

Figure 5-6. Healed Four Months

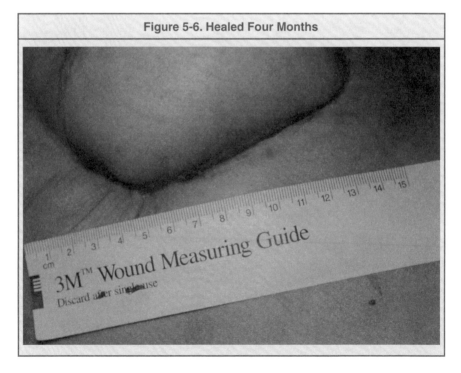

wound care, regardless of care setting, has been summarized by the mnemonic SPECIAL (Alvarez et al., 2007):

S = stabilize the wound
P = prevent new wounds
E = eliminate odor
C = control pain
I = infection prophylaxis
A = advanced, absorbent wound dressings
L = lessen dressing changes.

Alvarez et al. (2007) have published successful outcomes including wound closure using SPECIAL for palliative care patients. Controlling pain at the time of dressing change, as well as for fungating tumors, can be challenging. Alvarez et al., experts in palliative wound care, have reported good pain management by using a pharmacy-prepared topical formulation of 2.75% topical lidocaine in a cream vehicle containing zinc oxide. Topical metronidazole is helpful in controlling wound odor (Alvarez et al.; Finlay, Bowszyc, Ramlau, & Gwiezdzinski, 1996; McMullen, 1992). Dressings with carbon/charcoal layers or wound management systems also can be used to filter wound odors (Hess, 2000).

Debridement is an important part of treating wounds (Agency for Health Care Research and Quality, 1994; Wound, Ostomy and Continence Nurses Society, 2003). It is performed to remove necrotic tissue and other wound burdens, such as bacteria, from the wound bed. Even maintenance wounds may benefit from debridement. Wounds without adequate blood supply usually are not debrided. Although five methods of debridement exist, not all are used in patients with cancer. Surgical/sharp debridement is the most rapid way of removing nonviable tissue. Because it is painful, patients require either general anesthesia for large wounds or premedication when a scalpel is used to remove necrotic tissue from smaller wounds at the bedside.

Mechanical debridement uses force to rid the wound bed of the dead tissue. Traditionally, this was done by using wet-to-dry gauze dressings. The gauze was allowed to dry in the wound so that tissue would adhere to it, and then it was pulled out of the wound (Baranoski & Ayello, 2008). Not only was this very painful, but it also removed healthy tissue along with the necrotic tissue. Because of these disadvantages, its use is no longer recommended. *Hydrotherapy* (whirlpool) and *wound irrigation*, including using some of the newer equipment that delivers solutions under pressure, are also types of mechanical debridement.

Enzymatic or *chemical debridement* uses topical drugs (enzymes) to digest the necrotic tissue. Since a change in U.S. Food and Drug Administration ruling in September 2008, only one type of enzymatic debriding agent, collagenase, is available in the United States. The safety of using enzymes in cancerous wounds has not yet been clearly established (Ayello & Cuddigan, 2004).

Biological or *maggot debridement therapy* uses disinfected fly larvae (Sherman, 2002). In a study of 103 patients with pressure ulcers, 80% of maggot-treated wounds were completely debrided in five weeks compared to non-maggot-treated wounds (52%), which were not debrided (p = 0.021) (Sherman). Beginning evidence suggests that free-range technique may have better patient outcomes than contained maggots (Steenvoorde, Jacobi, & Oskam, 2005). Free-range maggots can move around in the wound because they are not contained (like loose tea), whereas contained maggots are not free to roam around in the wound (like tea in a tea bag).

Autolytic debridement is accomplished by using modern dressings to provide a moist environment that favors the body's own enzymes and white blood cells to remove the necrotic tissue (Ayello & Cuddigan, 2004). A discussion of different types of dressings follows.

Selected Wound Dressings

The following summary of wound dressings is not all-inclusive but represents the major products available for use in the palliative environment. The overall goal of palliative care should be to keep the patient comfortable and free from pain, manage infection, and protect the periwound area. The focus for these patients is not wound healing but rather optimizing their care.

Transparent Film Dressings

Transparent film dressings are thin polyurethane membranes. Transparent films adhere to the wound margins without sticking to the actual wound. Transparent films have no absorptive capacity but do transmit moisture vapor and are semipermeable. These dressings imitate the outer skin layer to provide a moist environment, similar to a blister. This covering allows epithelial cells to migrate over the surface of the wound (Baranoski & Ayello, 2008). Fluid may accumulate under these dressings; this is a normal occurrence. This fluid is sometimes mistaken for pus, a sign of infection. When excess fluid accumulates or leaks out from the sides of the dressing, the dressing needs to be changed. Maceration of periwound skin can occur if the transparent film dressing is not changed in a timely manner.

Transparent films can be used on a variety of wound types, such as stage I and II pressure ulcers, superficial wounds, minor burns, and lacerations, and over sutures, catheter sites, donor sites, and superficial dermal ulcers. Some of the newer transparent films on the market currently contain ionic silver. Ionic silver provides an antimicrobial effect to the film dressing. Transparent film dressings can be used on central lines, peripherally inserted central catheter lines, and infected wounds. These dressings may be useful in a palliative environment for skin tears and as protection against friction. They can stay on the wound for up to seven days, making them ideal for palliative care.

Hydrocolloid Dressings

Hydrocolloids are composed of opaque mixtures of adhesive, absorbent polymers, pectin gelling agents, and sodium carboxymethylcellulose. Hydrophilic particles within the dressing react with the wound fluid to wick fluid into the dressing, providing a soft gel over the wound bed (Baranoski & Ayello, 2008). Hydrocolloid dressings may have a noticeable odor during dressing changes. This is normal in the absence of clinical signs of infection. Some hydrocolloids also may leave residue in the wound bed. Always be sure to clean the wound before applying a new dressing. Hydrocolloid dressings are available in a variety of sizes, forms, and shapes to fit most wounds and locations. They are available in wafers, sheets, pastes, powders, and numerous sizes. Adhesive properties and ability to absorb exudate vary by product. Because some of these dressings are adhesive, care must be taken when using them on fragile skin. Some newer brands of hydrocolloid dressings do not strip the skin during removal and therefore are not as damaging to the skin. This is especially important for any patients who have completed radiation therapy, as their skin may be sensitive to adhesive products for several weeks after therapy is completed. Be sure to discuss dressing selection with the physician before using. For optimal dressing adherence, the dressing must extend at least 1 inch (2.5 cm) onto the healthy skin surrounding the wound. The dressing should be changed as recommended by the manufacturer. This could be from three to seven days and often depends on the amount of exudate.

Many of the newer hydrocolloids have other absorptive ingredients added, such as alginate, collagen, and sustained-released silver ions. Hydrocolloids are indicated for minimally to moderately exudating wounds, abrasions, skin tears, lacerations, pressure ulcers, dermal wounds, and granulating or necrotic wounds and for use under compression wraps. Some of the second-generation hydrocolloids are more absorptive and can be used in heavily exudating wounds. They also provide a moist environment conducive to autolytic debridement. Hydrocolloids often are used as a preventive dressing on high-risk areas (such as pressure points) and around surgical wounds to protect the skin from frequent tape removal.

Hydrogel Dressings

Hydrogel dressings have provided clinicians with a viable means to hydrate dry wound beds. *Amorphous hydrogel* dressings are water in a gel form or matrix. Their unique cross-linked polymer structure entraps water and reduces the temperature of the wound bed. The creation of a moist environment facilitates autolysis and removal of devitalized tissue (Baranoski & Ayello, 2008).

The main use for hydrogels is to hydrate dry wound beds and soften and loosen slough and necrotic wound debris. Hydrogels have a limited absorptive capacity because of their high water concentration. Some hydrogels have other ingredients, such as alginates, collagen, or starch, to enhance their absorptive capacity and will absorb low to moderate amounts of exudate. Absorptive capability varies by product and type of gel. They can be used for many types of wounds, including pressure ulcers, partial- and full-thickness wounds, and vascular ulcers. The sooth-ing and cooling properties make hydrogel dressings excellent choices for use in skin tears, dermabrasion, dermal wounds, donor sites, and radiation burns.

Maceration can be a concern for clinicians. Periwound skin areas need to be protected from excess hydration; thus, protective barriers often are rec-ommended. One of the benefits of a hydrogel is its ability to be used with top-ical medications or antibacterial agents. Hydrogels are packaged as sheets, tube gels, sprays, and impregnated gauze pads or strips for packing, tunnel-ing, and undermined areas within the wound bed. Some wounds require a secondary dressing to secure the hydrogel; new versions have adhesive bor-ders. Some newer versions also contain ionic silver.

Foam Dressings

Foam dressings are highly absorbent and usually are made from a polyure-thane base. Foam dressings are permeable to both gases and water vapor. The hydrophilic properties allow for absorption of exudate into the layers of the foam (Baranoski & Ayello, 2008).

Foam dressings are some of the most adaptable dressings for wound care. They are indicated for (Baranoski & Ayello, 2008)
• Wounds with moderate to heavy exudate
• Prophylactic protection over bony prominences or friction areas
• Partial- and full-thickness wounds
• Granular or necrotic wound beds
• Skin tears
• Donor sites
• Use under compression wraps
• Surgical or dermal wounds
• Use in combination with other primary dressings
• Wounds of any etiology.
Additionally, they can be used on infected wounds if changed daily. The sec-ond-generation foams also are available with ionic silver.

Foams should not be used on dry eschar wound beds. They could cause fur-ther desiccation of the wound site. Foams may be used in combination with topi-cal treatments and/or enzymatic debridement. Foams are available in many sizes and shapes and as cavity (pillow-type) dressings. Many types of foam do not have an adhesive border, so they will need to be secured with tape. This is an advantage for patients who have very fragile skin. New foam products have emerged that do have adhesive borders; be sure the patient's skin can handle an adhesive product.

Calcium Alginate Dressings

Calcium alginate dressings provide yet another choice for clinicians to use in managing highly exudative wounds. Alginate dressings are absorbent, nonad-herent, biodegradable, nonwoven fibers derived from brown seaweed. These specialized dressings are composed of calcium salts of alginic acid and man-nuronic and guluronic acids (Baranoski & Ayello, 2008).

When alginate dressings come in contact with sodium-rich solutions such as wound drainage, the calcium ions undergo an exchange for the sodium ions, forming a soluble sodium alginate gel. This gel maintains a moist wound bed that supports a therapeutic healing environment. Some alginates can absorb 20 times their weight; this may vary by particular product. They are extreme-ly beneficial in managing (Baranoski & Ayello, 2008)

- Large draining cavity wounds
- Pressure ulcers
- Vascular ulcers
- Surgical incisions
- Wound dehiscence
- Tunnels
- Sinus tracts
- Skin graft donor sites
- Exposed tendons
- Infected wounds.

Caregivers should be instructed that alginates have a distinctive odor that resembles seaweed so that they do not become alarmed during dressing chang-es. Alginates are contraindicated for dry wounds, eschar-covered wounds, sur-gical implantation, or third-degree burns. However, their hemostatic and ab-sorptive properties make them useful on minor bleeding wounds.

Alginates are available in sheet, pad, and rope formats, and in numerous siz-es. They are usually changed daily or as indicated by the amount of drainage. Early wound care interventions may warrant more frequent dressing chang-es because of a high volume of drainage. As fluid management is attained, the frequency of dressing changes can be decreased. Some newer versions of calcium alginate dressings also contain controlled-release ionic silver. Ionic silver dressings have antimicrobial properties, which can treat infection, are easy to remove, and can be changed less frequently.

Hydrofiber Dressings

A *hydrofiber* dressing is made from sodium carboxymethylcellulose, which interacts with wound fluid/exudate to form a gel (Baranoski & Ayello, 2008). It may also contain controlled-released ionic silver. These dressings are com-fortable, easy to remove, and very absorptive products.

Collagen Dressings

Collagen is a major protein of the body and is necessary for wound heal-ing and repair. Collagen dressings are derived from bovine hide (cowhide) (Baranoski & Ayello, 2008). Collagen dressings are either 100% collagen or may be combined with alginates or other products. They are highly absorptive hydrophilic moist wound dressings. Collagen powders, particles, and pads are useful in treating highly exudating wounds. If the wound has low to moderate exudate, use sheets. If the wound is dry, use gels. Collagen dressings can be used on granulating or necrotic wounds and partial- or full-thickness wounds.

A collagen dressing should be changed at a minimum of every seven days. If wound infection is present, then daily dressing change is recommended. Collagen dressings require a secondary dressing for securement.

Contact Layer Dressings

Contact layer dressings consist of a single layer of a woven net that acts as a low-adherence material when applied directly to a wound or wound bed. It acts as a protective interface between the wound and the secondary dressings. The main purpose of these dressings is to allow exudate to pass through the contact layer and into the secondary dressing (Baranoski & Ayello, 2008). Contact layer dressings often are used with ointments, creams, or other topical products such as growth factors or tissue-engineered skin substitutes. Contact layer dressings are not recommended for dry wounds or third-degree burns. The package inserts provide clarification as to which wounds the product can be used on. Various sizes and shapes are available. The frequency of dressing change depends on the etiology of the wound and the amount of exudate.

Gauze Dressings

Gauze dressings have been used in wound care for many years. They were once considered a standard of care (Baranoski & Ayello, 2008). Despite the pain and disruption of healthy tissue associated with using it as a primary dressing, gauze still remains one of the most widely used dressings. Numerous variations of woven and nonwoven gauze products are available. Many are used as packing agents, as primary and secondary dressings for infected wounds, or for mechanical debridement. Woven gauze may leave lint fibers in the wound bed contributing to inflammation and possible infection. Nonwoven gauze is absorbent and does not leave fibers in the wound. Dry gauze adhering to the wound bed can cause pain and discomfort during dressing changes.

Gauze is **not** considered to be a moist wound therapy intervention and is best used as a secondary dressing. Gauze does not create an optimal moist healing environment, even if moistened with saline. Gauze impedes healing, increases the risk of infection, and requires numerous dressing changes, and the Centers for Medicare and Medicaid Services (2004) considers it to have limited use in wound healing. The benefits of gauze dressings are overshadowed by the disadvantages. Roller and stretch gauze may be useful to secure other types of nonadhesive wound dressings.

Antimicrobial Dressings

Antimicrobial dressings have added a new dimension to the wound dressing arena. Clinicians now have several choices of dressings when dealing with wound infections. These new dressings are different than topical antibiotic therapy. They provide the combined benefit of an antimicrobial effect against bacteria with a moist environment for healing. The active ingredient may be silver ions, cadexomer iodine, or polyhexamethylene biguanide, to name a few. Silver dressings are recommended for moist wounds. The active ingredient (silver) needs to be moistened before it can be released into the wound bed. Antimicrobial dressings provide an adjunct in treating wound infections. They may not replace the need for systemic antibiotic therapy. As research continues and new products become available, this classification of wound dressing will expand. Antimicrobial dressings are available in a variety of forms, including transparent dressings, gauze, island dressings, foams, and absorptive fillers (Baranoski & Ayello, 2008). Some of these dressings can remain in place for seven days. Be sure the patient is not allergic or hypersensitive to silver or metallic products. When the wound is free from signs and symptoms of infection, these dressings should be discontinued. Additionally, silver dressings should be removed before performing magnetic resonance imaging procedures.

Negative Pressure Wound Therapy

Negative pressure wound therapy (NPWT) is the application of subatmospheric pressure to a wound using an electric pump to intermittently or continuously convey pressure through a connecting tube to a special wound dressing that is covered with a transparent film to create a sealed environment. Drainage is collected from the wound site into a canister. These dressings usually are changed three times a week. The number of types and products available to provide this valuable treatment have increased in the marketplace. It is very important to review the application techniques for these new NPWT products, as application varies greatly.

NPWT enhances granulation tissue formation, removes excess fluid from the wound bed, and aids in the contraction and maturation of the wound (Fife, 2004). NPWT has been used successfully on wounds that develop in patients with cancer, such as pressure ulcers and wound dehiscence. NPWT may be contraindicated in osteomyelitis, fistulas to organs or body cavities, placement directly over exposed veins or arteries, and malignancies.

Hyperbaric Oxygen Therapy

Hyperbaric oxygen therapy is a treatment in which a patient breathes in 100% oxygen while inside a chamber at atmospheric pressure higher than sea level. Chambers may be monoplace (for one person) or multiplace (two or more).

The chamber is pressurized with compressed air while the patient breathes in 100% oxygen via a mask, head hood, or endotracheal tube (Fife, 2004). Oxygen is a drug and has many known pharmacologic benefits. For oxygen to be delivered to hypoxic tissue, it must be administered systemically (i.e., it must be breathed) (Fife). There is no significant topical absorption of oxygen. Hyperbaric oxygen has been proved to be very effective as an adjunct therapy with wounds in heavily irradiated tissues (Fife).

Conclusion

Wound care is a critical component of oncology care. Successful management promotes both comfort as well as improved quality of life for patients and caregivers. Prevention of skin breakdown and infection are key to reducing the risk of a life-threatening complication. Unfortunately, not all wounds can be avoided or prevented, which results in a shift in paradigm to a focus on expediting the healing process without further damage or a focus on providing comfort when the probability of healing is unlikely (palliative care). Oncology nurses should be integrating the principles of wound care discussed in this chapter into their practice with each patient. Table 5-1 provides a review of the key components to effective wound care.

Table 5-1. Wound Care Knowledge at a Glance		
Wound Preparation	**Specific Procedures**	**Key Factors**
Methods of debridement	Surgical/sharp	• Rapid • Requires analgesia, as it is painful • Clinician licensure and skill vital
	Mechanical	• Can be very painful • Removes necrotic as well as healthy tissue • Wet-to-dry gauze dressings not recommended
	Biologic (maggots)	• Emotional acceptance varies by patient and clinician
	Enzymes	• Only collagenase is approved for Medicare part D • Enzymes not used in cancer wounds as research does not support use
	Autolytic	• Slower method • Uses modern dressings • Possibly painful dressing removal

(Continued on next page)

Table 5-1. Wound Care Knowledge at a Glance *(Continued)*		
Wound Preparation	**Specific Procedures**	**Key Factors**
Dressings	Transparent films	• Superficial wound • Little or no drainage • Softens dry eschar by moisture (autolysis)
	Foams	• Highly absorbent • Moderate to heavy drainage
	Hydrocolloids	• "Melt" or "swell" when exposed to moisture • Adhere to the surrounding skin, not the wound bed • Low to moderate drainage absorption • Available in many shapes and sizes • Can remain in place for several days; varies by specific brands
	Hydrogels	• Sheets or amorphous gel • Need a secondary dressing • Have cooling ability • Used with thermal or radiation burns or painful wounds • Add moisture to dry eschar or wound bed • Gels fill empty space in wound.
	Alginates	• Highly absorbent • "Seaweed" odor • Will desiccate nondraining wounds • Can be used to stop bleeding in wounds
	Antimicrobials	• Use with infected wounds—check if the patient is sensitive to silver or iodine. • Ionic silver needs moisture to work. It is not effective on a dry wound and requires a secondary dressing. • Magnetic resonance imaging is contraindicated when dressing is applied to wound.
	Gauze	• No longer considered for moist wound healing • Only used for mechanical debridement (wet to dry), not in clean granulating wounds • If used as packing, never use on the surface of wound; do not let it dry out.

References

Agency for Health Care Policy and Research. (1994). *Treatment of pressure ulcers* [Clinical Guideline Number No. 15, AHCPR Publication No. 95-0652]. Rockville, MD: Author.

Alvarez, O.M., Kalinski, C., Nusbaum, J., Hernandez, L., Pappous, E., Kyriannis, C., et al. (2007). Incorporating wound healing strategies to improve palliation (symptom management) in patients with chronic wounds. *Journal of Palliative Medicine, 10*(5), 1161–1189.

Ayello, E.A., & Cuddigan, J.E. (2004). Conquer chronic wounds with wound bed preparation. *Nurse Practitioner, 29*(3), 8–25.

Baranoski, S., & Ayello, E.A. (2008). *Wound care essentials: Practice principles* (2nd ed.). Philadelphia: Lippincott Williams & Wilkins.

Centers for Medicare and Medicaid Services. (2004). *CMS manual for guidance to surveyors for long term care facilities.* Retrieved February 10, 2009, from http://www.cms.hhs.Gov/transmittals/Downloads/R4SOM.pdf

Ferris, F.D., Khateib, A.A.A., Fromantin, I., Hoplamazian, L., Hurd, T., Krasner, D.L., et al. (2007). Palliative wound care: Managing chronic wounds across life's continuum. A consensus statement from the International Palliative Wound Care Initiative. *Journal of Palliative Medicine, 10*(1), 37–39.

Fife, C. (2004). Hyperbaric oxygen therapy applications in wound care. In P.J. Sheffield, A.P.S. Smith, & C.E. Fife (Eds.), *Wound care practice* (pp. 661–684). Flagstaff, AZ: Best Publishing.

Finlay, I.G., Bowszyc, J., Ramlau, C., & Gwiezdzinski, Z. (1996). The effect of topical 0.75% metronidazole gel on malodorous cutaneous ulcers. *Journal of Pain and Symptom Management, 11*(3), 158–162.

Hess, C.T. (Ed.). (2000). *Clinical guide: Wound care* (5th ed.). Philadelphia: Lippincott Williams & Wilkins.

Hughes, E., & Van Onselen, J. (Eds.). (2001). *Dermatology nursing: A practical guide.* New York: Churchill Livingstone.

Kirshen, C., Woo, K., Ayello, E.A., & Sibbald, R.G. (2006). Debridement: A vital component of wound bed preparation. *Advances in Skin and Wound Care, 19*(9), 506–517.

McMullen, D. (1992). Topical metronidazole. Part II. *Ostomy/Wound Management, 38*(3), 42–46, 48.

Schultz, G.S., Sibbald, R.G., Falanga, V., Ayello, E.A., Dowsett, C., Harding, K., et al. (2003). Wound bed preparation: A systematic approach to wound management. *Wound Repair and Regeneration, 11*(Suppl. 1), S1–S28.

Sherman, R.A. (2002). Maggot versus conservative debridement therapy for the treatment of pressure ulcers. *Wound Repair and Regeneration, 10*(4), 208–214.

Steenvoorde, P., Jacobi, C.E., & Oskam, J. (2005). Maggot debridement therapy: Free-range or contained? An in-vivo study. *Advances in Skin and Wound Care, 18*(8), 430–435.

Wound, Ostomy and Continence Nurses Society. (2003). *Guideline for prevention and management of pressure ulcers* [WOCN Clinical Practice Guideline No. 2]. Glenview, IL: Author.

CHAPTER 6

Radiation-Induced Skin Reactions

Maurene McQuestion, RN, BA, BScN, MSc, CON(C)

Introduction

Alterations in skin integrity resulting from radiation treatment can cause significant acute and long-term consequences for patients. Acute radiation skin reactions may be experienced by more than 90% of patients receiving treatment and contribute to physical discomfort and pain, itching, difficulty with movement of a limb or ambulation, sleep impairment, and difficulty with wearing clothing; impact activities of daily living; and have the potential to affect an individual's quality of life (McQuestion, 2006). Additionally, patients may suffer from changes in body image and the visible unpleasant reactions from others.

Hidden and often unrecoverable costs are incurred as a result of the need to alter care and purchase over-the-counter or prescription treatments and dressing supplies to manage the skin reactions. The symptoms and consequences from radiation skin reactions often are experienced along with clusters of other symptoms related to the cancer and treatment. Severe skin reactions may have a dose-limiting impact on treatment, or treatment breaks may be required. Late effects may occur months to years after treatment as a result of extracellular matrix (ECM) alterations and the deposition of collagen during the healing phases.

This chapter will address the pathophysiology of acute and late radiation skin reactions, factors affecting the degree of reaction, assessment of skin reactions including clinical tools that are available for documentation, and the evidence-based management of skin reactions. Special populations will be discussed in relation to phototherapy, total body irradiation, total skin irradiation, hyperthermia, and the treatment of patients with special conditions, such as scleroderma.

Physiology of Radiation-Induced Skin Reactions

Acute Skin Reactions

Skin changes can be experienced by more than 90% of patients receiving radiation therapy for cancer treatment (Ratliff, 1990). Reactions resulting directly from the radiation occur most frequently within the first four weeks of treatment, with epidermal regeneration, healing, and resolution occurring within three to five weeks following treatment. Complete healing can take up to three months (Hymes, Strom, & Fife, 2006). The epidermis is a relatively radiosensitive organ, and a fixed percentage of basal cells are destroyed following an initial dose of radiation. A disruption occurs in the balance between the rate of cell renewal and the destruction of cells at the skin surface. Cells become cornified and shed more quickly. Although noncycling basal cells are then stimulated into a cycling phase, the accelerated rate of destruction of basal cells occurs from ongoing radiation treatment. The end result is inflammation, epidermal cell apoptosis, and a reduction and alteration in normal epithelial stem cells, as well as a potential for permanently altered fibroblasts. Collagen that is formed is immature or insufficient to meet the demands of normal wound healing (Hymes et al.; Tibbs, 1997).

An inflammatory response with the secretion of histamine and serotonin occurs, as well as a vascular response with extracapillary cell injury and capillary dilation. Transient erythema localized to the treatment field may occur within hours of commencing treatment. It begins as a result of cytokine-mediated capillary dilation in the dermis accompanied by edema caused by increased vascularity and obstruction (Denham & Hauer-Jensen, 2002; Hymes et al., 2006). The skin appears red and warm and may have a rash-like appearance. Patients may describe their skin as feeling sensitive and tight. Other changes in the skin as a result of radiation include changes in pigmentation, interrupted hair growth, and changes to the sweat and sebaceous glands. As a result of the cellular destruction, melanin cells are able to migrate to more superficial layers of the epidermis, causing hyperpigmentation. It may appear as a moderate tan, occurring after two to four weeks of treatment (Denham & Hauer-Jensen; Ratliff, 1990). Normal skin tone usually returns within three months following the last radiation treatment. Hair may fall out as a result of the follicles shedding the hair and moving into a cell cycle resting phase, thereby causing an interruption in the production of new hair. Total hair loss within the radiation field can occur with doses higher than 55 gray (Gy) and may take two to three months to regrow following the radiation treatment. Sweat and sebaceous glands may be permanently destroyed after a cumulative dose 30 Gy, leading to a reduction in skin lubrication and an increase in dryness and pruritus (Ratliff).

As a result of the radiation entering and exiting through the skin from multiple angles within the treatment field, including a dose of radiation being deposited at the skin surface, some reactions will be expected. In other cases, the dose deposited in the skin and the resulting skin changes may have a dose-limiting impact for the patient. Normal tissue repair and re-epithelialization caused by the migration of epithelial cells from the basal membrane through homeostatic stimulation, proliferation, and cellular differentiation begins about 10–14 days following the completion of treatment (Mendelsohn, Divino, Reis, & Kerstein, 2002). The migration of these cells across the irradiated field is improved with a moist wound-healing environment, which has been shown to heal wounds 50% faster than a non-moist wound-healing environment (Hom, Adams, Koreis, & Maisel, 1999; Winter, 1962).

Types and Severity of Acute Skin Reactions

Radiation skin reactions generally are described and graded by severity using terms such as erythema, dry desquamation, and moist desquamation, and in more severe situations, ulceration. *Desquamation* refers to the sloughing of the epithelium with potential exposure of the dermal layer of the skin. Many patients do not experience any discomfort or noticeable changes within the first two weeks of treatment with a daily fraction of 1.8–2 Gy. When the cumulative dose reaches 20 Gy, the patient may experience dryness, pruritus, flaking of the skin, or dry desquamation (Korinko & Yurick, 1997; Maddocks-Jennings, Wilkinson, & Shillington, 2005). At doses exceeding 30 Gy, extracapillary cell damage may occur, resulting in increased capillary blood flow and edema. If severe, there is epilation leading to moist desquamation characterized by arterial thrombi, fibrinous exudate, edema, and considerable pain. This can occur at doses of 40–60 Gy. *Staphylococcus aureus* overgrowth can contribute to increased cytokine production, inflammation, and damage (Hill, Hanson, Bogle, & Duvic, 2004; Hymes et al., 2006). Other factors increasing the risk of moist desquamation include friction, skinfolds, the use of bolus material (i.e., a tissue-equivalent material used to alter where the dose is deposited, thereby increasing the skin dose), and the addition of chemotherapy to the treatment plan. The dermis is exposed with moist desquamation, and the treatment field is moist and tender with oozing and leaking of serous fluid. Light or heavy exudate and crusting also may be present (Ratliff, 1990; Sparks, 2007). Ulcer formation, hemorrhage, and necrosis are less common but represent more severe changes.

Risk Factors Related to Acute Skin Reactions

Patients may be at risk for increased skin reactions because of treatment-related factors and patient-related factors. Treatment-related risk factors include (Porock, 2002)
- The location of the treatment field (e.g., head and neck region, breast, axilla, perineum, areas of skinfolds)

- A larger volume of tissue being treated
- The total dose of radiation
- A large fraction size (greater than 2 Gy per fraction)
- Accelerated fractionation treatments
- A longer treatment duration
- The type of energy used resulting in a higher skin dose (e.g., lower-energy photons and electrons)
- The use of tangential fields
- The use of tissue equivalent or bolus material.

Linear accelerators, or megavoltage units with higher energies, are used most frequently today for the delivery of external beam radiation. The energy of the particular unit will determine the skin reaction. *Photons* range from 6–18 MV, with higher energies delivering the maximal dose of radiation to tissues 1.5–3 cm below the skin surface and therefore sparing some dose to the skin (Noble-Adams, 1999a; Porock, 2002; Sitton, 1992). *Electron beams*, having a shorter wavelength, often are used as a boost or way of enhancing the dose to tumors or lymph nodes closer to the skin surface, thereby causing a greater amount of radiation to be deposited in the skin. The lower-energy cobalt 60 unit, in comparison, will deposit the maximum delivery dose 0.5 cm below the skin surface, potentially increasing the skin reaction (Khan, 2003).

Patient-related factors that affect the risk of an increased skin reaction include
- Areas of thin or smooth epidermis
- Areas of skin-to-skin contact (e.g., axilla, face, perineum)
- Previous lymphocele aspiration
- Areas of compromised skin integrity within the treatment field (burns, lesions, existing surgical incisions or scars or planned postoperative radiation)
- The presence of comorbidities (e.g., diabetes, renal failure)
- Poor nutritional status
- Older age
- The inclusion of drug therapy to the treatment plan (concurrent chemotherapy, immunotherapy, or targeted therapies)
- The individual's race.

Additionally, the individual's usual skin routine, chronic sun exposure, smoking, and environmental conditions can influence the degree of radiation-related skin reactions (Ryan et al., 2007; Sparks, 2007).

Radiation Recall

Radiation recall dermatitis (RRD) is an acute inflammatory response in a previously irradiated treatment field following the administration of an inciting systemic drug. The drugs associated with causing radiation recall include chemotherapy agents such as anthracyclines, taxanes, alkylating agents, 5-fluorouracil, methotrexate, and gemcitabine, as well as hormonal

Table 6-1. Drugs Associated With Radiation Recall Reactions			
Drug Classification	Examples of Specific Drugs Causing Radiation Recall Reactions	Range of Time to Onset of Reaction	Time Interval Between Radiation and Drug Administration
Chemotherapy agents	Anthracyclines	2 days to 5 weeks	Days to weeks
	Taxanes	4–11 days	3 days to 6 weeks
	5-fluorouracil	2 weeks	7 weeks
	Methotrexate	24 hours to 1 month	5–7 days
	Gemcitabine	3 days to 6 weeks	2 weeks to 6 months
Hormonal drugs	Tamoxifen	5 days	2 years
Immunotherapy	Interferon	6 days	5 days
Antimicrobials	Tuberculosis treatment Cefazolin	48 hours	10 months

drugs, immunotherapy, and antimicrobials (Azria, Magne, & Abderrahim, 2005) (see Table 6-1). RRD mostly frequently is associated with megavoltage radiation, and although it most commonly is observed on the skin within the previously treated field, it also can occur in the oral mucosa, muscles, and organs. On the skin, the recall reaction appears as dermatitis and may range from a mild erythema or pruritic rash to a severe exfoliative dermatitis (Kodym et al., 2005; Sparks, 2007). There may be days to years between the occurrence of a radiation recall reaction and the completion of radiation therapy, but once a recall-triggering agent is given, the recall reaction generally appears within days to one or two months (Caloglu et al., 2007; Camidge & Price, 2001). Although the etiology of RRD is not completely understood, it has been suggested that the surviving cells within the irradiated field "remember" the reaction and are stimulated by an inciting agent (Azria et al.). Another hypothesis is that the surviving epithelial cells have been genetically mutated and are unable to tolerate the effect of the recall-triggering drug (Azria et al.). It also has been suggested that RRD results from epithelial cell sensitivity or a drug hypersensitivity reaction causing a nonimmune inflammatory reaction in a host with an already lowered inflammatory response threshold (Azria et al.; Thomas & Stea, 2002; Yeo & Johnson, 2000). Treatment includes topical, oral, or IV corticosteroids, nonsteroidal anti-inflammatory drugs, opioids as required, and discontinuation of the triggering agent.

Late Effects

Consequential late effects may be identified as persistent, nonhealing acute skin reactions, whereas true late radiation-induced changes may take months or years to develop, become progressive, and vary in severity. These late effects may appear as transient edematous changes, hyperpigmentation and hypopigmentation (dyspigmentation) resulting from the destruction of melanocytes, and telangiectasia. Telangiectasia appears as reddened spider-like veins close to the skin surface within the treatment field. They are caused by damage to and stretching of the small vessels, likely associated with moist desquamation and exposure to inflammatory, infectious, or mechanical irritants (O'Sullivan & Levin, 2003). The patient also may experience photosensitivity, xerosis (dry skin), atrophy, fibrosis, ulceration, and necrosis (Hymes et al., 2006). These changes are indicative of chronic and more severe cutaneous injury. The reactions may continue or slowly improve. Late effects or chronic radiation injury are considered to be complex wounds involving structural and functional changes. The late effects have been associated with

- Larger total treatment dose and volume of irradiated tissue
- A dose per fraction greater than 2 Gy and higher daily dose
- Other therapies including chemotherapy
- The patient's age and general medical condition
- Comorbidities (e.g., diabetes, collagen vascular disorders)
- Individual genetic factors such as gene mutations
- Radiation fibrosis
- Atrophy
- Vascular and neural changes
- Endocrine and growth-related effects.

Fibrosis can result in altered tissue flexibility, strictures, pain, neuropathies, restricted range of motion, lymphedema, and reduced tissue strength (Bentzen, 2006; Hymes et al., 2006).

Normal wound healing, as explained in Chapter 1, involves the inflammatory phase, proliferative phase, and tissue remodeling phase (see Figure 6-1, above the timeline). Radiation induces other series of changes (see Figure 6-1, below the timeline) resulting in an upregulation and perpetual cascade of proinflammatory cytokines (tumor necrosis factor-alpha, interleukins, and growth factors) and fibroblasts leading to the development of an excessive ECM and collagen (Bentzen, 2006).

The late effect of radiation fibrogenesis results from a combination of processes (see Figure 6-2) including (1) the direct activation of the transforming growth factor-beta (TGF-β) by the ionizing radiation through the dissociation of the latency-associated peptide, (2) endothelial cell damage resulting in the release of profibrotic cytokines, and (3) the interference with the homeostatic control of the reactive oxygen and reactive nitrogen species. These three processes result in the activation of the TGF-β pathway and interference with the signaling pathway, leading to increased ECM and collagen deposition, vascular

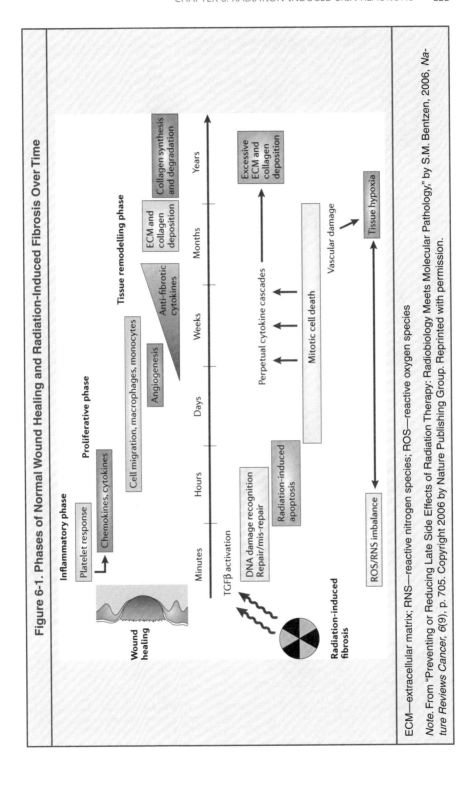

Figure 6-1. Phases of Normal Wound Healing and Radiation-Induced Fibrosis Over Time

ECM—extracellular matrix; RNS—reactive nitrogen species; ROS—reactive oxygen species

Note. From "Preventing or Reducing Late Side Effects of Radiation Therapy: Radiobiology Meets Molecular Pathology," by S.M. Bentzen, 2006, *Nature Reviews Cancer, 6*(9), p. 705. Copyright 2006 by Nature Publishing Group. Reprinted with permission.

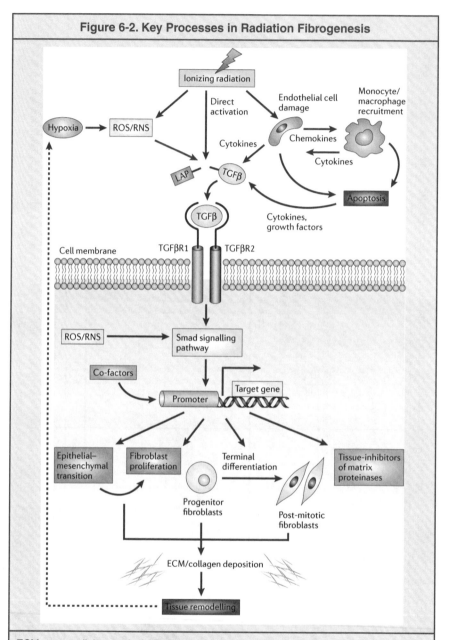

Figure 6-2. Key Processes in Radiation Fibrogenesis

ECM—extracellular matrix; LAP—latency-associated peptide; RNS—reactive nitrogen species; ROS—reactive oxygen species; TGFβ—transforming growth factor-beta; TGFβR—transforming growth factor-beta receptor

Note. From "Preventing or Reducing Late Side Effects of Radiation Therapy: Radiobiology Meets Molecular Pathology," by S.M. Bentzen, 2006, *Nature Reviews Cancer, 6*(9), p. 706. Copyright 2006 by Nature Publishing Group. Reprinted with permission.

damage, and uncontrolled tissue remodeling. This, in turn, leads to hypoxia, thereby creating a negative feedback cycle, which may further perpetuate the processes (Bentzen, 2006; O'Sullivan & Levin, 2003).

Surgical Complications Secondary to Radiation

Surgical complications following radiotherapy may occur as a result of a diminished blood supply in irradiated tissues, fibrosis and excessive collagen deposition, or the direct impact on the cellular reparative potential. Wound healing complications within irradiated tissues may include the following (Lin et al., 2005; Morgan, Randall, Suen, & Hanna, 2007):

- Delayed healing
- Dehiscence
- Abscesses
- Seromas
- Hematomas
- Fistulas
- Skin flap failures
- Anastomotic leaks.

Increased length of stays and need for transfusions also have been documented for patients undergoing surgical procedures following a course of radiation (O'Sullivan et al., 2002). Advantages of *preoperative* radiation include smaller treatment volumes and radiation fields, lower radiation doses (less tumor cell hypoxia), and surgery being performed on more normal blood vessels, resulting in fewer hypoxic and radioresistant cells. Disadvantages include increased wound complications and difficulties associated with interpreting postsurgical pathology specimens. Advantages of *postoperative* radiation include a lower risk of and fewer short-term wound complications and access to a full pathology report. Disadvantages include the need for a larger radiation treatment field and volume (the need to encompass the original tumor volume prior to surgery), concern that treatment may be compromised if there is a wide surgical disruption of tissues, the risk of enhanced late toxicity, and a higher risk of fractures (in patients with sarcoma) (O'Sullivan et al., 2002).

Preoperative radiotherapy has been shown to reduce the risk of recurrence in soft tissue sarcoma and improve survival rates in rectal cancer (Birgisson, Pahlman, Gunnarsson, Glimelius, & Swedish Rectal Cancer Trial Group, 2005; O'Sullivan et al., 2002). Although studies have supported the organ-sparing benefits of preoperative radiotherapy for patients with head and neck squamous cell carcinomas, there has been an increased need for regional myocutaneous flaps or free tissue transfers during the more extensive surgical procedures in situations of recurrence following primary radiation treatment (Lin et al., 2005; Morgan et al., 2007; Schwartz et al., 2004). Despite the concerns related to a 35% increase in wound complications (43% in the lower limb) for patients receiving preoperative radiation in the management of sarcoma and a 20% rate in patients with head and neck sarcomas, preoperative radiation has shown to reduce the rate of local recurrence (O'Sullivan et al., 2002, 2003). Other factors contributing to increased radiation skin doses include the thermoplastic material, polyurethane cradle foam, and the carbon fiber couch used for treatment immobilization because the materials may be within the radiation treatment field. These concerns have led to the development of innovative devices that provide immobilization outside the treatment fields, ensure a more stable and consistent treatment setup, and can be used for lengthy intensity modulated radiotherapy treatment with higher dose gradients created between critical and target tissues (Euler & Parent, 2007).

Assessment and Clinical Documentation Tools

A variety of grading or scoring tools are available to assess and document acute and late radiation skin reactions. Each incorporates the language used to identify skin reactions resulting from radiation treatment including erythema, dry desquamation, and moist desquamation. The following are the most commonly used assessment and grading tools.
- Radiation Therapy Oncology Group (RTOG) Acute Radiation Morbidity Scoring Criteria (Cox, Stetz, & Pajak, 1995)
- RTOG/ EORTC (European Organisation for Research and Treatment of Cancer) Late Radiation Morbidity Scoring Scheme (Cox et al., 1995)
- National Cancer Institute Cancer Therapy Evaluation Program (NCI CTEP) Common Terminology Criteria for Adverse Events (CTCAE) (NCI CTEP, 2009)
- Skin Toxicity Assessment Tool (STAT) (Berthelet et al., 2004)
- Oncology Nursing Society (ONS) Acute Skin Toxicity Scale utilizing NCI's Common Toxicity Criteria (Pollock, Catlin-Huth, & Haas, 2002)
- Radiation-Induced Skin Reaction Assessment Scale (RISRAS) (Noble-Adams, 1999a, 1999b)

Other methods less frequently used to assess radiation skin reactions include dielectric measurements using electromagnetic frequencies, ultrasound imaging, and reflectance spectrometry (Momm, Bartelt, Haigis, Grobe-Sender, & Witucki, 2005; Nuutinen et al., 1998; Warszawski, Rottinger, Vogel, & Warszawski, 1998; Wengstrom, Forsberg, Naslund, & Bergh, 2004).

Grading tools have consistently been used in the collection of data for clinical trials, but they can be used effectively in clinical practice to document the changes in individual patients and trends across patients with changing protocols and treatment modalities. The skin should be assessed at baseline and routinely at weekly review appointments. A thorough assessment should include an evaluation of changes in color, dryness, the presence of sloughing and patchy dry desquamation, open areas, patchy or confluent moist desquamation, and any drainage and odor. Although infection is not common, monitoring for the potential for infection is important. Patient-reported symptoms of pain and pruritus, as well as the impact of the skin reaction on daily living, quality of life, self-care ability, and costs incurred as a result of managing any skin reaction, should be assessed.

The RTOG Acute Radiation Morbidity Scoring Criteria, developed in 1985 (Cox et al., 1995), is a widely used and accepted grading tool utilized in clinical trials research and practice for the assessment of skin, other tissues, and organs. To date, reliability and validity testing has not been published. The RTOG scoring criteria for radiation skin reactions measures the intensity or severity of a reaction using an ordinal scale from 0 to 4, ranging from no change through degrees of skin desquamation to ulceration and necrosis. Major toxicities are graded as 3 or 4. Discrimination is made between signs resulting from treatment rather than disease. Although the RTOG scoring system captures a practitioner or observer physical assessment of the skin reaction, it does not address the patient perspective, including symptoms such as pain, distress, or the impact of the reaction upon the patient. Porock and Kristjanson (1999) modified the RTOG tool in their study of the evaluation of a method for predicting the severity of radiation skin reactions in women with breast cancer. The grade 2 category of skin reaction was subdivided into two categories based on results from an initial pilot study. Tender or bright erythema was scored as 2 and patchy moist desquamation as 2.5, providing more specificity to the tool by recognizing subjects reporting that any skin loss, regardless of being patchy rather than confluent, was worse than erythema.

The RTOG/EORTC grading tool (Cox et al., 1995) assesses the late complications of radiation treatment involving the skin and other tissues or organs. Reactions are identified as acute if they occur within 90 days of the first day of the radiation therapy and late if they occur after day 90 of treatment. The tool used to assess complications of radiation therapy affecting the *skin* utilizes an ordinal scale ranging from grade 1 to grade 4 including the criteria for late injury with ranges of atrophy, pigmentation changes, and hair loss. Additionally, the RTOG/EORTC tool identifies criteria for late subcutaneous tissue injury as including fibrosis and induration, loss, field contracture, and necrosis.

The NCI CTCAE (NCI CTEP, 2009), initially developed in 1990 and now in its fourth version, is a standard terminology used to report adverse events using a severity grading scale. The revised CTCAE documents grades of radiation dermatitis using an ordinal scale from 1 to 5, ranging from faint erythema or dry desquamation through higher degrees of erythema and desquamation to necrosis or ulceration and death. Similar to the RTOG grading tools, the descriptors reflect only an observer physical assessment. Version 2.0 has been incorporated into the ONS *Radiation Therapy Patient Care Record* for radiation dermatitis by the disease site (Pollock et al., 2002).

The STAT (Berthelet et al., 2004) was developed by a Canadian multidisciplinary team and includes three components of assessment. Included are patient and treatment characteristics potentially affecting the incidence and intensity of skin reactions (e.g., total dose and dose per fraction, treatment site, field size, boost, bolus, chemotherapy), an objective score ranging from erythema through grades of desquamation, and the identification of patient symptoms. In comparison to the RTOG, RTOG/EORTC, and CTCAE, the STAT includes the subjective symptoms experienced by patients in addition to the objective measurements by healthcare providers. The authors have reported preliminary reliability and validity results in a small pilot study (Berthelet et al.). Agreement ranged from 65%–97% on objective indicators and from 72%–92% on subjective indicators. The assessment tool is both easy to use in the clinical setting and quickly administered.

The RISRAS is a nursing assessment tool developed by a group of practitioners in New Zealand that incorporates the appearance of the skin as well as addressing the patient's perspective of the skin reaction (Noble-Adams, 1999a, 1999b). The tool was developed to provide a holistic assessment and measure subjective symptoms in addition to observable signs of a radiation skin reaction. Categories are weighted for scoring, and although there is an overall lower incidence of moist desquamation, it is recognized that the impact is greater on the patient; therefore, the category of moist desquamation was weighted higher than the categories of erythema or dry desquamation. Cumulative scores result from a combination of the patient symptom scale (tenderness, itch, burning, warmth, impact on activity) and the healthcare professional assessment (erythema, dry desquamation, moist desquamation, and necrosis). Face and content validity were reported. Photographs, rather than direct patient contact, were used to evaluate inter-rater reliability (coefficients ranged from 0.64–0.75) and intra-rater reliability involved a small group of nursing and physician experts (coefficients for nurses ranged from 0.75–0.94). Unfortunately, the scale has not been widely used in research or clinical practice but may have potential in the future.

Special Populations

Phototherapy/Photodynamic Therapy

Phototherapy or *photodynamic therapy* (PDT) has been used since the early 1900s. It is a treatment that involves the use of a cellular photosensitizing agent and artificial light to cause a cytotoxic reaction within cells. PDT has been used in the treatment of nonmelanoma skin cancers, lupus, and other dermatologic conditions, as well as in the management of refractory internal tumors and the palliative management of obstructive symptoms caused by esophageal and lung cancers (Bruner, Haas, & Gosselin-Acomb, 2005; Goodell, 2006). It involves a two-step process, including the administration of photosensitizing drug (e.g., porfimer sodium [Photofrin®, Axcan Pharma PDT Inc.]) with exposure to a nonthermal wavelength-specific laser light. Following administration, most of the drug is excreted in approximately 48 hours with the remaining drug retained within the malignant tumors, hence the requirement for the waiting period of 40–50 hours between the administration of the drug and the light activation. Debridement of the necrotic tumor may be required, followed by a second exposure of light and repeat debridement (Bruce, 2001; Bruner et al., 2005; Chen et al., 2002; Goodell). Cell death is caused by photooxidation, apoptosis, and tumor vascular thrombosis as a result of intracellular oxygen reactions caused by the interaction of the drug and the light (Webber, Herman, Kessel, & Fromm, 2000). Photosensitivity is the main side effect of PDT and can begin immediately after the drug is injected, ranging from mild erythema, swelling, and blistering to severe burn. It can continue for four to six weeks following the treatment. Patients must strictly adhere to instructions regarding the avoidance of light exposure and sun protection with the use of protective clothing, including long sleeves, full-length pants, gloves, hats, scarves, and sunglasses (Bruce). Sunscreen does not provide protection against photosensitivity related to PDT. Outdoor activities should be limited to after sunset. After one month, the patient can self-test to check for any photosensitivity reaction by placing his or her hand in a paper bag with a one-inch hole. If after 10 minutes of direct sunlight exposure no reaction occurs, the patient can gradually increase exposure to sunlight.

Total Body Irradiation

Total body irradiation (TBI) is used in conjunction with chemotherapy as a part of the conditioning protocol in preparation for bone marrow transplantation (BMT) in the treatment of leukemias, non-Hodgkin lymphoma, aplastic anemia, and other hematologic cancers. TBI delivers a uniform dose of radiation to the entire body, including the skin, underlying tissues, and organs, with the ability to shield or protect specific organs such as the lung, liver, kidneys, and eyes (Dunn & Lew, 2007). TBI may be delivered in either a single fraction of 8–10 Gy or as a fractionated treatment over three to six days. Skin reactions associated with TBI begin to appear within hours or days following the radiation and have a duration of 3–21 days. The skin reaction is typically generalized erythema, alopecia, and tanning or hyperpigmentation of the entire skin. Moist desquamation of the skin may occur after treatment. Patients also may experience chronic dry skin as a result of the radiation effects on sebaceous or sweat glands. Nails can become dystrophic. The hyperpigmentation usually fades within about a year of transplantation unless complicated by conditions such as graft-versus-host disease. Hair will regrow in about two to three months following TBI and BMT. Nail regrowth and replacement often takes up to a year (Bruner et al., 2005; McConn, 1987) (see Chapter 8 for more detailed information on BMT).

Total Skin Irradiation

Total skin irradiation (TSI), also referred to as *total skin electron beam therapy*, is used in the treatment of cutaneous T-cell lymphomas (CTCL), including mycosis fungoides and Sezary syndrome (immature T-lymphocytes invade the epidermis and dermis causing patchy plaques that can occur across large areas of the skin). TSI is administered to the entire skin surface using electrons and is the most effective treatment for CTCL. It also may be used as local treatment in unilateral or localized lymphomas or sarcomas and can be used alone or in combination with chemotherapy and biotherapy treatments (Maingon et al., 2002). Treatment is delivered using a lower-energy linear accelerator (e.g., 6 MeV) with a six-field technique (anterior, posterior, right and left anterior, and posterior oblique fields). The patient remains standing and is positioned for treatment to ensure homogeneity of the dose, with the distance between the patient and the source ranging from 3–8 meters. Typical doses for treatment of the skin are 30–60 Gy with 18–20 Gy for the hands and feet with treatment time ranging from 30–45 minutes per day (Gosselin-Acomb, 2007b). Shielding of the hands and feet and eye shields to protect the cornea and lens are used during the treatment. If required, the hands, feet, and scalp will be treated separately from the six-field treatment. Skin reactions may include erythema, pruritus, dry desquamation, and moist desquamation. Wrinkling of the skin, uneven pigmentation, alopecia, and hypohidrosis (abnormal decrease in sweating) can occur following treatment. Alopecia usually resolves in four to six months with hypohidrosis lasting 6–12 months (Kim & Hoppe, 1999; Maingon et al.). Late effects of TSI can include atrophy, fibrosis, telangiectasia, and permanent alopecia. Management of skin reactions follows the principles of general radiation skin reactions, but a special care bed may be required for patients with full body desquamation (Gosselin-Acomb, 2007b).

Hyperthermia

Hyperthermia, or the use of heat to destroy cells, has received intermittent attention since the 1970s. Although it has been used since the 1800s, it is still in the infancy stage of research and the evaluation of outcomes. Clinical trials employing hyperthermia treat several types of cancer, including breast, head and neck, rectal, and cervical cancers as well as brain tumors (glioblastoma multiforme), malignant melanomas, and sarcomas. Hyperthermia enhances the effects of radiation, especially when given prior to external beam radiation, and can be used with combination chemotherapy and radiation for tumor downstaging prior to surgery. It is effective on cells that have a low pH and with the hypoxic component of cells, with the radiation destroying the oxygen and nutrient-rich peripheral cells. Additionally, hyperthermia is associated with the inhibition of cellular repair caused by radiation damage (Gosselin-Acomb, 2007a). Treatment takes approximately 60–90 minutes, may be administered daily or once to twice a week, and often is planned according to the cycle of chemotherapy and radiation therapy for maximum cell kill. Hyperthermia can be given as local treatment (superficial tumors), as regional treatment (abdominal or pelvic tumors), or as whole-body hyperthermia, as well as being administered intraoperatively (Kouloulias et al., 2002). Nonionizing radiation using electromagnetic and ultrasound therapy is delivered to the tumor site and a margin of surrounding tissue or to the full body in situations of disseminated disease.

Contraindications to the use of hyperthermia include metallic foreign bodies such as prostheses, clips, and pacemakers, significant cardiac comorbidities, and pregnancy (Gosselin-Acomb, 2007a). Caution is required for patients with prior surgical procedures involving skin grafts or flaps and patients with peripheral neuropathies or altered sensory perceptions. Analgesics and anxiolytics need to be provided prior to the procedures, and deep sedation or general anesthetic is required for whole body hyperthermia. Side effects of the treatment may include pain, fatigue, risk of dehydration, skin reactions including first- or second-degree burns to the skin or subcutaneous tissue, peripheral neuropathy, and possible cardiac arrhythmias (Kouloulias et al., 2002).

The skin reactions may look similar to ionizing radiation skin reactions ranging from erythema to moist desquamation, with first- or second-degree burns occurring in about 5% of treatments (Bruner et al., 2005). Treatment of skin reactions is similar to that of irradiated skin reactions with similar goals of care to maintain skin integrity and cleanliness, maintain moisture, prevent infection, and promote comfort (Gosselin-Acomb, 2007a). Skin grafts may be required in the case of third-degree burns.

Patients With Scleroderma

Scleroderma, or *systemic sclerosis,* is a connective tissue disease that can affect the skin and internal organs. The diagnosis generally has been a contraindication to radiation therapy because of the perceived increased risks of acute and late effects. Concerns are related to the potential increased toxic effects in the tissues of the treatment field or the risk of progression of the scleroderma. Case reports from the early 1990s have documented fibrotic changes and edema in the skin and subcutaneous tissues, as well as fistulas in patients with scleroderma receiving radiation to the breast, pelvis, anal canal, and head and neck region (Abu-Shakra & Lee, 1993; Cooper & Denham, 1990; Robertson, Clarke & Prevzner, 1991; Varga, Haustein, Creech, Dwyer, & Jimenez, 1991). Results of a recent review also suggested that patients with collagen vascular disorders may be at a higher risk for late effects from radiation, although the authors did not report specifically on the risk associated with scleroderma (Holscher, Bentzen, & Baumann, 2006). Gold, Miller, Petersen, and Osborn (2007) conducted a retrospective study spanning a 23-year period involving 20 patients in one treatment center who were diagnosed with systemic scleroderma and received radiation treatment. Results showed that 75% of patients had acute effects, and 13 of the 20 (65%) patients had chronic toxic effects. In both groups, only three patients experienced grade 3 or higher acute or chronic toxicity. The retrospective design and small numbers in the study limit the conclusions that can be drawn, but this study may suggest that the prevalence of severe chronic toxicity (grade 3 or higher) may be less than anticipated for patients with scleroderma who received radiation therapy. Ongoing research is required to identify patients who will be at highest risk for fibrosis and chronic toxicity and whether some patients with scleroderma can, in the future, be safely treated with radiation.

Treatment of Skin Reactions: Evidence-Based Management

Few interventions used in clinical practice for the prevention or management of radiation skin reactions are supported by evidence. Significant differences in practice occur within interprofessional teams and across organizations as a result of historical practices and limited evidence to guide consistent practice (Bolderston, 2003). Several systematic reviews of the literature related to interventions to prevent or manage radiation skin reactions have been conducted in order to identify appropriate interventions for practice, to standardize the care of radiation skin reactions, and to establish consensus in the development of clinical practice guidelines (Bolderston et al., 2005, 2006; McQuestion, 2006; Naylor & Mallett, 2001; Nystedt et al., 2005; Wickline, 2004). Reviews conducted to date have identified several factors influencing the lack of evidence to guide practice, including the limited number of well-designed, sound, methodologic intervention studies. Problems identified with existing literature involve a focus on prevention versus management, small sample sizes or power calculations either not done or identified, a variety of measurement tools used across studies, and the range of outcomes measured (severity of skin reaction, time to erythema, mean and maximum erythema scores, mean severity scores, mean toxicity, time to dry desquamation, incidence and frequency of grades of skin reaction, pain, pruritus), all making comparison among studies difficult (Bolderston et al., 2006; McQuestion).

Despite the lack of evidence, clinicians recognize the need to intervene for purposes other than preventing or reducing the onset or duration of a skin reaction, including patient comfort and the reduction of pain, cleanliness, protection from trauma, and reducing the impact on self-image. Although some recommendations in practice are guided by evidence, others are guided by clinical experience, expert opinion and consensus, knowledge based on the principles of moist wound healing, and knowledge that a particular intervention will cause no harm. Figure 6-3 identifies unstudied or non-evidence-based clinical recommendations for patients who are receiving radiation treatment and expected to develop skin reactions.

Current interventions with supporting evidence include
- Washing with soap and water (Campbell & Illingworth, 1992; Roy, Fortin, & LaRochelle, 2001)
- Continued use of deodorant on intact skin

**Figure 6-3. Clinical Recommendations for General Skin Care
for Patients Receiving Radiation Therapy**

General Patient Instructions
- Wash skin using soap and lukewarm water in bath or shower.
- Use only a mild soap (e.g., Dove® [Unilever]) with thorough rinsing. Pat dry with a soft towel.
- Unscented, lanolin-free, hydrophilic (water-based) simple lubricant or moisturizing cream may be used on intact skin.
- Do not use cosmetic or perfumed products on irradiated skin.
- Use deodorant only on intact skin.
- Do not use cornstarch or baby power, especially in the area of skinfolds.
- Wear loose clothing made from cotton or a soft fabric.
- Protect the skin from the sun or cold wind; wear a hat or cover the area.
- Avoid the use of tapes, adhesives, or adhesive bandages within the treatment field to prevent mechanical injury.
- Do not use heating pads or ice packs on the area being treated.
- Use an electric razor if shaving is necessary.
- Avoid swimming in lakes and chlorinated pools or using hot tubs and saunas if dry desquamation is present.
- Use cool mist humidification only if required for other reasons.
- Avoid sun exposure and trauma following radiation treatment. Use sun protection, especially on irradiated areas. Use sunscreen with a sun protection factor of 30 or higher at all times.

Management of Moist Desquamation—Considerations for Nurses
- The use of specialized dressings for specific situations (e.g., moist desquamation, bleeding, exudates, drainage) should be considered.
- The choice of dressing should be based on principles of wound healing, patient assessment, patient comfort, need for and frequency of dressing changes, product evaluations, and cost.
- Available wound care products may include barriers, hydrogels, hydrocolloid dressings, film dressings, foam and absorbent dressings, calcium alginates, hypertonic dressings, silicone mesh dressings, and other specialty products.
- Topical or systemic antimicrobials should be considered in the presence of positive cultures and documented infection.

Note. Based on information from BC Cancer Agency, 2006; Bolderston et al., 2006; Mc-Question, 2006.

- Use of calendula cream in the prevention and/or reduction of grade 2 or higher dermatitis (supported by early evidence) (Pommier et al., 2004)
- Use of Cavilon™ No-Sting Barrier Film (3M) for prophylactic prevention of moist desquamation (Graham et al., 2004)
- Use of silver leaf nylon dressings for reduction in incidence of grade 3 and 4 reactions (Vuong et al., 2004).

Unfortunately, all other studies assessing lotions, creams, or emulsions (aloe vera, Biafine® [OrthoNeutrogena], hyaluronic acid cream, corticosteroids, sucralfate) either proved no benefit in preventing or managing radiation skin reactions or provided conflicting evidence (Bolderston et al., 2005; McQuestion, 2006; Wickline, 2004). See Chapter 5 for more detailed information on products.

Soap and Water

Current literature supports washing irradiated skin with lukewarm water and a mild soap. Campbell and Illingworth (1992) studied groups of women and compared no washing, washing with water alone, and washing with soap and water. Patients who washed with soap and water had a statistically significant reduction ($p < 0.05$) in itching, erythema, and desquamation scores. A study by Roy et al. (2001) found similar results with statistically significant increased incidence of moist desquamation in patients assigned to the no-washing arm of the study, as well as an insignificant greater incidence of pain, itching, and burning in the no-wash group. Although these studies have been conducted in groups of women with breast cancer, the recommendations regarding washing with soap and lukewarm water should be considered for all patients receiving treatment. It also is important to support patients to continue with normal and socially accepted hygiene practices during treatment to avoid adding unnecessary distress.

A variety of soaps often are recommended to patients with general guidance about avoiding irritating or highly aromatic products, but only one study has evaluated the irritant properties of a variety of soaps. A soap chamber method was used to assess the irritancy of 18 soaps, with Dove® (Unilever) being the only one identified as being mild (Frosch & Kligman, 1979).

Deodorant

The use of deodorant during treatment remains controversial because of different interpretations of the literature. Only one study is available that evaluated the potential bolus effects of deodorants (Burch, Parker, Vann, & Arazie, 1997). The authors used an ionizing chamber to compare and measure the surface dose of radiation following the application of 15 products including seven lotions, two powders, and six deodorants (roll-on, solid, spray); samples consisted of both metallic (magnesium, aluminum, zinc) and nonmetallic products. Normal application was compared to an application that was five times the thickness of a normal application. No increase in surface dose was reported for any product with the use of a normal thickness in application. Additionally, no difference was found between nonmetallic and metallic products. Any reactions to the products were determined to be caused by an irritating chemical ingredient rather than a bolus effect or increased surface dose.

Various agencies and authors have interpreted this data, resulting in continued variations in practice. Aistars (2006) identified the need for further research and evidence before changing the practice regarding advising patients to not use products, including deodorant, for four hours prior to the daily radiation treatment. Although the BC Cancer Agency (2006) did not address the use of deodorant in its online guideline and patient education booklet, other centers, including the Princess Margaret Hospital in Toronto, Canada (based on this author's clinical practice and institutional guidelines for radiation therapy skin reactions), have changed practice to support the application of deodorant on intact skin throughout treatment. No evidence exists to support or refute any practice recommendations related to restricting the time frame for the application of products prior to treatment.

Calendula Cream

Calendula officinalis is a medicinal herb with antimicrobial activity developed from the marigold plant. Only one study has been conducted, and it showed a statistically significant benefit in reducing grade 2 skin reactions (p < 0.001), pain reduction (p < 0.03), and reducing the number of treatment interruptions (Pommier et al., 2004). Adherence with use of the product was 84%, but one-third of the group of patients identified that product application was difficult because of the thickness of the cream. A new formulation with a petroleum jelly base has been developed and is under study, which may prove beneficial and therefore be more easily adopted into practice.

Occlusive Dressings

Occlusive dressings have been shown to reduce pain in skin reaction wounds, reduce the development of eschar, and improve epidermal regeneration and overall wound healing. Dressings with low water transmission rates retain moisture and support a moist wound-healing environment without increasing the incidence of infection (Alvarez, Mertz, & Eaglstein, 1983; Bolton, Monte, & Pirone, 2000; Brett, 2006; Hutchinson & McGuckin, 1990). Few intervention studies exist assessing the benefits of dressings such as hydrocolloids, semipermeable dressings, or moisture vapor permeable dressings, or they have not been conducted in the setting of radiation treatment. Dressings that have been evaluated during treatment, other than silver leaf dressings, have not shown statistical differences between various dressings for the outcomes measured (e.g., wound healing time) (Margolin et al., 1990; Shell, Stanutz, & Grimm, 1986). Evaluating dressing interventions during radiation treatment is problematic because the dressing may need to be removed daily to deliver the treatment and avoid any bolus effect, thereby hindering the potential benefit of the dressing designed to remain on for several days (Naylor & Mallett, 2001). Despite these challenges, occlusive dressings such as hydrocolloids may play a significant role in the management of radiation skin reactions because of the benefits they provide, including patient comfort and exudate and eschar management.

Cavilon No-Sting Barrier Film

Cavilon No-Sting Barrier Film has been shown to statistically reduce the frequency and duration of moist desquamation (p = 0.02) and pruritus (p = 0.011) with prophylactic use in women receiving radiation (50 Gy in 25 fractions) to the breast (Graham et al., 2004). The product is available in a cream or a saturated foam wipe and is easily applied to intact skin acting as a protective film or across a radiation skin reaction, providing both protection from further trauma and a moisture-retaining barrier, thereby creating a healing environment.

Silver Leaf Nylon Dressings

Slow-release silver leaf (silver hydrofiber) nonadherent rayon and polyester dressings have been used to manage a variety of acute and chronic wounds. The benefits of silver dressings include moisture retention, exudate management, improved comfort, and less disruption of the wound bed because of less frequent dressing changes. The antimicrobial effect from the silver ions in the dressing is a result of the cellular depletion of the electrolytes and fluids from microorganisms, causing DNA damage and cell death (Caruso et al., 2006). Although most studies have been conducted in vivo, in animal models, or found in the burn, venous ulcer, and chronic wound literature, one study has shown promising results in using silver dressings in the management of radiation skin reactions. Vuong et al. (2004) evaluated the use of silver dressings in 15 patients receiving radiation for gynecologic or anal canal cancers and found a statistically significant reduction (p < 0.0001) in the incidence of grades 3 and 4 moist desquamation (three grade-3 reactions versus 92 reactions in the control group).

Conclusion

Despite limited evidence to guide practice in the prevention and management of radiation skin reactions, the body of knowledge within the nursing, medical, and wound care literature is growing. Nurses must continue to address outcomes related to patient comfort, pain management, symptom relief, self-care, quality of life, and cost of interventions in order to support patients who will experience radiation skin reactions. Consistent documentation using both objective and subjective information will support patient care and communication between nurses and the interprofessional team. Future research will need to address improved treatment methods to reduce the incidence of reactions as well as the evaluation of products and dressings to manage the reactions.

References

Abu-Shakra, M., & Lee, P. (1993). Exaggerated fibrosis in patients with systemic sclerosis (scleroderma) following radiation therapy. *Journal of Rheumatology, 20*(9), 1601–1603.

Aistars, J. (2006). The validity of skin care protocols followed by women with breast cancer receiving external radiation. *Clinical Journal of Oncology Nursing, 10*(4), 487–492.

Alvarez, O.M., Mertz, P.M., & Eaglstein, W.H. (1983). The effect of occlusive dressings on collagen synthesis and reepithelialization in superficial wound. *Journal of Surgical Research, 35*(2), 142–148.

Azria, D., Magne, N., & Abderrahim, Z. (2005). Radiation recall: A well recognized but neglected phenomenon. *Cancer Treatment Reviews, 31*(7), 555–570.

BC Cancer Agency. (2006). *Care of radiation skin reactions* [Booklet]. Retrieved March 24, 2008, from http://www.bccancer.bc.ca/HPI/CancerManagementGuidelines/SupportiveCare/RadiationSkinReactions/default.htm

Bentzen, S.M. (2006). Preventing or reducing late side effects of radiation therapy: Radiobiology meets molecular pathology. *Nature Reviews Cancer, 6*(9), 702–713.

Berthelet, E., Truong, P.T., Musso, K., Grant, V., Kwan, W., Moravan, V., et al. (2004). Preliminary reliability and validity testing of a new skin toxicity assessment tool (STAT) in breast cancer patients undergoing radiotherapy. *American Journal of Clinical Oncology, 27*(6), 626–631.

Birgisson, H., Pahlman, L., Gunnarsson, U., Glimelius, B., & Swedish Rectal Cancer Trial Group. (2005). Adverse effects of preoperative radiation therapy for rectal cancer: Long-term follow-up of the Swedish Rectal Cancer Trial. *Journal of Clinical Oncology, 23*(34), 8697–8705.

Bolderston, A. (2003). Skin care recommendations during radiotherapy: A survey of Canadian practice. *Canadian Journal of Medical Radiation Therapy, 34*(1), 3–11.

Bolderston, A., Lloyd, N.S., Wong, R.K.S., Holden, L., Robb-Blenderman, L., & members of the Supportive Care Guidelines Group. (2005). *The prevention and management of acute skin reactions related to radiation therapy: A clinical practice guideline.* Retrieved March 24, 2008, from http://www.cancercare.on.ca/pdf/pebc13-7s.pdf

Bolderston, A., Lloyd, N.S., Wong, R.K.S., Holden, L., Robb-Blenderman, L., & Supportive Care Guidelines Group of Cancer Care Ontario Program in Evidence-Based Care. (2006). The prevention and management of acute skin reactions related to radiation therapy: A systematic review and practice guideline. *Supportive Care in Cancer, 14*(8), 802–817.

Bolton, L.L., Monte, K., & Pirone, L.A. (2000). Moisture and healing: Beyond the jargon. *Ostomy/Wound Management, 46*(Suppl. 1A), 51S–62S.

Brett, D.W. (2006). A review of moisture-control dressings in wound care. *Journal of Wound, Ostomy, and Continence Nursing, 33*(6), S3–S8.

Bruce, S. (2001). Photodynamic therapy: Another option in cancer treatment. *Clinical Journal of Oncology Nursing, 5*(3), 95–99, 108–109.

Bruner, D.W., Haas, M.L., & Gosselin-Acomb, T.K. (Eds.). (2005). *Manual for radiation oncology nursing practice and education* (3rd ed.). Pittsburgh, PA: Oncology Nursing Society.

Burch, S.E., Parker, S.A., Vann, A.M., & Arazie, J.C. (1997). Measurement of 6-MV X-ray surface dose when topical agents are applied prior to external beam irradiation. *International Journal of Radiation Oncology, Biology, Physics, 38*(2), 447–451.

Caloglu, M., Yurut-Caloglu, V., Cosar-Alas, R., Saynak, M., Karagol, H., & Uzal, C. (2007). An ambiguous phenomenon of radiation and drugs: Recall reactions. *Onkologie, 30*(4), 209–214.

Camidge, R., & Price, A. (2001). Characterizing the phenomenon of radiation recall dermatitis. *Radiotherapy and Oncology, 59*(3), 237–245.

Campbell, I.R., & Illingworth, M.H. (1992). Can patients wash during radiotherapy to the breast or chest wall? A randomized controlled trial. *Clinical Oncology, 4*(2), 78–82.

Caruso, D.M., Foster, K.N., Blome-Eberwein, S.A., Twomey, J.A., Herndon, D.N., Luterman, A., et al. (2006). Randomized clinical study of Hydrofiber dressing with silver or silver sulfadiazine in the management of partial-thickness burns. *Journal of Burn Care and Research, 27*(3), 298–309.

Chen, J., Keltner, L., Christophersen, J., Zheng, F., Krouse, M., Singhal, A., et al. (2002). New technology for deep light distribution in tissue or phototherapy. *Cancer Journal, 8*(2), 154–163.

Cooper, S.G., & Denham, J.W. (1990). Progressive systemic sclerosis (diffuse scleroderma) and radiotherapy. *British Journal of Radiology, 63*(754), 804–805.

Cox, J.D., Stetz, B.S., & Pajak, T.F. (1995). Toxicity criteria of the Radiation Therapy Oncology Group (RTOG) and the European Organization for Research and Treatment of Cancer (EORTC). *International Journal of Radiation Oncology, Biology, Physics, 31*(5), 1341–1346.

Denham, J.W., & Hauer-Jensen, M. (2002). The radiotherapeutic injury—A complex 'wound'. *Radiotherapy and Oncology, 63*(2), 129–145.

Dunn, J., & Lew, C.M.C. (2007). Total body irradiation and total lymphoid irradiation. In M.L. Haas, W.P. Hogle, G.J. Moore-Higgs, & T.K. Gosselin-Acomb (Eds.), *Radiation therapy: A guide to patient care* (pp. 444–487). St. Louis, MO: Elsevier Mosby.

Euler, C., & Parent, A. (2007). An innovative approach to immobilization for intensity modulated radiation therapy of extremity soft tissue sarcoma. *Canadian Journal of Radiation Medical Technology, 38*(2), 37–53.

Frosch, P.J., & Kligman, A.M. (1979). The soap chamber test: A new method for assessing the irritancy of soaps. *Journal of the American Academy of Dermatology, 1*(1), 35–41.

Gold, D.G., Miller, R.C., Petersen, I.A., & Osborn, T.G. (2007). Radiotherapy for malignancy in patients with scleroderma: The Mayo Clinic experience. *International Journal of Radiation Oncology, Biology, Physics, 67*(2), 559–567.

Goodell, T. (2006). Measuring subjective side effects and symptoms in palliative photodynamic therapy. *Oncology Nursing Forum, 33*(3), 647–650.

Gosselin-Acomb, T.K. (2007a). Hyperthermia. In M.L. Haas, W.P. Hogle, G.J. Moore-Higgs, & T.K. Gosselin-Acomb (Eds.), *Radiation therapy: A guide to patient care* (pp. 488–495). St. Louis, MO: Mosby Elsevier.

Gosselin-Acomb, T.K. (2007b). Total skin electron beam therapy. In M.L. Haas, W.P. Hogle, G.J. Moore-Higgs, & T.K. Gosselin-Acomb (Eds.), *Radiation therapy: A guide to patient care* (pp. 503–507). St. Louis, MO: Elsevier Mosby.

Graham, P., Browne, L., Capp, A., Fox, C., Graham, J., Hollis, J., et al. (2004). Randomized, paired comparison of No-Sting Barrier Film versus sorbolene cream (10% glycerine) skin care during postmastectomy irradiation. *International Journal of Radiation Oncology, Biology, Physics, 58*(1), 241–246.

Hill, A., Hanson, M., Bogle, M.A., & Duvic, M. (2004). Severe radiation dermatitis is related to Staphylococcus aureus. *American Journal of Clinical Oncology, 27*(4), 361–363.

Holscher, T., Bentzen, S.M., & Baumann, M. (2006). Influence of connective tissue diseases on the expression of radiation side effects: A systematic review. *Radiotherapy and Oncology, 78*(2), 123–130.

Hom, D., Adams, G., Koreis, M., & Maisel, R. (1999). Choosing the optimal wound dressing for irradiated soft tissue wounds. *Otolaryngology Head and Neck Surgery, 121*(5), 591–598.

Hutchinson, J.J., & McGuckin, M. (1990). Occlusive dressings: A microbiologic and clinical review. *American Journal of Infection Control, 18*(4), 257–268.

Hymes, S.R., Strom, E.A., & Fife, C. (2006). Radiation dermatitis: Clinical presentation, pathophysiology, and treatment 2006. *Journal of the American Academy of Dermatology, 54*(1), 28–46.

Khan, F.M. (2003). *The physics of radiation therapy* (3rd ed.). Philadelphia: Lippincott Williams & Wilkins.

Kim, Y.H., & Hoppe, R.T. (1999). Mycosis fungoides and the Sézary syndrome. *Seminars in Oncology, 26*(3), 276–289.

Kodym, E., Kalinska, R., Ehringfeld, C., Sterbik-Lamina, A., Kodym, R., & Hohenberg, G. (2005). Frequency of radiation recall dermatitis in adult cancer patients. *Onkologie, 28*(1), 18–21.

Korinko, A., & Yurick, A. (1997). Maintaining skin integrity during radiation therapy. *American Journal of Nursing, 97*(2), 40–44.

Kouloulias, V.E., Nikita, K.S., Kouvaris, J.R., Colematis, B.C., Uzunoglu, N.K., Mystakidou, K., et al. (2002). Intraoperative hyperthermia and chemoradiotherapy for inoperable pancreatic carcinoma. *European Journal of Cancer Care, 11*(2), 100–107.

Lin, S., Dutra, J., Keni, J., Dumanian, G.A., Fine, N., & Pelzer, H. (2005). Preoperative radiation therapy and its effects on outcomes in microsurgical head and neck reconstruction. *Otolaryngology—Head and Neck Surgery, 132*(6), 845–848.

Maddocks-Jennings, W., Wilkinson, J.M., & Shillington, D. (2005). Novel approaches to radiotherapy-induced skin reactions: A literature review. *Complementary Therapy in Clinical Practice, 11*(4), 224–231.

Maingon, P., Truc, G., Dalac, S., Barillot, I., Lambert, D., Petrella, T., et al. (2002). Radiotherapy of advanced mycosis fungoides: Indications and results of total skin electron beam and photon beam irradiation. *Radiotherapy and Oncology, 54*(1), 73–78.

Margolin, S.G., Breneman, J.C., Denman, D.L., LaChapelle, P., Weckbach, L., & Aron, B.S. (1990). Management of radiation-induced moist skin desquamation using hydrocolloid dressing. *Cancer Nursing, 13*(2), 71–80.

McConn, R. (1987). Skin changes following bone marrow transplantation. *Cancer Nursing, 10*(2), 82–84.

McQuestion, M. (2006). Evidence-based skin care management in radiation therapy. *Seminars in Oncology Nursing, 22*(3), 163–173.

Mendelsohn, F.A., Divino, C.M., Reis, E.D., & Kerstein, M.D. (2002). Wound care after radiation therapy. *Advances in Skin and Wound Care, 15*(5), 216–224.

Momm, F., Bartelt, S., Haigis, K., Grobe-Sender, A., & Witucki, G. (2005). Spectrophotometric skin measurements correlate with EORTC/RTOG-common toxicity criteria. *Strahlentherapie und Onkologie, 181*(6), 392–395.

Morgan, J.E., Randall, L.B., Suen, J.Y., & Hanna, E.Y. (2007). Surgical wound complications after intensive chemoradiotherapy for advanced squamous cell carcinoma of the head and neck. *Archives of Otolaryngology—Head and Neck Surgery, 133*(1), 10–14.

National Cancer Institute Cancer Therapy Evaluation Program. (2009). *Common terminology criteria for adverse events* (version 4.0). Bethesda, MD: National Cancer Institute. Retrieved July 23, 2009, from http://ctep.cancer.gov/protocolDevelopment/electronic_applications/docs/ctcaev4.pdf

Naylor, W., & Mallett, J. (2001). Management of acute radiotherapy induced skin reactions: A literature review. *European Journal of Oncology Nursing, 5*(4), 221–233.

Noble-Adams, R. (1999a). Radiation-induced skin reactions 2: Development of a measurement tool. *British Journal of Nursing, 8*(18), 1208–1211.

Noble-Adams, R. (1999b). Radiation-induced skin reactions 3: Evaluating the RISRAS. *British Journal of Nursing, 8*(19), 1305–1312.

Nuutinen, J., Lahtinen, T., Turunen, M., Alanen, E., Tenhunen, M., Usenius, T., et al. (1998). A dielectric method for measuring early and late reactions in irradiated human skin. *Radiotherapy and Oncology, 47*(3), 249–254.

Nystedt, K.E., Hill, J.E., Mitchell, A.M., Goodwin, F., Rowe, L.A., Wong, F.L., et al. (2005). The standardization of radiation skin care in British Columbia: A collaborative approach. *Oncology Nursing Forum, 32*(6), 1199–1205.

O'Sullivan, B., Davis, A.M., Turcotte, R., Bell, R., Catton, C., Chabot, P., et al. (2002). Preoperative versus postoperative radiotherapy in soft-tissue sarcoma of the limbs: A randomised trial. *Lancet, 359*(9325), 2235–2241.

O'Sullivan, B., Gullane, P., Irish, J., Nelligan, P., Gentili, F., Mahoney, J., et al. (2003). Preoperative radiotherapy for adult head and neck soft tissue sarcoma: Assessment of wound complication rates and cancer outcome in a prospective series. *World Journal of Surgery, 27*(7), 875–883.

O'Sullivan, B., & Levin, W. (2003). Late radiation-related fibrosis: Pathogenesis, manifestations, and current management. *Seminars in Radiation Oncology, 13*(3), 274–289.

Pollock, V., Catlin-Huth, C., & Haas, M.L. (Eds.). (2002). *Radiation therapy patient care record: A tool for documenting nursing care.* Pittsburgh, PA: Oncology Nursing Society.

Pommier, P., Gomez, F., Sunyach, M.P., D'Hombres, A., Carrie, C., & Montbarbon, X. (2004). Phase III randomized trial of *Calendula officinalis* compared with trolamine for the prevention of acute dermatitis during irradiation for breast cancer. *Journal of Clinical Oncology, 22*(8), 1447–1453.

Porock, D. (2002). Factors influencing the severity of radiation skin and oral mucosal reactions: Development of a conceptual framework. *European Journal of Cancer Care, 11*(1), 33–43.

Porock, D., & Kristjanson, L. (1999). Skin reactions during radiotherapy for breast cancer: The use and impact of topical agents and dressings. *European Journal of Cancer Care, 8*(3), 143–153.

Ratliff, C. (1990). Impaired skin integrity related to radiation therapy. *Journal of Enterostomal Therapy, 17*(5), 193–198.

Robertson, J.M., Clarke, D.H., & Prevzner, M.M. (1991). Breast conservation therapy: Severe breast fibrosis after radiation therapy in patients with collagen vascular diseases. *Cancer, 68*(3), 502–508.

Roy, I., Fortin A., & LaRochelle, M. (2001). The impact of skin washing with water and soap during breast irradiation: A randomized study. *Radiotherapy and Oncology, 58*(3), 333–339.

Ryan, J.L., Bole, C., Hickok, J.T., Figueroa-Moseley, C., Colman, L., Khanna, R.C., et al. (2007). Post-treatment skin reactions reported by cancer patients differ by race, not by treatment or expectations. *British Journal of Cancer, 97*(1), 14–21.

Schwartz, S.R., Yueh, B., Maynard, C., Daley, J., Henderson, W., & Khuri, S.F. (2004). Predictors of wound complications after laryngectomy: A study of over 2000 patients. *Otolaryngology—Head and Neck Surgery, 131*(1), 61–68.

Shell, J.A., Stanutz, F., & Grimm, J. (1986). Comparison of moisture vapor permeable (MVP) dressings to conventional dressings for management of radiation skin reactions. *Oncology Nursing Forum, 13*(1), 11–16.

Sitton, E. (1992). Early and late radiation-induced skin alterations. Part II. Nursing care of irradiated skin. *Oncology Nursing Forum, 19*(6), 907–912.

Sparks, S.G. (2007). Radiodermatitis. In M.L. Haas, W.P. Hogle, G.J. Moore-Higgs, & T.K. Gosselin-Acomb (Eds.), *Radiation therapy: A guide to patient care* (pp. 511–522). St. Louis, MO: Elsevier Mosby.

Thomas, R., & Stea, B. (2002). Radiation recall dermatitis from high-dose interferon alfa-2b. *Journal of Clinical Oncology, 20*(1), 353–357.

Tibbs, M.K. (1997). Wound healing following radiation therapy: A review. *Radiotherapy and Oncology, 42*(2), 99–106.

Varga, J., Haustein, U.F., Creech, R.H., Dwyer, J.P., & Jimenez, S.A. (1991). Exaggerated radiation-induced fibrosis in patients with systemic sclerosis. *JAMA, 265*(24), 3292–3295.

Vuong, T., Franco, E., Lehnert, S., Lambert, C., Portelance, L., Nasr, E., et al. (2004). Silver leaf nylon dressing to prevent radiation dermatitis in patients undergoing chemotherapy and external beam radiotherapy to the perineum. *International Journal of Radiation Oncology, Biology, Physics, 59*(3), 809–814.

Warszawski, A., Rottinger, E.M., Vogel, R., & Warszawski, N. (1998). 20 MHz ultrasonic imaging for quantitative assessment and documentation of early and late postradiation skin reactions in breast cancer patients. *Radiotherapy and Oncology, 47*(3), 241–247.

Webber, J., Herman, M., Kessel, D., & Fromm, D. (2000). Photodynamic treatment of neoplastic lesions of the gastrointestinal tract. Recent advances in techniques and results. *Langenbeck's Archives of Surgery, 385*(4), 299–304.

Wengstrom, Y., Forsberg, C., Naslund, I., & Bergh, J. (2004). Quantitative assessment of skin erythema due to radiotherapy—Evaluation of different measurements. *Radiotherapy and Oncology, 72*(2), 191–197.

Wickline, M.M. (2004). Prevention and treatment of acute radiation dermatitis: A literature review. *Oncology Nursing Forum, 31*(2), 237–244.

Winter, G. (1962). Formation of the scab and the rate of epithelialization of superficial wounds in the skin of the young domestic pig. *Nature, 193,* 293–294.

Yeo, W., & Johnson, P.J. (2000). Radiation-recall skin disorders associated with the use of antineoplastic drugs. Pathogenesis, prevalence, and management. *American Journal of Clinical Dermatology, 1*(2), 113–116.

CHAPTER 7

Systemic Therapy– Induced Skin Reactions

Vanna M. Dest, MSN, APRN-BC, AOCN®

Introduction

Skin-related toxicities are common in the oncology population and usually are related to systemic therapy, either treatment or supportive therapies. Most systemic therapies can cause a wide array of side effects, including cutaneous skin reactions. The skin and its constituents are rapidly dividing cells with epithelial, connective tissue, vascular, and neural components, which in turn can lead to skin manifestations present at diagnosis, during treatment, or as chronic effects of cancer and its treatment (Agha, Kinahan, Bennett, & Lacouture, 2007). Oncology nurses face the challenge of accurate assessment and differentiation of the etiology because of combined modality and multidrug approaches. Management strategies of skin-related toxicities vary and are dependent upon the causative agent. Early detection and treatment of these symptoms will assist with control, decrease morbidity, and permit continuation of therapy (Wyatt, Leonard, & Sachs, 2006). This chapter will review the potential skin toxicities seen in patients receiving chemotherapy/hormonal agents, targeted therapies, and supportive therapies. Patient assessment and management interventions for skin-related toxicities also will be reviewed.

Skin Assessment in the Oncology Patient

A thorough history is imperative, as well as assessment of skin problems, and should include exposure to infections, history of cancer treatments, current drug/medication profile, history of past skin disorders, and presence of current skin disorders or symptoms. Skin assessment should include the general characteristics of the skin, including the color, integrity, temperature, texture, and turgor. Assessment is not complete without documentation of the following:
- Presence of erythema

- Presence of purpura
- Presence of ecchymosis
- Presence of jaundice
- Presence of lesions (macular, papular, or vesicular)
- Presence of dry or moist desquamation
- Local erythema or inflammation at injection sites
- Pruritus
- Pain
- Alopecia.

Various skin assessment tools are available to distinguish skin disorders within the cancer population. These will be addressed in the corresponding sections.

Chemotherapy-Induced Skin Manifestations

Skin-related side effects are common in patients with cancer who are receiving antineoplastic therapy. The most rapidly dividing cells are most affected by the administration of chemotherapy. Examples of rapidly dividing cells include the cells of the gastrointestinal tract, bone marrow, gonadal, and, in particular, dermatologic cells, including the skin, hair follicles, and nail matrix. Chemotherapy targets the tissues with rapid proliferation and division leading to toxicities. The most common dermatologic side effects include the following (Alley, Green, & Schuchter, 2002; Wyatt et al., 2006):

- Alopecia
- Hyperpigmentation
- Hand-foot syndrome
- Maculopapular/morbilliform reaction
- Radiation recall
- Nail dystrophies
- Hypersensitivity
- Chemotherapy extravasation.

Each of these side effects will be discussed with focus on causative agents, incidence, pathophysiology, presentation, specific assessment, and management strategies.

Alopecia

Alopecia, or hair loss, is the most common skin manifestation of systemic chemotherapy (Fischer, Knobf, Durivage, & Beaulieu, 2003). It can be very distressing for both men and women, causing social and psychological ramifications and altered body image. Antineoplastic agents affect rapidly growing hair cells, also referred to as cells in the anagen phase. The degree of hair loss varies from thinning to total hair loss. About 85% of scalp hair follicles are in the anagen phase, and the most common area for hair loss is the scalp. Other hair follicles usually are less active and not as readily affected, such as the eyebrows, axilla, and pubic region (Camp-Sorrell, 2005; Wyatt et al., 2006).

Chemotherapy causes the hair shaft to become more fragile, resulting in breakage. Some chemotherapeutic agents or higher doses of chemotherapy can cause complete mitotic arrest, which results in atrophy of the hair root and loss of hair root bulb. Other drugs cause bulb deformity and narrowing of the hair shaft. Alopecia usually begins within two to three weeks of chemotherapy initiation, and hair loss is temporary and reversible. The mechanism of hair loss is spontaneous, or hair is lost with combing or shampooing. Hair loss may be asymptomatic with the exception of the psychological pain associated with alopecia. However, some patients may experience scalp itching and discomfort within one to two days prior to alopecia and during periods of hair loss. After completion or discontinuation of chemotherapy, regrowth of hair generally takes three to five months, but complete hair regrowth may take up to one to two years (Camp-Sorrell, 2005; Wyatt et al., 2006). As hair grows back, changes in hair color (lighter/darker), texture (thinner/coarser), and type (curly/straight) may be apparent. Alopecia depends on the type of chemotherapy given, combination of drugs, dosage, frequency of administration, route of administration, and pharmacokinetics. Alopecia has varying degrees described as minimal, moderate, or severe. Figure 7-1 lists agents that cause varying degrees of alopecia. Grading of alopecia is illustrated in Table 7-1. Route of administration is another predictor of degree of hair loss. The use of bolus IV chemotherapy agents produces immediate peak serum levels, which results in hair loss. IV infusions over several hours to days are associated with greater risk for alopecia. Low-dose IV infusions have a lesser risk for alopecia (Camp-Sorrell; Wyatt et al.).

Patient and family education about alopecia is essential and should be tailored to the patient's chemotherapy regimen and degree of alopecia expected. No preventive measures exist for alopecia, but many management strategies can ensure safety. Patients should not use dryers, straightening irons, hot rollers, or curling irons, as they may facilitate alopecia. The scalp needs to be protected from the sun by wearing sunscreen with or without protective covering. With total alopecia, the scalp must be cleaned and conditioned regularly. Because of associated body image changes, patients should be encouraged to use wigs, scarves, and hats. Some insurance companies will reimburse for wigs, also known as cranial prostheses. In addition, patients should be encouraged to call and attend the *Look*

Figure 7-1. Chemotherapy Agents Causing Alopecia

- Bleomycin
- Cyclophosphamide
- Cytarabine
- Dactinomycin
- Daunorubicin
- Docetaxel
- Doxorubicin
- Etoposide
- Fluorouracil
- Idarubicin
- Ifosfamide
- Irinotecan
- Mechlorethamine
- Methotrexate
- Mitoxantrone
- Paclitaxel
- Vincristine

Note. Based on information from Alley et al., 2003; Fischer et al., 2003.

Table 7-1. Grading of Alopecia (Scalp/Body)					
Adverse Event	**Grade**				
	1	**2**	**3**	**4**	**5**
Alopecia	Hair loss of up to 50% of normal for that individual that is not obvious from a distance but only on close inspection; a different hair style may be required to cover the hair loss but it does not require a wig or hair piece to camouflage	Hair loss of > 50% normal for that individual that is readily apparent to others; a wig or hair piece is necessary if the patient desires to completely camouflage the hair loss; associated with psychosocial impact	–	–	–

Definition: A disorder characterized by a decrease in density of hair compared to normal for a given individual at a given age and body location.

Note. From *Common Terminology Criteria for Adverse Events* (Version 4.0), by National Cancer Institute Cancer Therapy Evaluation Program, 2009. Retrieved July 23, 2009, from http://ctep.cancer.gov/protocolDevelopment/electronic_applications/docs/ctcaev4.pdf

Good . . . Feel Better® program (see www.lookgoodfeelbetter.org). This program is designed to provide patients with support and education for body image changes including alopecia (Camp-Sorrell, 2005; Fischer et al., 2003).

Hyperpigmentation

Hyperpigmentation or discoloration of the skin, nails, and mucous membranes is another common skin manifestation seen with the use of some chemotherapy agents. The mechanism for hyperpigmentation is thought to be related to the toxic effects of chemotherapy on melanocytes. The degree of hyperpigmentation can be classified as local or generalized. Local hyperpigmentation occurs at the site of administration. Hyperpigmentation is common in dark-skinned individuals. The antimetabolites, especially fluorouracil, commonly cause hyperpigmentation. Approximately 24% of patients treated with fluorouracil will develop hyperpigmentation (Agha et al., 2007). See Figure 7-2 for an example of hyperpigmented skin. A common site of hyperpigmentation is the nail surface, either transversely or longitudinally. Discoloration of the teeth can also be seen. Fluorouracil commonly causes hyperpigmented streaking of veins used for infusion without evidence of extravasation or chemical phlebitis. This generally occurs in 2%–5% of patients (Agha et al.). Busulfan commonly causes a generalized hyperpigmentation often referred to as the "busulfan tan" (Alley et al., 2002). The hyperpigmentation may persist after discontinuation of the drug and may exacerbate with sun exposure. Bleomycin has been found to cause hyperpigmentation that manifests itself in linear streaks. This occurs in 8%–38% of patients and reverses itself after the drug is discontinued (Wyatt et al., 2006). Table 7-2 lists the common chemotherapeutic drugs that

Figure 7-2. Hyperpigmentation

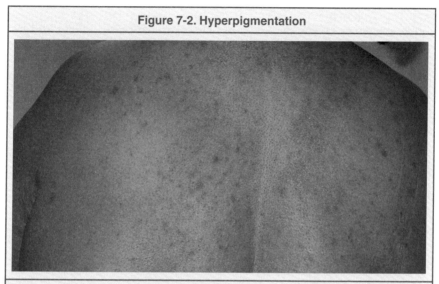

Note. From "Clinical Presentation and Pathophysiology of EGFR1 Dermatologic Toxicities," by E.P. Mitchell, R. Perez-Soler, E. Van Cutsem, and M.E. Lacouture, 2007, *Oncology, 21*(11, Suppl. 5), p. 8. Copyright 2007 by CMPMedica. Reprinted with permission.

Table 7-2. Chemotherapy Agents Causing Hyperpigmentation

Drug	Skin Pigmentation Manifestation
Bleomycin	Linear hyperpigmentation
Busulfan	Generalized
Carmustine	Localized
Cyclophosphamide	Generalized
Dactinomycin	Generalized
Daunorubicin	Generalized
Doxorubicin	Generalized
Fluorouracil	Localized; vein hyperpigmentation
Hydroxyurea	Generalized
Methotrexate	Generalized
Thiotepa	Localized

Note. Based on information from Agha et al., 2007; Alley et al., 2003.

cause hyperpigmentation. Table 7-3 addresses the grading of hyperpigmentation. Management recommendations include avoidance of sunlight and use of sunscreen. Other interventions may include the application of topical retinoids, topical hydroquinone, and corticosteroids. If no treatment is utilized, hyperpigmentation will resolve over time once the drug is discontinued (Agha et al.; Alley et al.; Camp-Sorrell, 2005; Fischer et al., 2003; Wyatt et al., 2006).

		Grade			
Adverse Event	**1**	**2**	**3**	**4**	**5**
Skin hyperpigmentation	Hyperpigmentation covering < 10% BSA; no psychosocial impact	Hyperpigmentation covering > 10% BSA; associated psychosocial impact	–	–	–

Table 7-3. Grading System for Hyperpigmentation

Definition: A disorder characterized by darkening of the skin due to excessive melanin deposition.

Note. From *Common Terminology Criteria for Adverse Events* (Version 4.0), by National Cancer Institute Cancer Therapy Evaluation Program, 2009. Retrieved July 23, 2009, from http://ctep.cancer.gov/protocolDevelopment/electronic_applications/docs/ctcaev4.pdf

Hand-Foot Syndrome

Hand-foot syndrome is commonly referred to as palmar-plantar erythrodysesthesia or acral erythema. The pathophysiology is not completely understood, but it is thought to be caused by a direct toxic effect on the vasculature of the epidermis and dermis or by the accumulation of the chemotherapeutic agent in eccrine structures leading to erythema of the palms and soles (Wilkes & Doyle, 2005). Chemotherapeutic agents with sustained serum levels are most likely to cause this syndrome. They include liposomal doxorubicin and capecitabine and occur in up to 48% of patients (Wilkes & Doyle). It is estimated that more than 40% of patients receiving fluorouracil infusion develop this syndrome (Lokich, 2007). This syndrome is not just dose-related but is related to duration of exposure. It is rare to see this manifestation if the patient is receiving fluorouracil boluses. The syndrome is characterized by demarcated, tender erythematous plaques on the palms of the hands and/ or soles of the feet. It generally begins with pain and tingling of the hands and feet and then progresses to edema, erythema, tenderness to touch, and desquamation. The pain can range from mild to moderate. See Figure 7-3 for further description. Severe hand-foot syndrome can decrease one's quality of life secondary to pain and inability to wear shoes, ambulate, or hold various objects (Agha et al., 2007; Lokich; Wilkes & Doyle; Wyatt et al., 2006).

The grading system for hand-foot syndrome toxicity is listed in Table 7-4. The management of symptoms focuses on comfort measures. Topical ointments that are recommended to aid in skin hydration and to maintain skin in-

Figure 7-3. Hand-Foot Syndrome

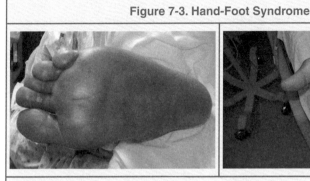
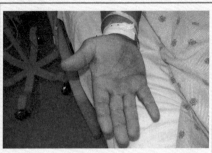

Note. Photos courtesy of Carol Viele, RN, University of California, San Francisco. Used with permission.

Table 7-4. Grading System for Hand-Foot Syndrome

Adverse Event	Grade 1	2	3	4	5
Palmar-plantar erythrodyses-thesia syndrome	Minimal skin changes or dermatitis (e.g., erythema, edema, or hyperkeratosis) without pain	Skin changes (e.g., peeling, blisters, bleeding, edema, or hyperkeratosis) with pain; limiting instrumental ADL	Severe skin changes (e.g., peeling, blisters, bleeding, edema, or hyperkeratosis) with pain; limiting self care ADL	–	–

Definition: A disorder characterized by redness, marked discomfort, swelling, and tingling in the palms of the hands or the soles of the feet.

Note. From *Common Terminology Criteria for Adverse Events* (Version 4.0), by National Cancer Institute Cancer Therapy Evaluation Program, 2009. Retrieved July 23, 2009, from http://ctep.cancer.gov/protocolDevelopment/electronic_applications/docs/ctcaev4.pdf

tegrity include Bag Balm® (Dairy Association Co., Inc.), Biafine® (OrthoNeutrogena), and Aquaphor® (Beiersdorf, Inc.). The use of topical corticosteroids or anesthetics is not recommended because they may exacerbate symptoms (Agha et al., 2007; Viele & Dest, 2007; Wilkes & Doyle, 2005).

Maculopapular/Morbilliform Reaction

Certain chemotherapeutic agents can cause an ill-defined erythematous, maculopapular rash with associated pruritus. These agents include docetaxel and paclitaxel. The toxicity grading system for rash is addressed in Table 7-5. Management of these rashes includes the use of topical and/or systemic corticosteroids (Agha et al., 2007; Wright, 2006).

Table 7-5. Grading System for Maculopapular Rash					
Adverse Event	Grade				
	1	2	3	4	5
Rash maculopapular	Macules/papules covering < 10% BSA with or without symptoms (e.g., pruritus, burning, tightness)	Macules/papules covering 10%–30% BSA with or without symptoms (e.g., pruritus, burning, tightness); limiting instrumental ADL	Macules/papules covering > 30% BSA with or without associated symptoms; limiting self care ADL	–	–

Definition: A disorder characterized by the presence of macules (flat) and papules (elevated). Also known as morbillform rash, it is one of the most common cutaneous adverse events, frequently affecting the upper trunk, spreading centripetally and associated with pruritus.

Note. From Common Terminology Criteria for Adverse Events (Version 4.0), by National Cancer Institute Cancer Therapy Evaluation Program, 2009. Retrieved July 23, 2009, from http://ctep.cancer.gov/protocolDevelopment/electronic_applications/docs/ctcaev4.pdf

Radiation Sensitivity and Recall

The integument is very sensitive to the effects of radiation therapy because of its rapid mitosis. When radiation therapy is used concurrently with certain chemotherapy agents, those effects are enhanced. These agents or chemicals also are referred to as *radiosensitizers*. Common radiosensitizers include bleomycin, carboplatin, cisplatin, dactinomycin, docetaxel, doxorubicin, etoposide, fluorouracil, gemcitabine, hydroxyurea, ifosfamide, methotrexate, mitomycin, paclitaxel, vinblastine, and vinorelbine (Gosselin-Acomb, 2005). Enhanced skin manifestations include erythema, hyperpigmentation, dry desquamation, and/or moist desquamation. See Table 7-6 for the grading system for radiation or chemoradiation skin changes. Management strategies for chemoradiation-related skin toxicities are based upon the toxicity grading. Topical ointments such as Aquaphor, Eucerin® (Beiersdorf, Inc.), and steroid-based ointments can be used. Other interventions include soft silicone dressings, hydrogel sheets, and dressings moistened with aluminum acetate astringent such as Domeboro® (Bayer Consumer Care Products) solution (Sparks, 2007) (see Table 7-7).

Table 7-6. Grading System for Radiation Dermatitis

Adverse Event	Grade 1	2	3	4	5
Dermatitis radiation	Faint erythema or dry desquamation	Moderate to brisk erythema; patchy moist desquamation, mostly confined to skin folds and creases; moderate edema	Moist desquamation in areas other than skin folds and creases; bleeding induced by minor trauma or abrasion	Life-threatening consequences; skin necrosis or ulceration of full thickness dermis; spontaneous bleeding from involved site; skin graft indicated	Death

Definition: A finding of cutaneous inflammatory reaction occurring as a result of exposure to biologically effective levels of ionizing radiation.

Note. From *Common Terminology Criteria for Adverse Events* (Version 4.0), by National Cancer Institute Cancer Therapy Evaluation Program, 2009. Retrieved July 23, 2009, from http://ctep.cancer.gov/protocolDevelopment/electronic_applications/docs/ctcaev4.pdf

Table 7-7. Combined Chemoradiation Skin Care Algorithm

Grade	Grade 1	Grade 2	Grade 3	Grade 4
Appearance	Faint erythema; dry desquamation	Moderate to brisk erythema	Moist desquamation	Skin necrosis or ulceration

Note. From *Challenging Management of Skin Problems With Combined Chemoradiation*, by M. Haas, D. Doughty, and A. Hatcher, November 2007. Presented at Oncology Nursing Society Institutes of Learning, Chicago, IL. Used with permission.

Radiation recall is another skin manifestation that can occur when certain treatments are administered. These agents include chemotherapeutic agents such as the anthracyclines, alkylating agents, antimetabolites, nucleoside analogs, taxanes, and tamoxifen, as well as antituberculosis agents, antibiotics, simvastatin, and exposure to ultraviolet light. It is an inflammatory skin reaction that occurs at a previously irradiated site. Radiation recall is not entirely understood, and its mechanism is unknown. This inflammatory response can cause an array of skin manifestations, which include maculopapular eruptions with erythema, vesicular development, and desquamation within the previously irradiated site (see Table 7-6). Management interventions for radiation recall include use of corticosteroids and nonsteroidal anti-inflammatory medications, as well as withdrawing the causative agent (Agha et al., 2007; Alley et al., 2002; Sparks, 2007; Wyatt et al., 2006). See Figures 7-4 through 7-5 for skin-related chemoradiation toxicities and Figure 7-6 for radiation recall.

Figure 7-4. Grade 3 Chemoradiation Skin Reaction

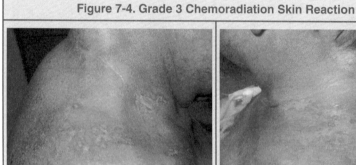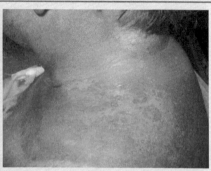

Note. Photos courtesy of the Department of Radiation Oncology at the Hospital of Saint Raphael, New Haven, CT. Used with permission.

Figure 7-5. Grade 4 Chemoradiation Skin Reaction

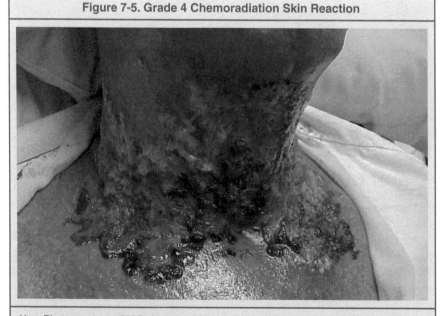

Note. Photo courtesy of M.D. Anderson Cancer Center, Memorial Healthcare, and Mountain Radiation Oncology. Used with permission.

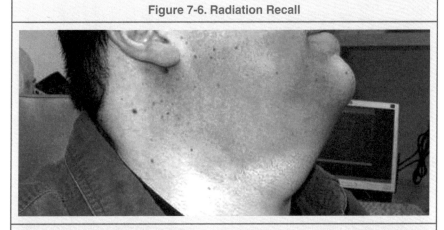

Figure 7-6. Radiation Recall

Note. Photo courtesy of the Department of Radiation Oncology at the Hospital of Saint Raphael, New Haven, CT. Used with permission.

Nail Dystrophies

Nail changes of the fingers and toes are very common in patients receiving chemotherapy. Nail growth is generally affected by chemotherapy. Chemotherapy-induced nail changes are transient and resolve slowly after treatment is discontinued. Complete resolution may take up to six months. Hyperpigmentation is common and occurs most often in black individuals. The pattern of pigmentation generally is at the base of the nail and causes transverse ridges. Hyperpigmentation may be accompanied by nail raising and paronychia. *Paronychia* is defined as an inflammation of the nail fold, which is frequently caused by bacteria or fungus, especially *Staphylococcus aureua* and *Candida albicans* (see Figure 7-7). Causative chemotherapy agents include paclitaxel, docetaxel, doxorubicin, and cyclophosphamide. The EGFR inhibitors also cause paronychia in 10%–15% of patients (Mitchell, Perez-Soler, Van Cutsem, & Lacouture, 2007). Up to 44% of patients who receive docetaxel will experience nail changes including onycholysis, subungual hyperkeratosis, Beau's lines, and dyschromia (Agha et al., 2007). *Onycholysis*, or partial separation of the nail plate, commonly occurs with fluorouracil, doxorubicin, paclitaxel, docetaxel, and bleomycin (Alley et al., 2002; Fischer et al., 2003; Marrs & Newton, 2004; Wyatt et al., 2006).

Assessment of nail changes is imperative, and a grading system was developed by the National Cancer Institute Cancer Therapy Evaluation Program (2006) (see Table 7-8). Patient and family education is important for best nail care practices. Patients should be encouraged to keep nails short, use good daily hygiene, and avoid exposure to harmful chemicals and detergents. Patients should keep nails and hands moisturized and protect hands from irritants by wearing gloves and avoiding trauma or injury. Artificial or acrylic

Figure 7-7. Paronychia

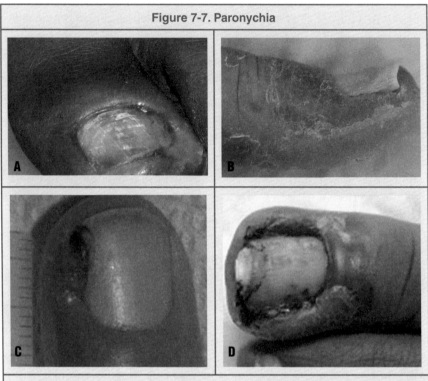

A and B show grade 1; C shows grade 2, and D shows grade 3.

Note. From "Clinical Presentation and Pathophysiology of EGFR1 Dermatologic Toxicities," by E.P. Mitchell, R. Perez-Soler, E. Van Cutsem, and M.E. Lacouture, 2007, *Oncology, 21*(11, Suppl. 5), p. 6. Copyright 2007 by CMPMedica. Reprinted with permission.

Table 7-8. Grading System for Nail Changes

Adverse Event	Short Name	Grade 1	2	3	4	5
Nail changes	Nail changes	Discoloration, ridging (koilonychias), pitting	Partial or complete loss of nail(s); pain in nail bed(s)	Interfering with ADL	–	–

ADL—activities of daily living

Note. From *Common Terminology Criteria for Adverse Events* (Version 3.0), by National Cancer Institute Cancer Therapy Evaluation Program, 2006. Retrieved April 1, 2008, from http://ctep.cancer.gov/protocolDevelopment/electronic_applications/docs/ctcaev3.pdf

nails should be avoided because of an increased risk of injury or infection. Patients can use nail polish, but using nail polish remover may be harmful to nail surface. Biotin, a water-soluble B-complex vitamin, may improve overall nail condition. Recommended dose is 5 mg/day (Marrs & Newton, 2004; Wyatt et al., 2006).

Hypersensitivity

Hypersensitivity reactions associated with chemotherapy administration are infrequent but can be life threatening when they occur. Type I hypersensitivity reactions can cause urticaria, angioedema, or anaphylaxis. Common chemotherapeutic agents that are associated with hypersensitivity reactions include paclitaxel, asparaginase, docetaxel, cisplatin, carboplatin, mechlorethamine (nitrogen mustard), oxaliplatin, and etoposide. Asparaginase reactions most commonly cause acute urticaria in about 10%–20% of patients (Camp-Sorrell, 2005; Fischer et al., 2003). Hypersensitivity reactions with paclitaxel are manifested by rash, hypotension, dyspnea, and bronchospasms. Measures to minimize a hypersensitivity reaction with the administration of paclitaxel include premedication with an antihistamine, a corticosteroid, and an H_2 receptor antagonist. Docetaxel also is associated with hypersensitivity reactions, including skin rash, anaphylaxis, and fluid retention. Measures to minimize a hypersensitivity reaction with the administration of docetaxel include premedication with dexamethasone, which is continued for three days after treatment (Camp-Sorrell; Wyatt et al., 2006).

Chemotherapy Extravasation

Chemotherapy or vesicant extravasation is an infrequent side effect of chemotherapy administration and occurs in approximately 0.1%–6% of patients receiving peripheral IV chemotherapy and 0.3%–4.7% of patients with central venous access devices (Ener, Meglathery, & Styler, 2004; Sauerland, Engelking, Wickham, & Corbi, 2006). Vesicant extravasation can lead to impaired quality of life and survival and can also significantly increase healthcare costs. *Extravasation* is defined as the inadvertent leakage of a drug or solution from a vein or unintentional injection into surrounding healthy, normal tissues (Sauerland et al.). Leakage of chemotherapeutic agents can lead to skin and tissue damage. The sequelae of vesicant extravasation can range from mild to severe tissue destruction, including erythema, pain, necrosis, and sloughing of skin. Figure 7-8 shows an example of vesicant extravasation. Chemotherapeutic drugs are divided into three categories, which include nonvesicant agents, irritant agents, and vesicant agents (see Figure 7-9). Additionally, some nonchemotherapeutic agents have been reported to be vesicants (see Figure 7-10). The most damaging drugs are called *vesicants*, and these drugs can cause pain, erythema, and ulceration. Another ramification of vesicant extravasation is full-thickness skin necrosis with damage to the underlying tendons, muscles, and neurovascular structures. The pathophysiology of chemotherapy extravasation is caused by direct cellular toxicity, but the exact sequence of injury is unknown and may be different for various chemothera-

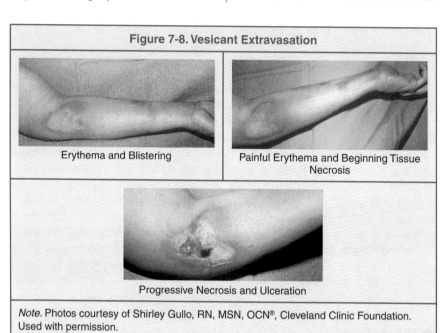

Figure 7-8. Vesicant Extravasation

| Erythema and Blistering | Painful Erythema and Beginning Tissue Necrosis |

Progressive Necrosis and Ulceration

Note. Photos courtesy of Shirley Gullo, RN, MSN, OCN®, Cleveland Clinic Foundation. Used with permission.

Figure 7-9. Chemotherapy Agents Classified by Degree of Tissue Damage (Extravasation)

Nonvesicant Agents	Irritant Agents	Vesicant Agents
• Asparaginase	• Carmustine	• Cisplatin*
• Bleomycin	• Cisplatin*	• Dactinomycin
• Cladribine	• Dacarbazine	• Daunorubicin
• Cyclophosphamide	• Daunorubicin liposomal	• Doxorubicin
• Cytarabine	• Docetaxel	• Epirubicin
• Fludarabine	• Doxorubicin liposomal	• Idarubicin
• Gemcitabine	• Etoposide	• Mechlorethamine
• Gemtuzumab	• Floxuridine	• Melphalan
• Ifosfamide	• Irinotecan	• Mitomycin
• Interleukin-2	• Mitoxantrone	• Paclitaxel
• Methotrexate	• Oxaliplatin	• Vinblastine
• Pentostatin	• Topotecan	• Vincristine
• Rituximab		• Vindesine
• Thiotepa		• Vinorelbine
• Trastuzumab		

*Vesicant if greater than 20 ml of 0.5 mg/ml concentration extravasates

Note. Based on information from Sauerland et al., 2006; Wickham et al., 2006.

Figure 7-10. Nonchemotherapeutic Agents Considered to Be Vesicants

- Calcium chloride 5.5%
- Calcium gluconate 10%
- Central venous nutrition
- Dobutamine
- Dopamine
- Epinephrine
- Glucose (> 10%)
- Mannitol 15%
- Penicillin
- Phenytoin
- Potassium chloride 7.45%
- Radiograph contrast media
- Sodium bicarbonate (4.2%–8.4%)
- Sodium chloride 10%
- Vancomycin
- Vasopressin

Note. Based on information from Wickham et al., 2006.

---

peutic agents (Sauerland et al.). One of the most common drugs extravasated is doxorubicin. It is theorized that as the affected cells die, the drug is released and taken up by surrounding normal cells. This leads to tissue damage over a period of weeks to months. Other factors that determine degree of tissue damage include drug concentration, amount of chemical infiltrated, and duration of tissue exposure. In addition, assessment and expedient management strategies must be instituted to decrease cellular damage. It is thought that delayed interventions may cause increased injury, pain, and disability. Risk factors for extravasation include administration device, type of treatment, patient-related characteristics, and clinician-related characteristics (Ener et al.; Hayden & Goodman, 2005; Sauerland et al.; Schulmeister, 2005; Wyatt et al., 2006).

Assessment and differentiation of an extravasation versus *localized reaction* is imperative for oncology nurses administering chemotherapeutic agents with the potential for extravasation. Patients with irritant reactions generally experience aching, pain, or tightness with administration. Visible changes may include erythema and hyperpigmentation of the vein with associated swelling at the site and loss of blood return. Localized hypersensitivity skin reactions are rare but can occur with anthracyclines or nitrogen mustard. They may cause localized pruritus with the development of erythematous streaks or hives along the vein pathway. These reactions usually resolve within one to two hours after administration (Hayden & Goodman, 2005; Schulmeister, 2005; Wickham, Engelking, Sauerland, & Corbi, 2006; Wyatt et al., 2006). Signs of chemotherapy extravasation include complaints of pain or burning, erythema, swelling at site, and loss of blood return. For some extravasations, no signs are apparent for hours to days later. Management of a suspected or actual extravasation should include the following (Ener et al., 2004; Fischer et al., 2003; Hayden & Goodman; Schulmeister; Wickham et al.; Wyatt et al.).

- Have an extravasation kit readily available.
- Stop infusion of chemotherapy.
- Disconnect IV tubing, and aspirate any residual chemotherapy.
- Apply ice for all chemotherapeutic agents except vinca alkaloids. Apply ice for 15–20 minutes at least four times per day, and elevate the affected extremity. Apply heat if extravasation was caused by a vinca alkaloid.
- Consider an antidote, if applicable (see Table 7-9).
- Document the event, including photographs.
- Perform patient follow-up for at least two weeks, with referral to a plastic surgeon and physical therapist.

Hormonal Agents and Associated Skin Manifestations

Hormonal agents are used in the treatment of breast and prostate cancers and produce skin-related manifestations. The agents that most commonly

Table 7-9. Vesicant Chemotherapeutic Antidotes	
Chemotherapy Agent	**Suggested Antidote**
Cisplatin	Sodium thiosulfate
Daunorubicin	Topical dimethyl sulfoxide (DMSO) 99%; dexrazoxane
Docetaxel	Hyaluronidase; topical DMSO 99%
Doxorubicin	Topical DMSO 99%; dexrazoxane
Epirubicin	Topical DMSO 99%
Idarubicin	Topical DMSO 99%
Mechlorethamine	Sodium thiosulfate
Oxaliplatin	Sodium thiosulfate
Paclitaxel	Topical DMSO 99%
Vinblastine	Hyaluronidase
Vincristine	Hyaluronidase
Vinorelbine	Hyaluronidase

Note. Based on information from Wickham et al., 2006.

cause skin changes are luteinizing hormone-releasing hormone antagonists, which include leuprolide acetate and goserelin. Dermatitis, local skin reaction at injection site, pruritus, and hyperpigmentation are common. The agents used in the treatment of breast cancer, such as antiestrogens or aromatase inhibitors, rarely cause skin changes (Fischer et al., 2003).

Biotherapy-Induced Skin Manifestations

Biotherapy is used in the treatment of cancers such as renal cell carcinoma and melanoma to stimulate one's immune system in the hope of attacking and killing the cancer cells. *Cytokines* are the messengers within the immune system that help communication between the macrophages and lymphocytes. Interleukin (IL)-2 and interferon alfa are classified as cytokines. IL-2 is a cytokine that causes T-cell proliferation in response to an antigen, whereas interferon alfa targets uninfected host cells and is able to inhibit viral replication (Corwin, 2000; Esper, Gale, & Muehlbauer, 2007; Fischer et al., 2003; Newton, Jackowski, & Marrs, 2002; Sandstrom, 1996; Viele & Moran, 1993).

Side effects of both these agents are caused by the proinflammatory response to cytokines. Common side effects include fatigue, flu-like symptoms, fever, arthralgias, myalgias, rigors, hypotension, capillary leak syndrome, and skin manifestations. Common skin manifestations with IL-2 usually begin within a few days after the start of therapy and may include flushing, pruritus, and development of an erythematous rash (see Figure 7-11). Sloughing of the skin also can occur with IL-2 therapy. Skin manifestations may last 7–10 days after the last dose was administered. Common skin manifestations with interferon alfa include pruritus, rash, mild alopecia, and increased eyelash growth, as well as exacerbation of known dermatologic and autoimmune disorders (Corwin, 2000; Esper et al., 2007; Newton et al., 2002; Fischer et al., 2003; Sandstrom, 1996; Viele & Moran, 1993).

History taking and assessment are most important and should include
- History of skin disorders
- Presence of skin lesions or rashes
- Characteristics of rash including color, appearance, and location.

Patient and family education are essential. Patients should be instructed to keep skin hydrated with moisturizers. Skin products should be alcohol-free, odor-free, and water-based. Interventions to minimize pruritus include using nondrying soaps such as oatmeal-based soap and pharmacologic agents such as diphenhydramine and hydroxyzine. Patients are advised to avoid sun exposure and wear sunscreen. Topical corticosteroid ointments also are contraindicated in patients receiving biologic agents. Because of the suppression of the immune system by steroids, the use of topical steroids could affect the antitumor effects of biotherapy drugs (Corwin, 2000; Esper et al., 2007; Newton et al., 2002; Fischer et al., 2003; Sandstrom, 1996; Viele & Moran, 1993).

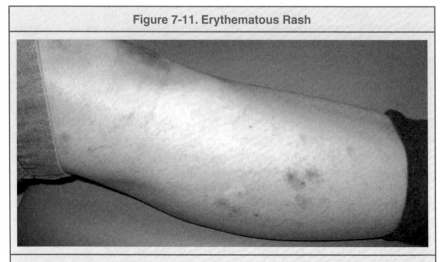

Figure 7-11. Erythematous Rash

Note. Photo courtesy of the Department of Radiation Oncology at the Hospital of Saint Raphael, New Haven, CT. Used with permission.

Targeted Therapies and Associated Skin Manifestations

Targeted therapies are the newest novel agents used in the treatment of cancer. These therapies have emerged because of a better understanding of cellular processes, in particular, tumor growth and development. Targeted therapy agents assist in preventing tumors from growing, metastasizing, and interfering with one's immune system. They can be used as monotherapy or in combination with conventional chemotherapy. The mechanism of action is targeted toward cell membrane receptors, signaling pathways and proteins, enzymatic activity, and regulatory cell growth. It is thought that these factors are aberrant or more prevalent in cancer cells than normal cells (Herbst, 2004; Lacouture, 2007). The human epidermal growth factor receptor, also referred to as HER1/EGFR, plays a role in normal differentiation and development of epidermal keratinocytes, stimulating epidermal growth, inhibiting differentiation and inflammation, protecting against ultraviolet damage, and assisting in quicker would healing. EGFR is expressed on normal epidermal and follicular keratinocytes, basal layers of the epidermis, outer root of the hair follicles, sebaceous epithelium, eccrine epithelium, and some connective tissues. EGFR also plays a key role in the tumorigenic process of epithelial cancers. HER1/EGFR is overexpressed in 30%–100% of cancers. These include head/neck, colorectal, breast, cervical, renal, esophageal and lung cancers (Esper et al., 2007).

Skin manifestations are common in therapies that target epidermal growth factor signaling and pathways. The exact mechanism of skin manifestations with targeted agents is unknown but is thought to be related to the inhibition of human keratinocytes, leading to alterations in proliferation, differentiation, and migration. Both monoclonal antibodies and small-molecule tyrosine kinase inhibitors interfere with EGFR. Examples of monoclonal antibodies that interfere with EGFR include cetuximab and panitumumab. Examples of EGFR tyrosine kinase inhibitors include gefitinib, erlotinib, sunitinib, and sorafenib (Esper et al., 2007; Herbst, 2004; Lacouture, 2007). In 2009, the National Comprehensive Cancer Network (NCCN) Task Force met to discuss recommendations in the management of skin toxicities with EGFR inhibitors. Skin manifestations in patients receiving EGFR inhibitors are correlated to a good therapeutic response (Mulcahy, 2009).

Dermatologic side effects of targeted therapies include papulopustular reaction, xerosis/pruritus, acral erythema, subungual splinter hemorrhages, fissures, telangiectasia, hyperpigmentation, hair changes, and paronychia with pyogenic granuloma. The most common side effect of targeted therapies is the development of a papulopustular reaction. The rash appears to be dose dependent and occurs in 45%–100% of patients (Lacouture, 2007). It occurs in more seborrheic areas and generally appears on the face, neck, shoulders, upper trunk, and scalp (see Figure 7-12). The rash is characterized by the presence of papulopustular lesions, but these are very different from comedones or lesions associated with acne vulgaris. The EGFR-related rash does not have the same clinical features as acne vulgaris (Lorusso, 2009). Some clinicians may refer to this rash as *acneform* in nature, which many experts consider incorrect. For grading of acneform rash, see Table 7-10. The rash contributes to the symptomatology as well as functional and emotional well-being of the patient (Lorusso). Perez-Soler et al. (2005) and others have proposed that the etiology and pathology of these rashes is unclear, so clinicians need to describe rash in terms of the appearance and location. Recommended terminology includes *pustular/papular rash, pustular eruption,* or *follicular* and *intrafollicular eruption.* The rash also is associated with pruritus (see Table 7-11). The rash typically appears within one to three weeks of initiation of therapy and reaches its peak within three to five weeks. The severity of the rash depends on the agent and dosage. The incidence of rash with EGFR monoclonal antibodies is slightly higher than the incidence of rash with small-molecule EGFR tyrosine kinase inhibitors (Esper et al., 2007; Lorusso, 2009; Robert et al., 2005).

Management of papulopustular rash continues to be studied with limited evidence-based research available; however, some practice guidelines have been instituted. The research literature is limited regarding evidence-based practice in the management of cutaneous toxicities associated with targeted therapies. Recently, some randomized clinical trials have been developed and are ongoing to evaluate management strategies of these skin toxicities (Esper et al., 2007; Lorusso, 2009). Treatment of rash should be based upon symptoms and their effect on the patient's quality of life, as well as clinical recommendations. It is recommended that the skin stay moisturized and hydrated as well as protected from injury. Emollient creams and ointments should be utilized. The following products have been recommended in the literature

(Dick & Crawford, 2005; Esper et al.; Lorusso; Perez-Soler et al., 2005; Robert et al., 2005):

- Eucerin
- Cetaphil® (Galderma Laboratories, Inc.)
- Aquaphor
- Bag Balm
- Neutrogena Norwegian Formula® (Neutrogena).

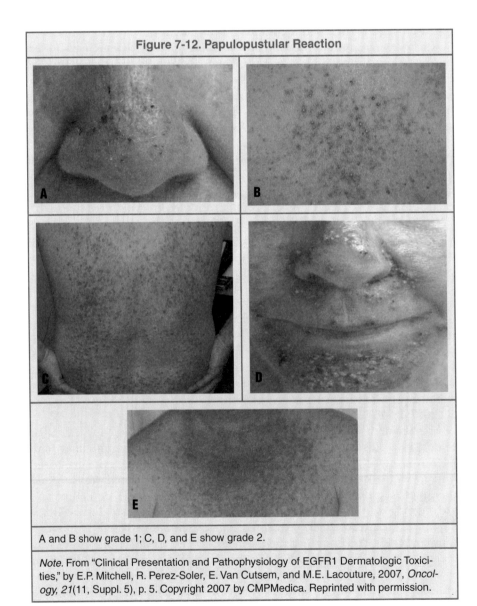

Figure 7-12. Papulopustular Reaction

A and B show grade 1; C, D, and E show grade 2.

Note. From "Clinical Presentation and Pathophysiology of EGFR1 Dermatologic Toxicities," by E.P. Mitchell, R. Perez-Soler, E. Van Cutsem, and M.E. Lacouture, 2007, *Oncology, 21*(11, Suppl. 5), p. 5. Copyright 2007 by CMPMedica. Reprinted with permission.

Patients should be advised not to use moisturizing products that contain alcohol, perfumes, or dyes because of increased dryness and irritation (Dick & Crawford, 2005; Lynch et al., 2007). A pruritic rash can be treated with emollient creams as mentioned previously (Lynch et al.; Perez-Soler et al., 2005; Robert et al., 2005). If emollient creams are not effective, patients may require antihistamine therapy with diphenhydramine or hydroxyzine. Patients are encouraged to used water-based cleansers such as Cetaphil (Esper et al., 2007; Lynch et al.). No evidence-based information is available about the prophylactic use of topical or systemic antibiotics. The incidence of infection increases when lesions develop honey-crusted scabs or purulent drainage. The most common causes of infection are *Staphylococcus aureus.* Treatment of suspected infection should include the use of topical antibiotics such as 1% clindamycin, benzoyl peroxide, or erythromycin, or the use of systemic antibiotics. Most appropriate antibiotics include minocycline, doxycycline, and tetracycline. Oral isotretinoin at 30–40 mg daily with metronidazole gel has been shown to reduce EGFR-induced rash by week 4 of therapy (Mulcahy, 2009).

Topical cyclosporine analogs and topical and oral corticosteroids are recommended to alleviate inflammation (Esper et al., 2007; Lacouture, 2007;

Table 7-10. Grading System for Acneform Rash					
Adverse Event	**Grade**				
	1	**2**	**3**	**4**	**5**
Rash acneiform	Papules and/or pustules covering < 10% BSA, which may or may not be associated with symptoms of pruritus or tenderness	Papules and/or pustules covering 10-30% BSA, which may or may not be associated with symptoms of pruritus or tenderness; associated with psychosocial impact; limiting instrumental ADL	Papules and/or pustules covering > 30% BSA, which may or may not be associated with symptoms of pruritus or tenderness; limiting self care ADL; associated with local superinfection with oral antibiotics indicated	Papules and/or pustules covering any % BSA, which may or may not be associated with symptoms of pruritus or tenderness and are associated with extensive superinfection with IV antibiotics indicated; lifethreatening consequences	Death

Definition: A disorder characterized by an eruption of papules and pustules, typically appearing in face, scalp, upper chest and back.

Note. From *Common Terminology Criteria for Adverse Events* (Version 4.0), by National Cancer Institute Cancer Therapy Evaluation Program, 2009. Retrieved July 23, 2009, from http://ctep.cancer.gov/protocolDevelopment/electronic_applications/docs/ctcaev4.pdf

Table 7-11. Grading System for Pruritus

Adverse Event	Grade				
	1	2	3	4	5
Pruritus	Mild or localized; topical intervention indicated	Intense or widespread; intermittent; skin changes from scratching (e.g. edema, papulation, excoriations, lichenification, oozing/crusts); oral intervention indicated; limiting instrumental ADL	Intense or widespread; constant; limiting self care ADL or sleep; oral corticosteroid or immunosuppressive therapy indicated	–	–

Definition: A disorder characterized by an eruption of papules and pustules, typically appearing in face, scalp, upper chest and back.

Note. From *Common Terminology Criteria for Adverse Events* (Version 4.0), by National Cancer Institute Cancer Therapy Evaluation Program, 2009. Retrieved July 23, 2009, from http://ctep.cancer.gov/protocolDevelopment/electronic_applications/docs/ctcaev4.pdf

Lorusso, 2009; Lynch et al., 2007; Perez-Soler et al., 2005; Yamamoto, Viale, & Zhao, 2004; Mitchell et al., 2007). Patients are also encouraged to use sunscreen containing zinc oxide or titanium dioxide with sun protection factor of 15 or greater (Lorusso; Lynch et al.).

Xerosis, or dry skin with flaking, occurs in approximately 12%–58% of all patients receiving erlotinib or gefitinib (Mulcahy, 2009; Perez-Soler et al., 2005). Patients can experience increased skin fragility, bruising, and swelling over joints with associated fissures leading to increased tenderness. Management of dryness includes use of emollient creams such as Aquaphor, Bag Balm, Eucerin, Kerasal® (Alterna, LLC), and Neutrogena Norwegian Formula. Telangiectasia also may occur and generally appears behind the ears, on the face, on the chest, and on extremities. This skin manifestation usually fades with time but may result with some hyperpigmentation. Hyperpigmentation after resolution of a papulopustular rash or eczema is common. Acral erythema is common in patients undergoing treatment with sunitinib and sorafenib. It generally occurs on the palms of the hands and soles of the feet. It is characterized by erythema with associated edema and pain. Formation of hyperkeratosis and desquamation also may occur, which differentiates it from handfoot syndrome. Nail changes are less frequent than rash but occur in 10%–15% of patients (Mitchell et al., 2007). They usually become evident within four to eight weeks from the initiation of therapy and are considered a late effect. The nail fold of the thumb and great toe usually become inflamed and may develop into a pyogenic granuloma, also referred to as paronychia. The NCCN Task Force recommends bacterial and fungal culturing and treatment with oral antibiotics. For fissuring, they recommend Monsel's solution, silver nitrate, or zinc oxide cream (Mulcahy, 2009). Another nail manifestation is the formation of *subungual splinter hemorrhage,* which is a mass of blood that develops under the nail bed. This is particularly common in patients receiving sunitinib, sorafenib, and imatinib. Hair changes have been reported as occurring within four to eight weeks of therapy and include changes in scalp hair texture, which usually manifests with curlier, more brittle hair, and dry, pruritic scalp. Occasionally, alopecia occurs but is less common. The growth of facial hair and eyelashes may increase. Increased eyelash growth is referred to as *trichomegaly*. Patients may exhibit curling, lengthening, and rigidity of eyelashes, as well as thickening and rigidity of eyebrows (Agha et al., 2007; Esper et al., 2007; Lorusso, 2009; Mitchell et al.; Mulcahy, 2009; Wood, 2007).

Supportive Therapy–Induced Skin Manifestations

Some supportive therapies also can cause skin manifestations in the oncology population. These include chronic steroid usage, administration of certain colony-stimulating factors such as granulocyte macrophage–colony-stimulating factor (GM-CSF), and administration of amifostine (Ethyol®, MedImmune, LLC) subcutaneously as a radioprotectant. The use of prednisone or dexamethasone can cause thin, fragile skin that bruises easily. Agents such as GM-CSF, a colony-stimulating factor to stimulate granulocytes within the bone marrow, can cause localized reactions at the injection site. Most commonly seen are local erythema, skin rash, alopecia, and pruritus. Amifostine is a cytoprotectant agent that has been shown to cause skin manifestations when given subcutaneously. These skin reactions are seen locally at the injection site or generalized in the form of an erythematous, maculopapular rash, which may be associated with a fever (see Figures 7-13 and 7-14). The presentation of amifostine-related skin reactions was evaluated by the Ethyol Cutaneous Treatment Advisory Panel (ECTAP) (Boccia et al., 2004). It is estimated that 6–9 cases occur per 10,000 patients receiving amifostine with radiation therapy and an estimated 0.8–1 cases per 10,000 patients receiving amifostine with chemotherapy (Boccia et al.). Most skin reactions occurred 10 days after initiation of treatment. ECTAP recommendations for skin assessment with amifostine include daily assessment for any rash or ulceration involving the lips or the mucosa that is not known to be attributable to another etiology, such as radiation or herpes simplex. In addition, assessment for erythematous, edematous, or bullous lesions on the palms of the hands, soles of the feet, or other cutaneous reactions on the trunk is advised (Boccia et al.). Generalized rash may be associated with the presence of fever. Management recommendations for localized reactions include rotation of injection sites and application of corticosteroid ointment to injection sites if erythema develops. It is recommended that amifostine be discontinued if the skin reaction begins to extend outside of radiation fields, or if the cutaneous skin reaction resembles erythema multiforme, such as toxic epidermal necrolysis, Stevens-Johnson syndrome, or exfoliative dermatitis (Boccia et al.; Hockett, 2004; Viele & Dest, 2007).

Figure 7-13. Amifostine Localized Reaction

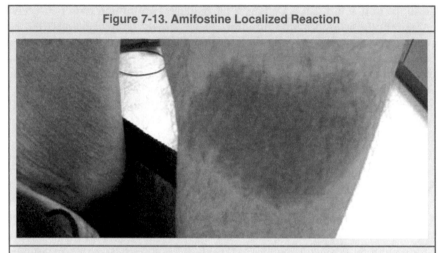

Note. Photo courtesy of the Department of Radiation Oncology at the Hospital of Saint Raphael, New Haven, CT. Used with permission.

Figure 7-14. Amifostine Generalized Rash

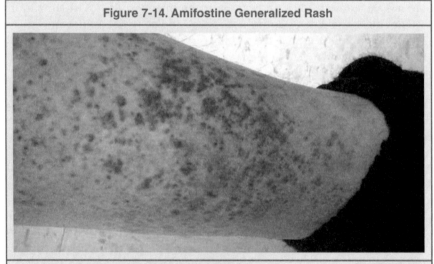

Note. Photo courtesy of the Department of Radiation Oncology at the Hospital of Saint Raphael, New Haven, CT. Used with permission.

Conclusion

Many dermatologic manifestations, as evidenced by this chapter, may be exhibited after the administration of systemic agents used in the treatment of cancer. Oncology nurses must be able to recognize and, even more importantly, differentiate amongst the various skin manifestations. Another challenge is in the management of these dermatologic manifestations. More evidence-based practice guidelines are needed for patient management and continuity of care, as well as for improved quality of life, both physically and psychologically.

References

Agha, R., Kinahan, K., Bennett, C., & Lacouture, M. (2007). Dermatologic challenges in cancer patients and survivors. *Oncology, 21*(12), 1462–1493.

Alley, E., Green, R., & Schuchter, L. (2002). Cutaneous toxicities of cancer therapy. *Current Opinion in Oncology, 14*(2), 212–216.

Boccia, R., Anne, P., Bourhis, J., Brizel, D., Daly, C., Holloway, N., et al. (2004). Assessment and management of cutaneous reactions with amifostine administration: Findings of the Ethyol Cutaneous Treatment Advisory Panel (ECTAP). *International Journal of Radiation Oncology, Biology, Physics, 60*(1), 302–309.

Camp-Sorrell, D. (2005). Chemotherapy toxicities and management. In C.H. Yarbro, M.H. Frogge, & M. Goodman (Eds.), *Cancer nursing: Principles and practice* (6th ed., pp. 412–457). Sudbury, MA: Jones and Bartlett.

Corwin, E. (2000). Understanding cytokines part I: Physiology and mechanism of action. *Biological Research for Nursing, 2*(1), 30–40.

Dick, S.E., & Crawford, G.H. (2005). Managing cutaneous side effects of epidermal growth factor receptor (HER1/EGFR) inhibitors. *Community Oncology, 2*(6), 492–496.

Ener, R.A., Meglathery, S.B., & Styler, M. (2004). Extravasation of systemic hemato-oncological therapies. *Annals of Oncology, 15*(6), 858–862.

Esper, P., Gale, D., & Muehlbauer, P. (2007). What kind of rash is it? Deciphering the dermatologic toxicities of biologic and targeted therapies. *Clinical Journal of Oncology Nursing, 11*(5), 659–666.

Fischer, D., Knobf, M., Durivage, H., & Beaulieu, N. (2003). *The cancer chemotherapy handbook* (6th ed.). Philadelphia: Mosby.

Gosselin-Acomb, T. (2005). Principles in radiation therapy. In C.H. Yarbro, M.H. Frogge, & M. Goodman (Eds.), *Cancer nursing: Principles and practice* (6th ed., pp. 229–249). Sudbury, MA: Jones and Bartlett.

Hayden, B., & Goodman, M. (2005). Chemotherapy: Principles of administration. In C.H Yarbro, M.H. Frogge, & M. Goodman (Eds.), *Cancer nursing: Principles and practice* (6th ed., pp. 412–457). Sudbury, MA: Jones and Bartlett.

Herbst, R.S. (2004). Review of epidermal growth factor receptor biology. *International Journal of Radiation Oncology, Biology, Physics, 59*(Suppl. 2), 21–26.

Hockett, K. (2004). Stevens-Johnson syndrome and toxic epidermal necrolysis: Oncologic considerations. *Clinical Journal of Oncology Nursing, 8*(1), 27–30.

Lacouture, M.E. (2007). Insights into the pathophysiology and management of dermatologic toxicities to EGFR-targeted therapies in colorectal cancer. *Cancer Nursing, 30*(4, Suppl. 1), S17–S26.

Lokich, J. (2007). The three most common chemotherapy-related skin reactions. *Oncology, 21*(12), 1473–1476.

Lorusso, P. (2009). Toward evidence-based management of the dermatologic effects of EGFR inhibitors. *Oncology, 23*(2), 186–198.

Lynch, T.J., Jr., Kim, E.S., Eaby, B., Garey, J., West, D.P., & Lacouture, M.E. (2007). Epidermal growth factor receptor inhibitor-associated cutaneous toxicities: An evolving paradigm in clinical management. *Oncologist, 12*(5), 610–621.

Marrs, J., & Newton, S. (2004). Chemotherapy-induced nail changes: An unsightly nuisance. *Clinical Journal of Oncology Nursing, 8*(5), 527–528.

Mitchell, E.P., Perez-Soler, R., Van Cutsem, E., & Lacouture, M.E. (2007). Clinical presentation and pathophysiology of EGFR1 dermatologic toxicities. *Oncology, 21*(11, Suppl. 5), 4–9.

Mulcahy, N. (2009). *NCCN 2009: Recommendations on managing skin toxicities with EGFR inhibitors.* Retrieved March 21, 2009, from http://www.medscape.com/viewarticle/589714

National Cancer Institute Cancer Therapy Evaluation Program. (2009). *Common terminology criteria for adverse events* (version 4.0). Bethesda, MD: National Cancer Institute. Retrieved July 23, 2009, from http://ctep.cancer.gov/protocolDevelopment/electronic_applications/docs/ctcaev4.pdf

Newton, S., Jackowski, C., & Marrs, J. (2002). Biotherapy skin reactions. *Clinical Journal of Oncology Nursing, 6*(3), 181–182.

Perez-Soler, R., Delord, J.P., Halpern, A., Kelly, K., Krueger, J., Sureda, B.M., et al. (2005). HER1/EGFR inhibitor-associated rash: Future directions for management and investigation outcomes from the HER1/EGFR inhibitor rash management forum. *Oncologist, 10*(5), 345–356.

Robert, C., Soria, J., Spatz, A., Le Cesne, A., Malka, D., Pautier, P., et al. (2005). Cutaneous side effects of kinase inhibitors and blocking antibodies. *Lancet Oncology, 6*(7), 491–500.

Sandstrom, S.K. (1996). Nursing management of patients receiving biological therapy. *Seminars in Oncology Nursing, 12*(2), 152–162.

Sauerland, C., Engelking, C., Wickham, R., & Corbi, D. (2006). Vesicant extravasation part I: Mechanisms, pathogenesis, and nursing care to reduce risk. *Oncology Nursing Forum, 33*(6), 1134–1141.

Schulmeister, L. (2005). Managing extravasations. *Clinical Journal of Oncology Nursing, 9*(4), 472–475.

Sparks, S. (2007). Radiodermatitis. In M.L. Haas, W.P. Hogle, G.J. Moore-Higgs, & T.K. Gosselin-Acomb (Eds.), *Radiation therapy: A guide to patient care* (pp. 511–522). St. Louis, MO: Elsevier Mosby.

Viele, C., & Dest, V. (2007). *Do you want to be an oncology nurse idol?: The synergy of nursing mentorship and patient advocacy in improving supportive cancer care* [CE monograph]. Chester, CT: Center for Medical Knowledge LLC.

Viele, C., & Moran, T. (1993). Nursing management of the non-hospitalized patient receiving recombinant interleukin-2. *Seminars in Oncology Nursing, 9*(3), 20–24.

Wickham, R., Engelking, C., Sauerland, C., & Corbi, D. (2006). Vesicant extravasation part II: Evidence-based management and continuing controversy. *Oncology Nursing Forum, 33*(6), 1143–1150.

Wilkes, G., & Doyle, D. (2005). Palmar-plantar erythrodysesthesia. *Clinical Journal of Oncology Nursing, 9*(1), 103–106.

Wood, L. (2007). Targeted therapies for advanced renal cell carcinoma: Part I—Sunitinib. *Oncology Nursing News, 1*(3), 19–26.

Wright, L. (2006). Maculopapular skin rashes associated with high-dose chemotherapy: Prevalence and risk factors. *Oncology Nursing Forum, 33*(6), 1095–1103.

Wyatt, A.J., Leonard, G.D., & Sachs, D.L. (2006). Cutaneous reactions to chemotherapy and their management. *American Journal of Clinical Dermatology, 7*(1), 45–63.

Yamamoto, D.S., Viale, P.H., & Zhao, G. (2004). Severe acneiform rash. *Clinical Journal of Oncology Nursing, 8*(6), 654–656.

CHAPTER 8

Cutaneous Effects of Blood and Marrow Transplantation

Theresa M. Latchford, RN, MS, AOCN®

Introduction

Since the late 1960s, blood and bone marrow transplantation (BMT) has been used with curative intent to treat a variety of hematologic and solid organ malignancies, nonmalignant stem cell disorders, and certain genetic disorders in both children and adults. Several different types of transplantations exist. *Autologous* transplantation is the use of high-dose therapy aimed at curing the underlying malignancy. In autologous transplantation, the patient provides his or her own graft. The graft is collected prior to the high-dose therapy and is administered to rescue the bone marrow suppression caused by the high-dose therapy. If the graft is from a donor, the transplant is called *allogeneic* transplantation. The donor may be a sibling or an unrelated volunteer. A third and rare type of transplantation is called *syngeneic* transplantation. The graft for a syngeneic transplant is an identical twin. Grafts may be collected from the peripheral blood, bone marrow, or umbilical cord.

Traditionally, allogeneic transplantation required the patient to receive a myeloablative conditioning regimen consisting of moderate to high doses of chemotherapy and/or radiation therapy to eradicate malignant cells, leading to considerable transplantation-related morbidity and mortality. Because of the intensity of myeloablative conditioning regimens, this approach was limited to young and otherwise healthy individuals. However, over the past decade, "reduced intensity" or nonmyeloablative treatment conditioning regimens have been developed. Reduced intensity transplantations work by weakening recipients' immune system, allowing donor engraftment (Schaffer, 2006). The potential for cure comes from the donor's immune system recognizing and destroying residual malignancy. This effect is called *graft-versus-tu-mor*, *graft-versus-leukemia*, or *graft-versus-malignancy*, which is the primary benefit of allogeneic transplantation. Nonmyeloablative transplantation allows older recipients or recipients with other comorbid health conditions to have access to this potentially curative treatment option.

Tremendous progress in the field of BMT has resulted in improved survival and decreased morbidity. However, many challenges remain for nurses caring for BMT recipients. This chapter will discuss common cutaneous toxicities observed in BMT recipients and the nursing assessment and management of these toxicities. The focus of this chapter will be the cutaneous manifestations of acute graft-versus-host disease (aGVHD), chronic graft-versus-host disease (cGVHD), and palmar-plantar erythrodysesthesia (PPE).

Acute Graft-Versus-Host Disease

GVHD is a significant cause of morbidity and mortality following allogeneic BMT. Although aGVHD occurs in up to 90% of allogeneic transplant recipients, clinically significant disease occurs in approximately 50% of patients (Aractingi & Chosidow, 1998; Jacobsohn & Vogelsang, 2007). Survival for patients with mild aGVHD approaches 60% and greater; however, for patients with severe aGVHD, the prognosis is grave (Bacigalupo, 2007). The incidence and severity of aGVHD may depend on several factors, including (Aractingi & Chosidow; Bacigalupo; Schaffer, 2006)

- Age of the recipient
- GVHD prophylaxis
- Degree of donor and recipient human leukocyte antigen (HLA) matching
- Intensity of the conditioning regimen
- Composition of the graft
- Donor gender (higher risk of GVHD for male recipients with female donors)
- The use of donor lymphocyte infusions (DLI).

DLI have been used to treat leukemia relapse after allogeneic transplantation, enhancing the donors' immune response against the underlying malignancy. Donor lymphocytes are collected by leukaphereses and infused into the BMT recipient. The goal of DLI is to induce remission. Unfortunately, almost half of the patients experience severe aGVHD after the DLI infusion (Collins et al., 1997).

GVHD is initiated when immunocompetent T cells from the graft react against the recipients' tissue via recognition of alloantigens displayed by host *antigen-presenting cells* (APCs) (Schaffer, 2006). Acute GVHD disease is a multistep process. The first step involves inflammation and damage to host tissues from the preparative chemotherapy and/or radiotherapy regimen as well as prior therapies, the underlying disease, and infections. Damage to host tissues stimulates the release of inflammatory cytokines (interleukin [IL]-1, IL-

6, tumor necrosis factor alpha). In the second step, both recipient and donor APCs, in the setting of inflammatory cytokines released in step one, present antigens to donor T cells resulting in donor T-cell activation. Activated donor T cells then proliferate and secrete additional inflammatory cytokines such as IL-2, IL-12, and interferon gamma. In the third step, the effector phase, activated donor T cells kill target host cells either directly or by the release of cytokines. The ongoing tissue damage results in additional cytokine production that further contributes to host tissue damage. The abundant production of cytokines is called a *cytokine storm*. The tissue damage occurring in step three is seen clinically as aGVHD (Jacobsohn & Vogelsang, 2007).

Acute GVHD commonly occurs two to five weeks after allogeneic BMT and affects three systems: integument, liver, and gastrointestinal (GI) tract (Iwasaki, 2004). Traditionally, the onset of aGVHD was described as occurring in the first 100 days after transplantation. However, newer conditioning regimens, as well as the increased use of DLI, have blurred the time frame for the onset of aGVHD, resulting in the diagnosis of aGVHD occurring after day 100 (Hymes, Turner, Champlin, & Couriel, 2006). In 2005, the National Institutes of Health Consensus Project defined several categories of aGVHD. *Classic aGVHD* is defined as occurring before day 100, whereas aGVHD occurring after day 100 is categorized as *persistent, recurrent,* or *late-onset acute* (Filipovich et al., 2005). Table 8-1 summarizes the categories of aGVHD. Manifestations of aGVHD after day 100 are occasionally seen after the withdrawal of immunosuppressive agents.

Table 8-1. Categories of Acute and Chronic Graft-Versus-Host Disease			
Category	Time of Symptoms After HCT or DLI	Presence of Acute GVHD Features	Presence of Chronic GVHD Features
Acute GVHD			
• Classic acute GVHD	≤ 100 d	Yes	No
• Persistent, recurrent, or late-onset acute GVHD	> 100 d	Yes	No
Chronic GVHD			
• Classic chronic GVHD	No time limit	No	Yes
• Overlap syndrome	No time limit	Yes	Yes

DLI—donor lymphocyte infusions; GVHD—graft-versus-host disease; HCT—hematopoietic cell transplantation

Note. From "National Institutes of Health Consensus Development Project on Criteria for Clinical Trials in Chronic Graft-Versus-Host Disease: I. Diagnosis and Staging Working Group Report," by A.H. Filipovich, D. Weisdorf, S. Pavletic, G. Socie, J.R. Wingard, S.J. Lee, et al., 2005, *Biology of Blood and Marrow Transplantation, 11*(12), p. 951. Copyright 2005 by American Society for Blood and Marrow Transplantation. Reprinted with permission.

Cutaneous aGVHD is often the initial site of involvement. The manifestation typically presents as a morbilliform (maculopapular) eruption, sometimes preceded by a sensation of burning or pruritus. Acute GVHD can present as a scarlatiniform rash with confluent erythema that may eventually desquamate, leaving areas of hyperpigmentation. If aGVHD is severe, fluid-filled bullae will be seen, which eventually desquamate. See Figure 8-1 for a picture of grade III aGVHD skin rash and Figure 8-2 for grade IV aGVHD with bullae on the abdomen.

The skin in severe aGVHD is similar to that of a burn patient. See Figure 8-3 for severe aGVHD. Initially, the aGVHD rash appears on the palms and soles, outer ear, cheeks, lateral neck, and upper back (Schaffer, 2006). Less commonly, aGVHD presents as a clinical picture suggestive of varicella (Aractingi & Chosidow, 1998).

The GI tract and the liver are the other two systems affected by aGVHD. Liver or GI tract involvement usually is associated with concomitant cutaneous aGVHD. In some cases, isolated liver or GI tract involvement may be present. The principal manifestation of aGVHD of the liver is hyperbilirubinemia. Manifestations of aGVHD of the GI tract include nausea, abdominal cramping, abdominal pain, and copious diarrhea (Jacobsohn & Vogelsang, 2007).

Differential diagnoses for acute cutaneous GVHD include drug eruption, viral exanthem, return of the white blood cell count (*engraftment syndrome*), and infections. A skin biopsy is helpful in establishing the diagnosis. The his-

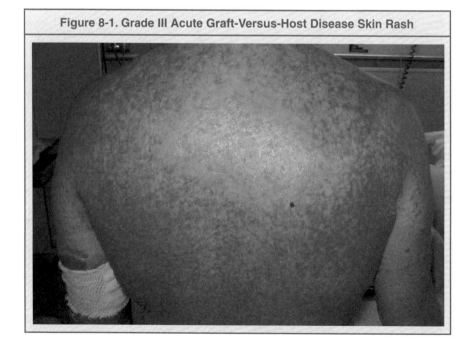

Figure 8-1. Grade III Acute Graft-Versus-Host Disease Skin Rash

Figure 8-2. Grade IV Acute Graft-Versus-Host Disease With Bullae on the Abdomen

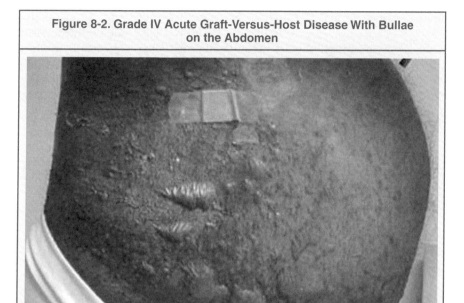

Figure 8-3. Severe Acute Graft-Versus-Host Disease

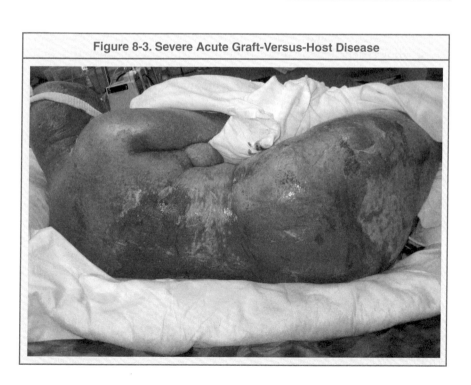

tologic aspects of aGVHD include lymphocytic infiltration and cytopathic changes of keratinocytes (Aractingi & Chosidow, 1998). The infiltrating lymphocytes are present in the dermis and epidermis. Characteristically, infiltrating lymphocytes are present around dead keratinocytes, referred to as *satellite cell necrosis*—considered a hallmark of aGVHD (Jacobsohn & Vogelsang, 2007). The histologic signs are classified into four grades (see Table 8-2) (Aractingi & Chosidow).

Table 8-2. Histologic Signs of Acute Graft-Versus-Host Disease	
Grade	**Signs**
Grade I	Basal cell vacuolization
Grade II	Basal cell vacuolization and single necrotic keratinocytes
Grade III	Superepidermal clefts and numerous necrotic keratinocytes
Grade IV	Necrosis of the entire epidermis and complete separation of the dermis
Note. Based on information from Aractingi & Chosidow, 1998.	

Clinical Staging of Acute Graft-Versus-Host Disease

Acute GVHD is staged by the number and extent of organ involvement. The grading system helps to divide patients into prognostic categories. In this system, patients are divided into one of four grades (I–IV) depending on the stage of involvement in each of the three organs: skin, liver, and GI tract. The skin is staged by calculating the percentage of body surface involved; the liver is staged by the degree of hyperbilirubinemia; and the GI tract is staged by the volume of diarrhea. Table 8-3 shows the staging and grading system for aGVHD organ involvement.

Prevention and Management of Acute Graft-Versus-Host Disease

Acute GVHD prophylaxis and treatment mainly consists of immunosuppressive agents. Prevention of aGVHD is paramount, as the treatment of aGVHD with additional immunosuppressive agents increases the risk of infectious complications. Immunosuppressive agents commonly used for prophylaxis include
- Cyclosporine
- Corticosteroids
- Tacrolimus
- Methotrexate.

Table 8-3. Extent of Organ Involvement			
Stage	Skin	Liver (bilirubin)	Gut (stool output/day)
0	No GVHD rash	< 2 mg/dl	< 500 ml/day or persistent nausea
1	Maculopapular rash < 25% BSA	2–3 mg/dl	500–999 ml/day
2	Maculopapular rash 25%–50% BSA	3–6 mg/dl	1,000–1,500 ml/day
3	Maculopapular rash > 50% BSA	6–15 mg/dl	Adult > 1,500 ml/day
4	Generalized erythroderma plus bullous formation	> 15 mg/dl	Severe abdominal pain with or without ileus
Grade			
I	Stage 1–2		None
II	Stage 3 or		Stage 1
III	–	Stage 2–3 or	Stage 2–4
IV	Stage 4 or	Stage 4	–

BSA—body surface area; GVHD—graft-versus-host disease

Note. Reprinted from "Acute Graft Versus Host Disease," by D.A. Jacobsohn and G.B. Vogelsang, September 2007, *Orphanet Journal of Rare Diseases, 2*, 35. Copyright 2007 by Jacobsohn and Vogelsang; licensee BioMed Central Ltd. Open access article distributed under the terms of the Creative Commons Attribution License (http://creativecommons .org/licenses/by/2.0). Retrieved September 24, 2008, from http://www.ojrd.com/content/ pdf/1750-1172-2-35.pdf

Newer agents used for prophylaxis include mycophenolate mofetil and sirolimus. Cyclosporine plus methotrexate is the most common combination for GVHD prophylaxis (Iwasaki, 2004). All of these immunosuppressive medications increase the risk of infections. Ex vivo or in vivo T-cell depletion with the use of antithymocyte globulin or alemtuzumab also has been used to prevent GVHD. See Table 8-4 for a review of immunosuppressive medications used for prevention and treatment of GVHD, as well as nursing implications in the administration of these agents.

Chronic Graft-Versus-Host Disease

Chronic GVHD is not only a life-threatening complication but also results in long-term sequelae, which can negatively affect physical functioning and quality of life. The incidence of cGVHD in allogeneic BMT recipients approaches 80% and is dependent on multiple risk factors (Filipovich et al., 2005). The

Table 8-4. Side Effects and Nursing Implications of Immunosuppressive Medications Used in Allogeneic Transplantation

Agent/Drug	Mechanism of Action	Dosing/ Administration	Side Effects	Nursing Implications
Cyclosporine A (Sandimmune®, Neoral®, Novartis Pharmaceuticals)	Prevents interleukin (IL)-2 gene expression, thus impairs IL-2 synthesis and activation of T lymphocytes	Total daily dose is usually 1.5 mg/kg IV q 12h, 0.75 mg/kg q 6h, or 3 mg/kg/day as a continuous infusion, with dosage adjusted to achieve therapeutic levels. IV to PO conversion is approximately 1:3. Dosage is dependent on achieving and sustaining therapeutic blood levels based on laboratory evaluation. Therapeutic monitoring is not required once drug is being tapered.	Metabolic: hyperkalemia and hyperglycemia, hypomagnesemia, hyperlipidemia, hyperuricemia, diabetes mellitus Neurotoxicity: headache, tremors, insomnia, paresthesia, dizziness, seizures Gastrointestinal (GI): diarrhea, nausea, constipation, anorexia, vomiting, abdominal pain, ascites, elevated liver function tests Renal: elevated creatinine, nephrotoxicity Cardiovascular: hypertension, chest pain Hematologic: anemia Cutaneous: acneform rash, striae Other: peripheral edema, infection, impaired wound healing, osteoporosis, gingival hyperplasia, flushing, sweating, hirsutism	• Bioavailability differs between oral solution and capsule formulation. Once a regimen is established, patients should be instructed not to change their formulation or brand. • Take with food. • Instruct patient about importance of strict adherence to the administration schedule and to notify the healthcare team immediately if unable to take medication because of GI side effects. • Monitor serum creatinine, blood urea nitrogen (BUN), potassium, magnesium, glucose, and triglyceride levels. • Avoid potassium-sparing diuretics. • Replete electrolytes as indicated. • Coadministration with grapefruit juice may increase cyclosporine A levels and should be avoided. • Drug-drug interactions can lead to subtherapeutic or toxic cyclosporine A levels. Drugs that inhibit or induce cytochrome P450 are most responsible. • Cyclosporine A trough levels to be drawn prior to the administration of the morning dose. Therefore, doses are usually timed for 10 am and 10 pm to allow trough blood draw at morning clinic visit. Instruct patient to bring dose to clinic and to administer once trough level is drawn.

(Continued on next page)

Table 8-4. Side Effects and Nursing Implications of Immunosuppressive Medications Used in Allogeneic Transplantation (Continued)

Agent/Drug	Mechanism of Action	Dosing/ Administration	Side Effects	Nursing Implications
				• Should not be used simultaneously with tacrolimus. • Tacrolimus should be discontinued 24 hours prior to starting cyclosporine A. In the presence of increased tacrolimus levels, initiation of cyclosporine A should be further delayed. • Doses should be adjusted for renal dysfunction. • Monitor levels carefully in patients with renal or hepatic dysfunction.
Tacrolimus (Prograf®, Fujisawa)	Impairs synthesis of IL-2; prevents T lymphocyte proliferation; interferes with the gene transcription for a variety of cytokines including interferon (IFN)-γ, tumor necrosis factor-α	Total daily dose is usually 1–2 mg PO q 12h; 0.05–0.1 mg/kg/day as a continuous infusion, with dosage adjusted to achieve therapeutic levels. IV to PO conversion is approximately 1:4. Dosage is dependent on achieving and sustaining therapeutic blood levels based on laboratory evaluation.	Metabolic: hyperkalemia and hypokalemia, hyperglycemia, hypomagnesemia, hyperlipidemia, hypophosphatemia, diabetes mellitus Neurotoxicity: headache, tremors, insomnia, paresthesia, dizziness, seizures GI: diarrhea, nausea, constipation, anorexia, vomiting, abdominal pain, ascites, elevated liver function tests Renal: elevated creatinine, nephrotoxicity	• Take on an empty stomach. • Instruct patient on importance of strict adherence to the administration schedule and to notify the healthcare team immediately if unable to take because of GI side effects. • Monitor serum creatinine, BUN, potassium, magnesium, phosphorus, glucose, and triglyceride levels. • Avoid potassium-sparing diuretics. • Replete electrolytes as indicated. • Coadministration with grapefruit juice may increase tacrolimus levels and should be avoided. • Drug-drug interactions can lead to subtherapeutic or toxic tacrolimus levels. Drugs that inhibit or induce cytochrome P450 are most responsible.

(Continued on next page)

Table 8-4. Side Effects and Nursing Implications of Immunosuppressive Medications Used in Allogeneic Transplantation *(Continued)*

Agent/Drug	Mechanism of Action	Dosing/ Administration	Side Effects	Nursing Implications
		Therapeutic monitoring is not required once drug is being tapered.	Cardiovascular: hypertension, chest pain Hematologic: anemia, leukocytosis, thrombocytopenia Cutaneous: pruritus, acneform rash Pulmonary: pleural effusion, atelectasis, dyspnea Other: peripheral edema, infection, impaired wound healing, osteoporosis	• Tacrolimus trough levels to be drawn prior to administration of morning dose. Therefore, doses are usually timed for 10 am and 10 pm to allow trough blood draw at morning clinic visit. Instruct patient to bring dose to clinic and to administer once trough level is drawn. • Should not be used simultaneously with cyclosporine A. • Tacrolimus should be discontinued 24 hours prior to starting cyclosporine A. In the presence of increased cyclosporine A levels, initiation of tacrolimus should usually be further delayed. • Doses should be adjusted for renal dysfunction. • Monitor levels carefully in patients with renal or hepatic dysfunction.
Steroids	The immunosuppressive properties of steroids are related to their ability to decrease cytotoxic T-cell proliferation, inhibit	Dosage varies according to institutional protocols. Dosage ranges from 0.5–2 mg/kg/day q 12h with tapering schedule based on starting dose and patient response.	Metabolic: fluid and electrolyte imbalance, diabetes mellitus, hyperlipidemia Neurotoxicity: tremors, seizures, headache, difficulty concentrating, insomnia GI: GI irritation Cardiovascular: hypertension, arrhythmias	• Usually used in combination with cyclosporine A or tacrolimus. • Consult physical therapy for proximal muscle strengthening exercise program. • Instruct patient in strategies to prevent or treat hyperglycemia and in diabetic self-management. • Administer oral corticosteroids with food/milk to minimize GI upset. • Administer H_2 blockers as ordered.

(Continued on next page)

Table 8-4. Side Effects and Nursing Implications of Immunosuppressive Medications Used in Allogeneic Transplantation *(Continued)*

Agent/Drug	Mechanism of Action	Dosing/ Administration	Side Effects	Nursing Implications
	production of IL-1 and IFN-γ, prevent production of IL-2, and inhibit neutrophil function by stabilization of leukocyte lysosomal membranes and inhibiting chemotaxis.		Cutaneous: bruising, fragile skin Neurotoxicity: tremors, seizures, headache Other: hunger, peripheral edema, infection, impaired wound healing, hirsutism, osteoporosis, weight gain, steroid myopathy, cataracts/glaucoma, Cushingoid changes, psychiatric disturbances (steroid psychosis, mood changes, confusion)	• May increase tacrolimus or cyclosporine A levels. • Report complaints of visual changes and consult ophthalmology. • For patients on long-term steroids or otherwise at risk for experiencing osteopenia (e.g., patients with acute lymphocytic leukemia, postmenopausal), ensure regular dual-energy X-ray absorptiometry scans, calcium and vitamin D supplementation, and specific treatment for osteopenia with antiresorptive agents such as pamidronate and alendronate. • A tapering calendar specifying the dosage to be taken each day can help to facilitate adherence in patients who are on tapering doses of steroids or an alternate-day steroid regimen.
Mycophenolate mofetil (MMF) (CellCept®, Roche)	Antimetabolite that selectively inhibits the proliferation of T and B lymphocytes by interfering with purine nucleotide synthesis	Dosage ranges from 1–1.5 g IV or PO every 12 hours depending upon institutional guidelines.	Metabolic: hyperkalemia and hypokalemia, hyperlipidemia, hypophosphatemia, hyperglycemia Neurotoxicity: headache, insomnia, tremors, seizures GI: diarrhea, nausea, constipation, anorexia, vomiting, abdominal pain, hepatotoxicity	• MMF should be taken on an empty stomach. • Monitor complete blood count at regular intervals, and adjust dosage for pancytopenia, as ordered. • Monitor liver function tests (bilirubin and serum transaminases) at regular intervals, and adjust dosage for liver function abnormalities, as ordered. • Monitor serum levels of the MMF metabolic to guide treatment in patients with renal dysfunction.

(Continued on next page)

Table 8-4. Side Effects and Nursing Implications of Immunosuppressive Medications Used in Allogeneic Transplantation *(Continued)*

Agent/Drug	Mechanism of Action	Dosing/ Administration	Side Effects	Nursing Implications
			Renal: elevated creatinine, nephrotoxicity Cardiovascular: hypertension, hypotension, arrhythmias Hematologic: anemia, leukocytosis, thrombocytopenia Cutaneous: acneform rash Pulmonary: cough, dyspnea Other: fever, edema, pain, infection, muscle weakness, anxiety, depression	• In the setting of renal impairment, or when coadministered with probenecid, acyclovir, or ganciclovir, the drug concentrations of MMF and of these drugs may increase. • There may be decreased MMF absorption when coadministered with magnesium oxide, aluminum- or magnesium-containing antacids, or cholestyramine.
Methotrexate	Antimetabolite that inhibits dihydrofolate reductase, thereby hindering DNA synthesis and cell reproduction, and thus inhibiting lymphocyte proliferation	Institutional protocols vary. Usual dose is 5–15 mg/m² given IV on days +1, +3, +6, and +11 after transplantation.	Myelosuppression, mucositis, photosensitivity, interstitial pneumonitis, hepatotoxicity, nephrotoxicity	• Doses may be adjusted or held for severe mucositis and renal or liver insufficiency. • Doses may need to be adjusted for hypoalbuminemia. • Wait at least 24 hours following stem cell infusion to give day +1 dose.

(Continued on next page)

Table 8-4. Side Effects and Nursing Implications of Immunosuppressive Medications Used in Allogeneic Transplantation *(Continued)*

Agent/Drug	Mechanism of Action	Dosing/ Administration	Side Effects	Nursing Implications
Antithymocyte globulin (ATG) (ATGAM®, Pfizer Inc., equine; Thymoglobulin®, SangStat, rabbit)	Polyclonal immunoglobulin composed of horse or rabbit antibodies capable of destroying human leukocytes	Institutional protocols vary; usual dose is 10–40 mg/kg/day for equine ATG and 2.5 mg/kg/day for rabbit ATG	Adverse reactions include fever, chills, seizures, laryngospasm, anaphylaxis, pulmonary edema, leukopenia, and thrombocytopenia. Because ATG is a foreign xenogeneic protein and an antibody, serum sickness can occur, including myalgias, arthralgias, and hand and facial edema.	• Monitor patient closely, both during and following infusion, for signs of serum sickness and anaphylaxis. Consider premedication with corticosteroids, acetaminophen, and H_1 and H_2 blockers. • Medications for treating hypersensitivity reactions (e.g., acetaminophen, antihistamines, corticosteroids, epinephrine) and supplemental oxygen should be available for immediate use in the event of a reaction. • Because transient and at times severe thrombocytopenia may occur following ATG administration in patients with platelets counts less than 100,000, monitor platelet count one hour following ATG administration and transfuse platelets as indicated.
Alemtuzumab (Campath-1®, Berlex Laboratories)	Monoclonal antibody directed against the cell surface antigen CD52, which is expressed on B and T lymphocytes	Institutional protocols vary; usual dose is 20 mg/day IV given over several hours for five days, beginning before transplantation.	Infusional toxicities may be severe and include fever and rigors in more than 80% of patients. Other adverse effects include neutropenia, anemia, thrombocytopenia, nausea, vomiting, rash, fatigue, and hypotension.	• Premedicate patient with acetaminophen and diphenhydramine. • Medications for treating hypersensitivity reactions (e.g., acetaminophen, antihistamines, corticosteroids, epinephrine) and supplemental oxygen should be available for immediate use in the event of a reaction. • Consider treatment with meperidine to control infusional rigors. • Administer fluid bolus as ordered to treat hypotension.

(Continued on next page)

Table 8-4. Side Effects and Nursing Implications of Immunosuppressive Medications Used in Allogeneic Transplantation *(Continued)*

Agent/Drug	Mechanism of Action	Dosing/ Administration	Side Effects	Nursing Implications
				• Produces profound and rapid lymphopenia; therefore, patients require broad antifungal, antibacterial, antiviral, and antiprotozoal prophylaxis for at least four months following treatment and ongoing surveillance for cytomegalovirus and adenovirus infection.
Rapamycin (Sirolimus®, Wyeth Laboratories)	Structurally similar to tacrolimus and cyclosporine A; however, it has a distinct immunosuppressant activity. Sirolimus inhibits response of B and T lymphocytes to cytokine stimulation by IL-2 and inhibits antibody production by B cells.	Long half-life permits once-daily dosing. Monitor trough blood levels.	Hyperlipidemia, thrombocytopenia, leucopenia, headache, nausea, anorexia, dizziness	• May suppress hematopoietic recovery if used in patients who have recently undergone high-dose therapy • Oral bioavailability is variable and is improved with high-fat meals. • Like tacrolimus and cyclosporine A, it is metabolized through the cytochrome P450-3A system.

Note. From "Graft Versus Host Disease" (pp. 100–104), by S.A. Mitchell in S.E. Ezzone (Ed.), *Hematopoietic Stem Cell Transplantation: A Manual for Nursing Practice,* 2004, Pittsburgh, PA: Oncology Nursing Society. Copyright 2004 by Oncology Nursing Society. Adapted with permission.

incidence is rising secondary to an increased use of DLI, a growing number of older transplant recipients and donors, the types of transplantations being performed, and an increase in the number of BMT survivors.

Risk factors for the development of cGVHD include (Filipovich et al. 2005)

- Prior aGVHD
- Older patient age
- The use of female donors for male recipients
- The use of DLI
- The use of unrelated or HLA-mismatched donors
- The use of peripheral blood grafts.

The pathophysiology of cGVHD is not completely understood but is thought to be similar to autoimmune diseases. Chronic GVHD is thought to be the result of autoreactive T cells that have escaped negative selection in the thymus because of thymic damage by the conditioning regimen, aGVHD, or age-related thymic atrophy. The autoreactive T cells promote the synthesis of autoantibodies against host tissues (Iwasaki, 2004). The role of various T-cell subsets, the interaction of T cells with B cells, and the role of various cytokines are all areas of active inquiry into the pathophysiology of cGVHD (Baird & Pavletic, 2006).

Chronic GVHD can affect almost any tissue. Systems commonly affected include the skin, eyes, oral cavity, GI tract, and liver. Less commonly, cGVHD will involve the lungs, nails, scalp and body hair, genitalia, muscles, fascia, and joints. Chronic GVHD may affect a single organ or tissue or multiple tissues. Chronic GVHD has features that resemble autoimmune or immunologic disorders, including (Filipovich et al., 2005)

- Scleroderma
- Sjögren syndrome
- Primary biliary cirrhosis
- Wasting syndrome
- Bronchiolitis obliterans
- Cytopenias
- Chronic immunodeficiency.

Symptoms usually present within the first year following BMT. The majority of BMT recipients that experience cGVHD have had prior aGVHD (Jacobsohn & Vogelsang, 2007). Chronic GVHD may occur after a period of recovery from aGVHD, without a history of prior aGVHD, or as an abrupt onset involving multiple systems with manifestations of both acute and chronic GVHD (Schaffer, 2006; Vogelsang & McDonough, 2004). Depending on the systems involved, cGVHD can have debilitating effects, such as limited joint function because of skin or muscle involvement and restrictive lung disease because of lung involvement. Immunosuppressive therapies used to treat cGVHD frequently lead to recurrent and life-threatening infections. The leading cause of nonrelapse mortality after day 100 following transplantation is cGVHD and associated infections (Filipovich et al., 2005). The three-year survival rate for cGVHD is 60% (Baird & Pavletic, 2006; Pavletic et al., 2005). Chronic GVHD is one of the most common and significant problems affecting long-term survivors and was correlated with poor quality-of-life scores (Lee et al., 2006).

Chronic GVHD may take on several forms and patterns and may exhibit a variety of different stages. Similar to aGVHD, cutaneous involvement is the most commonly involved system (Aractingi & Chosidow, 1998). Cutaneous manifestations of cGVHD are divided into the following five main subtypes (Filipovich et al., 2005):

- Poikiloderma
- Lichen planus–like eruptions
- Deep sclerotic features
- Morphea-like features or
- Lichen sclerosus–like features.

Poikiloderma presents as pigmentary changes with variegated colors. Poikiloderma skin changes may present with areas of hypo- or hyperpigmentation. The epidermis becomes thin with a cigarette-paper appearance. Poikilodermatous changes are a hallmark sign of cutaneous cGVHD. Poikilodermatous changes are commonly seen on the face, lateral neck, and trunk (Hausermann, 2008). See Figure 8-4 for poikiloderma cutaneous changes.

Lichen planus–like changes resemble an inflammatory skin condition appearing as a confluent rash or raised bumps that can be isolated appearing in a linear or folliculocentric pattern or even across a dermatome (Hymes, Turner, Champlin, & Couriel, 2006). The rash may reveal vesicles. Lichen planus-like changes may begin with dry skin that resembles fish scales, called *ichthyosis*. Lichen planus–like lesions often appear erythematous or as viola-

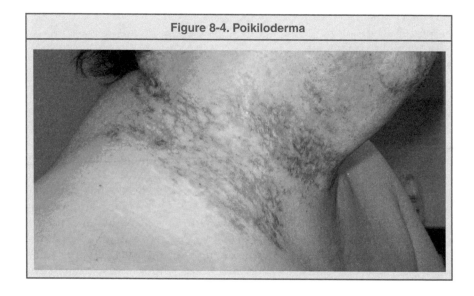

Figure 8-4. Poikiloderma

ceous papules commonly occurring on the dorsal aspect of the hands, forearms, and trunk. Lichen planus–like lesions are commonly seen and may overlap with lichen sclerosis-like lesions (Hymes et al.). See Figure 8-5 for lichen planus–type cutaneous changes.

Deep, sclerotic features of cGVHD involve the dermis and/or the muscular fascia. The skin may appear smooth, waxy, indurated, thickened, or tight. The tightness and thickness are attributable to deep and diffuse sclerosis over a wide area (Filipovich et al., 2005). See Figure 8-6 for cGVHD sclerotic skin changes. Skin may be hidebound or fixed to underlying tissue and is unable to be pinched (Pavletic, Lee, Socie, & Vogelsang, 2006). Joint contractures and stiffness from sclerosis or hidebound skin can drastically reduce physical mobility, independence, and quality of life. See Figure 8-7 for joint contractures associated with cGVHD fasciitis and sclerosis. Deep, sclerotic changes in the lower extremities can result in thin legs with the appearance of "pipestem" legs. An additional problem is the possibility of neuropathy further reducing mobility (Hymes et al., 2006).

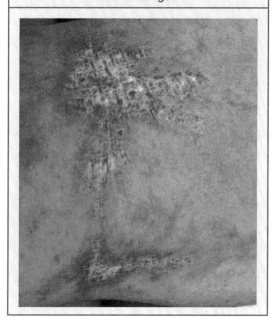

Figure 8-5. Lichen Planus–Type Skin Changes

Morphea-like superficial sclerotic features include a localized patchy area of moveable smooth or shiny skin with a leathery appearance. Lichen sclerosus–like lesions are discrete or coalescent, gray to white in color, with moveable plaques with a shiny appearance and a leather consistency (Filipovich et al., 2005). Chronic GVHD may take on a cellulite appearance with ripples or dimples occurring in the skin. Pain and edema often precede the development of the cellulite appearance. There may be a "groove sign" or depression along the course of a vein, between muscle groups, or both. These signs are evidence of fibrosis of the fascia and subcutaneous septae (Schaffer, 2006).

Additional cutaneous changes associated with cGVHD include loss of pigmentation, areas of alopecia, sweat gland destruction, and blistering. The palms and soles may develop vesicles and a scaly appearance similar to eczema. Ulcers may develop, placing the patient at risk for secondary infections that can be life threatening (Hymes et al., 2006). See Figures 8-8 and 8-9 for cGVHD with ulcer development.

Chronic GVHD of the skin is diagnosed based on clinical features; however, skin biopsy is helpful in confirming the diagnosis (Shulman et al., 2006). His-

Figure 8-6. Chronic Graft-Versus-Host Disease Sclerotic Skin Changes

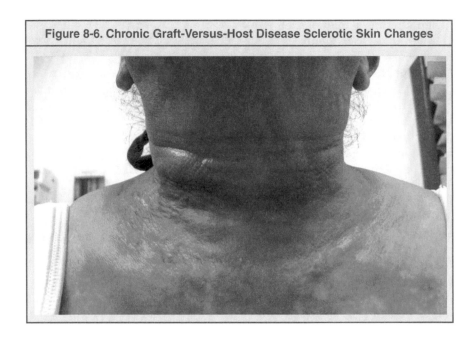

Figure 8-7. Joint Contractures Associated With Chronic Graft-Versus-Host Disease Fasciitis and Sclerosis

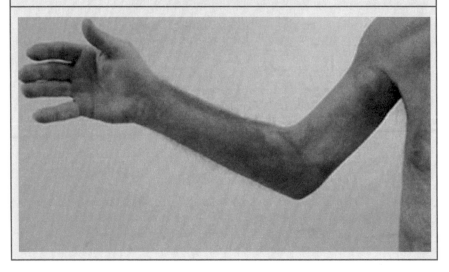

Figure 8-8. Chronic Graft-Versus-Host Disease (GVHD) With Ulcers

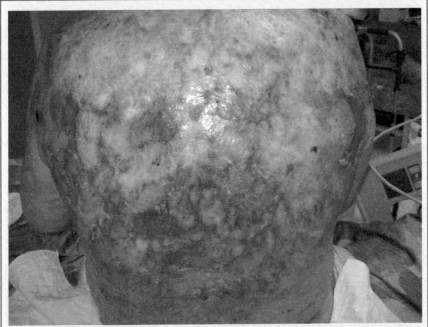

Patient two years and four months after a nonmyeloablative allogeneic transplant with chronic GVHD. Severe chronic GVHD of the skin with diffuse erythema, and sclerotic changes. Multiple raw areas of desquamation and ulcers.

Current immunosuppression: ECP twice a week, prednisone 20 mg daily, Prograft 1 mg daily

tologic interpretation of biopsies is confounded by immunosuppressive agents, concurrent infections, drug reactions, and change in histologic characteristics over time, as well as the site and timing of the biopsies (Shulman et al.). Table 8-5 reviews the histologic criteria for diagnosing cutaneous cGVHD.

The National Institutes of Health (NIH) Working Group recommends that the diagnosis of cutaneous cGVHD require at least one diagnostic manifestation of cGVHD or at least one distinctive manifestation with a confirmed diagnosis by pertinent biopsy, laboratory test, or radiology test (Filipovich et al., 2005). Diagnostic signs and symptoms refer to those manifestations that establish the presence of cGVHD without the need for further testing or evidence of other organ involvement. The presence of poikiloderma, lichen planus–like features, morphea-like features, and lichen sclerosus–like features are diagnostic features that would establish a diagnosis of cGVHD. Distinctive signs and symptoms of cGVHD refer to those manifestations that are not ordinarily found in aGVHD but are not considered sufficient to establish an unequivocal diagnosis of cGVHD without further testing or additional organ involvement (Filipovich, 2008). A distinctive feature of cutaneous cGVHD would be depigmentation.

Clinical Staging of Chronic Graft-Versus-Host Disease

The initial grading system for cGVHD consisted of limited or extensive disease according to clinical characteristics and laboratory features. However, in 2005, NIH proposed new consensus criteria to grade cGVHD to better predict outcomes. GVHD diagnosed after day 100 was classified as cGVHD. However,

Figure 8-9. Chronic Graft-Versus-Host Disease (GVHD) With Healed Ulcers

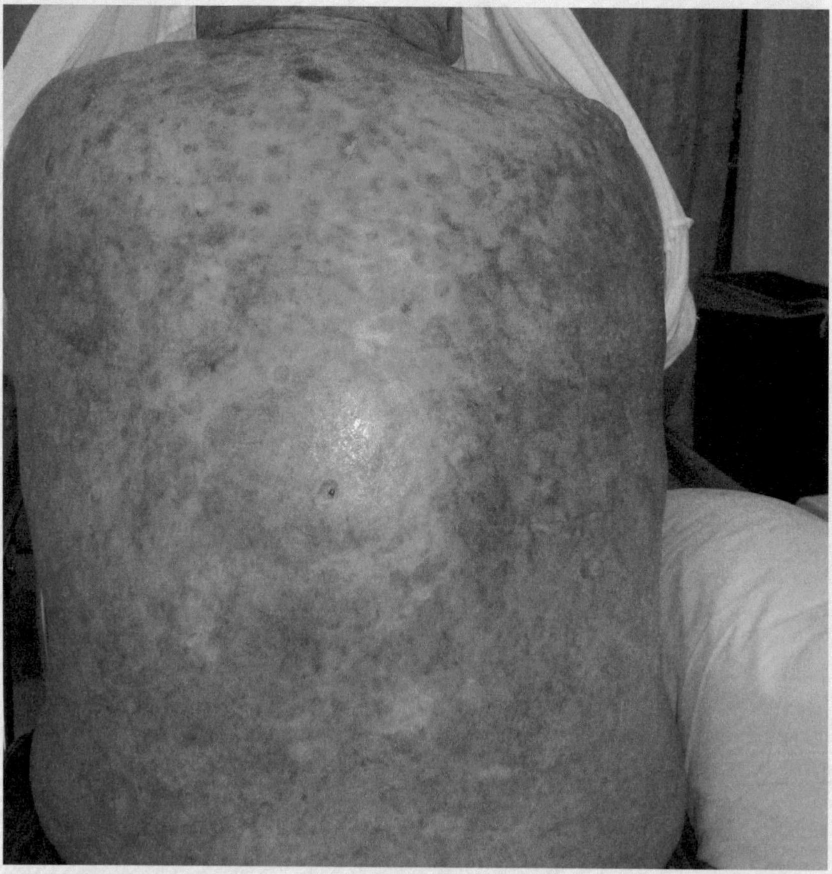

Patient three years and six months after a nonmyeloablative allogeneic transplant with chronic GVHD. Severe chronic GVHD of the skin with erythematous ashy violaceous patches, plaques, and sclerodermatous changes with hidebound skin.

Current immunosuppression: Prednisone 15 mg alternating every other day with 20 mg, ECP twice every four weeks.

Table 8-5. Cutaneous Histologic Criteria for Graft-Versus-Host Disease (GVHD)

Organ or System	Minimal Criteria for Active* GVHD	Specific Criteria for Chronic[†] GVHD
Skin, any stage	Apoptoses in epidermal basal layer or lower malphigian layer or outer root sheath of hair follicle or acrosyringium ± lichenoid inflammation ± vacuolar change ± lymphocytic satellitosis	–
Skin lichen planus–like	–	Combination of epidermal orthorkeratosis, hypergranulosis, and acanthosis with lichenoid changes ± syringitis of eccrine units ± panniculitis
Skin sclerotic	–	Collagenous deposition with thickening throughout the papillary dermis, or pan-dermal collagenosis ± panniculitis
Skin morpheic	–	Clinically focal or localized lesion predominated by sclerosis in the lower reticular dermis or along the dermal-hypodermal border ± epidermal and appendigeal involvement
Skin fasciitis	–	Fibrous thickening of fascial septa with adjacent inflammation ± panniculitis

* Conditions that result in lesser degrees of change include immunosuppressive treatment, biopsy very soon after the onset of signs, suboptimal or small tissue sample, insufficient serial sectioning, confounding infection, drug reaction, or inflammatory conditions.

[†]Once the diagnosis of chronic GVHD has been established or after immunosuppressive treatment, the histologic manifestations of active disease may meet only minimal diagnostic criteria for activity.

Note. From "Histopathologic Diagnosis of Chronic Graft-Versus-Host Disease: National Institutes of Health Consensus Development Project on Criteria for Clinical Trials in Chronic Graft-Versus-Host Disease: II. Pathology Working Group Report," by H.M. Shulman, D. Kleiner, S.J. Lee, T. Morton, S.Z. Pavletic, E. Farmer, et al., 2006, *Biology of Blood and Marrow Transplantation, 12*(1), p. 34. Copyright 2006 American Society for Blood and Marrow Transplantation. Adapted with permission.

this distinction of before day 100 and after day 100 is no longer clear cut, as characteristics of cGVAD and aGVHD have been found to appear outside of the indicated time frame. Factors contributing to blurring of the time frame for the occurrence of cGVHD include increased utilization of nonmyeloablative conditioning regimens and DLI (Hymes et al., 2006; Penas, Fernandez-Herrera, & Garcia-Diez, 2004).

cGVHD may now be categorized as *classic cGVHD* (features of cGVHD only) or *overlap* (features of acute and chronic) without a time limit after the transplantation date or DLI infusion (Filipovich et al., 2005). Table 8-1 describes the categories of cGVHD. The consensus global scoring system for cGVHD is based on both the severity and the functionality of each involved system. The scoring system considers the clinical manifestations, laboratory findings, and functionality of the target organ (Filipovich et al., 2005). *Mild* cGVHD involves one or two organs or sites (excluding the lungs) with no functional impairment. *Moderate* cGVHD involves at least one organ or site with clinically significant but no major disability. *Severe* cGVHD indicates major disability in any organ or site. Table 8-6 reviews the scoring system for *cutaneous* cGVHD. As this new scoring system is validated and adopted more widely, it will provide a common language for classifying cGVHD and direct therapy to the population that is at the highest risk of mortality. Standardized grad-

Table 8-6. Consensus Scoring System for Cutaneous Chronic Graft-Versus-Host Disease

Skin—Clinical Features	Score 0	Score 1	Score 2	Score 3
• Maculopapular rash • Lichen planus–like features • Papulosquamous lesions or ichthyosis • Hyperpigmentation • Hypopigmentation • Keratosis pilaris • Erythema • Erythroderma • Poikiloderma • Sclerotic features • Pruritus • Hair involvement • Nail involvement	No symptoms	< 18% BSA with disease signs but no sclerotic features	19%–50% BSA or involvement with superficial sclerotic features "not hidebound" (able to pinch)	> 50% BSA or deep sclerotic features "hidebound" (unable to pinch) or impaired mobility, ulceration or severe pruritus

Note. From "National Institutes of Health Consensus Development Project on Criteria for Clinical Trials in Chronic Graft-Versus-Host Disease: I. Diagnosis and Staging Working Group Report," by A.H. Filipovich, D. Weisdorf, S. Pavletic, G. Socie, J.R. Wingard, S.J. Lee, et al., 2005, *Biology of Blood and Marrow Transplantation, 11*(12), p. 952. Copyright 2005 by American Society for Blood and Marrow Transplantation. Adapted with permission.

ing also will facilitate the interpretation of cGVHD clinical trial results (Jagasia et al., 2007).

Prevention and Management of Chronic Graft-Versus-Host Disease

Therapies for the management of cGVHD rely on the same immunosuppressive medications used to prevent and treat aGVHD. However, the duration of therapy is different, often lasting months to years. Initial management of cGVHD usually involves systemic steroids. Grade II or higher GVHD is initially treated with steroids dosed at 2 mg/kg/day and then tapered as the mainstay of treatment (Jagasia et al., 2007). The duration and dosing of steroids is not standardized but usually continues until symptoms of cGVHD have resolved or stabilized. Although steroids are considered the mainstay of treatment, not all patients respond. Steroid resistance or steroid dependence may develop. *Steroid resistance* is defined as occurring when cGVHD does not respond to a certain dose of steroids over a defined period of time. *Steroid dependence* is defined as the inability to wean the steroid dose without a flare in symptoms (Scarisbrick et al., 2008). Calcineurin inhibitors (tacrolimus, cyclosporin) are given in conjunction with systemic steroids for clinically significant cGVHD (Jagasia et al.). A variety of immunosuppressant therapies have been tested, but no clear advantage of any one agent has been demonstrated. Mycophenolate mofetil and sirolimus are newer agents being evaluated for their use in cGVHD and generally are used in conjunction with both a calcineurin inhibitor and prednisone. Low-dose methotrexate also has been used to treat refractory cGVHD in small studies (Baird & Pavletic, 2006).

Patients with minimal cutaneous cGVHD may be treated with topical steroids or tacrolimus (Jagasia et al., 2007; Schaffer, 2006). It is difficult to evaluate the effectiveness of topical agents, as the literature includes only case studies or studies with small sample sizes and unclear response criteria (Choi & Nghiem, 2001).

Extracorporeal photopheresis (ECP) has been used for cGVHD therapy for more than 20 years and is now being evaluated in aGVHD. The mechanism of action of ECP is poorly understood, although it is known to affect the balance between T helper cells and dendritic cells. Through the process of apheresis, the mononuclear cells are exposed to ultraviolet light and methoxypsoralen, which shifts cytokines and destroys T lymphocytes (Baird & Pavletic, 2006; Schaffer, 2006). ECP commonly is used for steroid-refractory cGVHD. Many of the studies evaluating ECP had small sample sizes, differing treatment schedules, different response criteria, and varying definitions of cGVHD. Thus, the benefit of ECP in the literature is difficult to interpret (Couriel et al., 2006). In general, the response rate appears to be favorable, especially for skin but also for liver, eye, and oral manifestations (Baird & Pavletic, 2006; Couriel et al.; Scarisbrick et al., 2008). ECP is a safe and well-tolerated treatment option for patients with cutaneous GVHD compared to the alternative of long-term immunosuppressive therapy. Current treatment frequency and time to best response are unknown, although the majority of patients show some response after three to four months of treatment (Scarisbrick et al.).

Palmar-Plantar Erythrodysesthesia

PPE is also known as hand-foot syndrome (see Figure 8-10). It is a painful erythematous rash that occurs most often on the palms of the hands and soles of the feet; less commonly, the changes occur in skinfolds or the groin area. PPE is not well described in the BMT literature; however, it is a well-documented problem associated with various chemotherapy agents, including liposomal doxorubicin, capecitabine, docetaxel, cytarabine, and 5-fluorouracil (Remlinger, 2003). In the myeloablative transplantation setting, PPE is associated with the combination of high-dose chemotherapies used in preparative regimens, particularly etoposide (Murphy, Harden, & Herzig, 1993; Wright, 2006). The pathophysiology of PPE in the BMT setting is not well understood, but it is hypothesized to be a direct effect of chemotherapy agents on the dermal structures where there is a high concentration of eccrine glands (Murphy et al.).

PPE begins as erythema and edema and eventually progresses to desquamation. As the desquamation occurs, the affected area may develop a secondary fungal infection—especially in the skinfolds and groin area where moisture accumulates. Topical antifungals can be used for both the prevention and treatment of secondary fungal infection (Haisfield-Wolfe & Rund, 2000). Patients experience sensitivity to touch and potentially paresthesia. PPE is of-

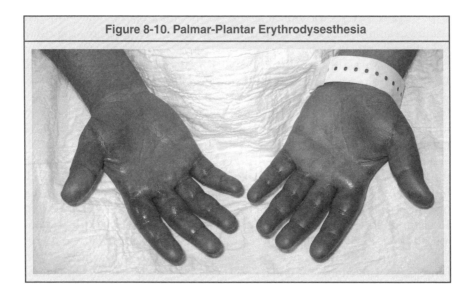

Figure 8-10. Palmar-Plantar Erythrodysesthesia

ten associated with pain, and pain management is a key component of nursing care. PPE resolves in approximately two weeks, typically with the return of the white blood cell count or engraftment. No known preventive strategies exist for PPE; therefore, nursing care focuses primarily on symptom management measures. Corticosteroids may help to relieve symptoms (Murphy et al., 1993). Maintaining a clean and dry environment where areas of desquamation occur is of utmost importance in preventing secondary infections.

Nursing Implications for Cutaneous Graft-Versus-Host Disease and Palmar-Plantar Erythrodysesthesia

The successful care of a BMT recipient experiencing cutaneous changes relies on an astute nursing team who recognizes early changes, proceeds with interventions and infection prophylaxis, and prioritizes patient education. Daily, thorough cutaneous assessment is crucial for patients undergoing BMT. Assessing the face, extremities, torso, palms, soles of the feet, and perineum for dryness, erythema, rashes, lesions, or bullae on a daily basis can help with early detection and implementation of interventions. Delayed healing is common in this patient population because of the effects of chemotherapy and immunosuppressive medications. Immunosuppressive medications, especially steroids, contribute to infectious risks and preventing wound healing, leading to an increased risk of mortality. Therefore, it is critical for BMT nurses to continually reinforce meticulous hygiene and other infection prevention measures.

Often, the cutaneous changes seen in GVHD take weeks to months to heal. It is beneficial to have a consistent assessment team follow the patient's progress. If a clinical nurse specialist or wound care nurse is not available to follow the patient on a consistent basis, establishing unit-based nursing experts on skin care is an alternative. Unit-based nursing experts can be created from self-selected nurses who exhibit interest and motivation in developing their expertise on a specific transplant-related complication. Developing a core group of unit-based nursing experts who focus primarily on skin care has the potential to improve the quality of care for BMT recipients suffering from cutaneous complications of transplantation. The unit-based nursing experts also can help less experienced staff learn principles of good wound care and assist with complicated dressing changes for patients with severe skin toxicities. Effective nursing management of skin toxicities requires consistent assessment, symptom management, meticulous skin care, and patient/family education. Photographing changes at regular intervals to provide documentation is helpful in monitoring response to treatment. These photographs are particularly important when multiple practitioners and disciplines are providing care.

Patient education is essential for the prevention and treatment of skin toxicities. Nursing patient education must include methods to prevent skin breakdown and infection. Aggressive use of moisturizers, daily cleansing, specialty beds, administration of antimicrobial and antiviral agents, pain management, thermal regulation, exudate management, and the diligent use of sunscreen are important factors not only for BMT recipients at risk for cutaneous changes but also for patients who are experiencing cutaneous GVHD or have wounds. Nurses must involve the multidisciplinary team in the patient's care. Proper nutrition and physical therapy are essential components to the recovery of BMT recipients experiencing cutaneous changes. Allogeneic transplant recipients must be taught to avoid direct sunlight and use sunscreen to prevent GVHD triggered by sunlight exposure. Furthermore, all patients must be taught to report skin changes such as rashes, dryness, lesions, and blisters to the BMT team as early as possible.

No evidence-based practice guidelines, standards of care, or recommendations have been published on the nursing management of cutaneous GVHD and PPE in the BMT population. Therefore, proactive nursing management of these unique cutaneous changes is vital in order to achieve a positive outcome.

Conclusion

For BMT recipients, cutaneous manifestations are significant problems that range from mild to severe and often are associated with pain, altered mobility, changes in body image, and lengthy hospitalization. The consequences of severe cutaneous changes can be life-threatening and negatively affect quality of life. Nurses play a key role in coordinating the complex care that is necessary for BMT recipients experiencing cutaneous toxicity. A great deal of research interest exists regarding the prevention and treatment of GVHD; however, little effort has been aimed at establishing standards of practice for the management of the complex cutaneous toxicities seen in BMT recipients. Nurses are in a pivotal position to establish standards of care as well as to develop research that is designed to test interventions for the best management for cutaneous toxicities seen in BMT recipients. While awaiting evidence-based practice guidelines, the development of unit-based nursing experts is one strategy for improving the management of cutaneous toxicities following BMT.

References

Aractingi, S., & Chosidow, O. (1998). Cutaneous graft-versus-host disease. *Archives of Dermatology, 134*(5), 602–612.

Bacigalupo, A. (2007). Management of acute graft-versus-host disease. *British Journal of Haematology, 137*(2), 87–98.

Baird, K., & Pavletic, S.Z. (2006). Chronic graft versus host disease. *Current Opinion in Hematology, 13*(6), 426–435.

Choi, C.J., & Nghiem, P. (2001). Tacrolimus ointment in the treatment of chronic cutaneous graft-versus-host disease: A case series of 18 patients. *Archives of Dermatology, 137*(9), 1202–1206.

Collins, R.H., Shpilberg, O., Drobyski, W., Porter, D., Giralt, S., Champlin, R., et al. (1997). Donor leukocyte infusions in 140 patients with relapsed malignancy after allogeneic bone marrow transplantation. *Journal of Clinical Oncology, 15*(2), 433–444.

Couriel, D., Hosing, C., Saliba, R., Shpall, E.J., Andelini, P., Popat, U., et al. (2006). Extracorporeal photopheresis for acute and chronic graft-versus-host disease: Does it work? *Biology of Blood and Marrow Transplantation, 12*(1, Suppl. 2), 37–40.

Filipovich, A.H. (2008). Diagnosis and manifestations of chronic graft-versus-host disease. *Best Practice and Research Clinical Haematology, 21*(2), 251–257.

Filipovich, A.H., Weisdorf, D., Pavletic, S., Socie, G., Wingard, J.R., Lee, S.J., et al. (2005). National Institutes of Health Consensus Development Project on criteria for clinical trials in chronic graft-versus-host disease: I. Diagnosis and Staging Working Group Report. *Biology of Blood and Marrow Transplantation, 11*(12), 945–956.

Haisfield-Wolfe, M.E., & Rund, C. (2000). A nursing protocol for the management of perineal-rectal skin alterations. *Clinical Journal of Oncology Nursing, 4*(1), 15–21.

Hausermann, P., Walter, R.B., Halter, J., Biedermann, B.C., Tichelli, A., Itin, P., et al. (2008). Cutaneous graft-versus-host disease: A guide for the dermatologist. *Dermatology, 216*(4), 287–304.

Hymes, S.R., Turner, M.L., Champlin, R.E., & Couriel, D.R. (2006). Cutaneous manifestations of chronic graft-versus-host disease. *Biology of Blood and Marrow Transplantation, 12*(11), 1101–1113.

Iwasaki, T. (2004). Recent advances in the treatment of graft-versus-host disease. *Clinical Medicine and Research, 2*(4), 243–252.

Jacobsohn, D.A., & Vogelsang, G.B. (2007, September). Acute graft versus host disease. *Orphanet Journal of Rare Diseases, 2,* 35.

Jagasia, M., Giglia, J., Chinratanalab, W., Dixon, S., Chen, H., Frangoul, H., et al. (2007). Incidence and outcome of chronic graft-versus-host disease using National Institutes of Health consensus criteria. *Biology of Blood and Marrow Transplantation, 13*(10), 1207–1215.

Lee, S.J., Kim, H.T., Ho, V.T., Cutler, C., Alyea, E.P., Soiffer, R.J., et al. (2006). Quality of life associated with acute and chronic graft-versus-host disease. *Bone Marrow Transplantation, 38*(4), 305–310.

Murphy, C.P., Harden, E.A., & Herzig, R.H. (1993). Dose-related cutaneous toxicities with etoposide. *Cancer, 71*(10), 3153–3155.

Pavletic, S.Z., Lee, S.J., Socie, G., & Vogelsang, G. (2006). Chronic graft-versus-host disease: Implications of the National Institutes of Health consensus development project on criteria for clinical trials. *Bone Marrow Transplantation, 38*(10), 645–651.

Pavletic, S.Z., Smith, L.M., Bishop, M.R., Lynch, J.C., Tarantolo, S.R., Vose, J.M., et al. (2005). Prognostic factors of chronic graft-versus-host disease after allogeneic blood stem-cell transplantation. *American Journal of Hematology, 78*(4), 265–274.

Penas, P.F., Fernandez-Herrera, J., & Garcia-Diez, A. (2004). Dermatologic treatment of cutaneous graft-versus-host disease. *American Journal of Clinical Dermatology, 5*(6), 403–416.

Remlinger, K.A. (2003). Cutaneous reactions to chemotherapy drugs: The art of consultation. *Archives of Dermatology, 139*(1), 77–81.

Scarisbrick, J.J., Taylor, P., Holtick, U., Makar, Y., Douglas, K., Berlin, G., et al. (2008). U.K. consensus statement on the use of extracorporeal photopheresis for treatment of cutaneous T-cell lymphoma and chronic graft-versus-host disease. *British Journal of Dermatology, 158*(4), 659–678.

Schaffer, J.V. (2006). The changing face of graft-versus-host disease. *Seminars in Cutaneous Medicine and Surgery, 25*(4), 190–200.

Shulman, H.M., Kleiner, D., Lee, S.J., Morton, T., Pavletic, S.Z., Farmer, E., et al. (2006). Histopathologic diagnosis of chronic graft-versus-host disease: National Institutes of Health Consensus Development Project on criteria for clinical trials in chronic graft-versus-host disease: II. Pathology Working Group Report. *Biology of Blood and Marrow Transplantation, 12*(1), 31–47.

Vogelsang, G.B., & McDonough, C.H. (2004). Chronic graft-versus-host disease after transplantation. In R. Soiffer (Ed.), *Stem cell transplantation for hematologic malignancies* (pp. 185–200). Totowa, NJ: Humaba Press.

Wright, L.G. (2006). Maculopapular skin rashes associated with high-dose chemotherapy: Prevalence and risk factors. *Oncology Nursing Forum, 33*(6), 1095–1103.

CHAPTER 9

Impact of Chronic Disease on Wound Healing

Pamela Savage, RN, MAEd, CON(C), and Claudia Ganson, RN, BScN, ET

Introduction

The world's population is aging, and while people are living longer, they often do so with a host of chronic diseases. Diseases such as heart disease, cancer, and diabetes are the leading causes of death and disability in the United States, accounting for 70% of the 1.7 million deaths that occur each year. In 2005, 133 million people—almost half of all Americans—lived with at least one chronic condition (Centers for Disease Control and Prevention [CDC], 2008). *Chronic disease* is characterized by a longer duration, often months or years, and usually is associated with symptoms of less severe intensity than those associated with acute disease. Chronic disease is much more prevalent with advanced age. Currently, vaccines are not available for the prevention of most chronic diseases; however, lifestyle changes and medical treatment may alter the course of some diseases. Consequently, oncology clinicians are likely to treat patients who have chronic diseases in addition to their cancer diagnosis. A number of diseases are classified as chronic, including the following (MedicineNet.com, 2004):
- Diabetes
- Chronic pulmonary disease
- Chronic renal failure
- Arthritis
- Obesity
- Cardiovascular and peripheral vascular disease
- Some cancers.

It is important to recognize that patients with these conditions are at a higher risk for developing myriad skin conditions and chronic wounds (see Table 9-1). This chapter will focus on the impact of the most common chronic diseases and their relationship to wound healing.

Table 9-1. Ulcer Type and Chronic Diseases							
Ulcer Type	**Diabetes**	**Chronic Obstructive Pulmonary Disease**	**Chronic Kidney Disease**	**Arthritis**	**Cardiovascular Disease**	**Peripheral Arterial and Venous Diseases**	**Obesity**
Arterial ulcers	X					X	
Diabetic foot ulcers	X		X			X	X
Pressure ulcers related to decreased mobility		X	X	X	X	X	X
Venous ulcers						X	X
X identifies the types of ulcers that are commonly associated with the chronic disease.							

The disrupting effect of chronic disease on wound repair is not restricted to the pathology related to the disease alone but can be further complicated by the medications and treatments that are required to treat the disease. This complex relationship of disease pathologies and their respective treatments can potentially impact the risk of wound development as well as impede wound healing. In fact, such comorbidities may cause the disruption in any one or all of the phases of the normally orderly sequence of wound healing. Cancer treatments such as systemic chemotherapy and radiation are known to disrupt one or all of the phases of wound healing. Unfortunately, this disruption results in some individuals living their entire life with an open, non-healing chronic wound. It is important for clinicians to have a fundamental understanding of wound healing and to consider what phase of wound healing may be affected by chronic disease and the treatment for cancer (see Table 9-2).

Overview of Wound Healing

Normal wound healing consists of four phases and is analogous to the construction of a house, as the process is one of order and predictability (Kane, 2007). This orderly process is essential for the success of the restructuring and closure of the broken skin. A protracted delay in wound healing is referred to as a *chronic wound*. Chronic wounds are the result of interrupted tissue repair and reconstruction. The reasons for the delay or interruption may not be known but commonly are thought to be the result of any or a combi-

Table 9-2. Phases of Wound Healing Affected by Chronic Diseases				
Disease	Phase 1 Hemostasis	Phase 2 Inflammatory	Phase 3 Proliferation	Phase 4 Remodeling
Arthritis	X		X	
Cardiovascular disease	X	X	X	X
Chronic kidney disease	X	X	X	X
Chronic obstructive pulmonary disease			X	X
Diabetes	X	X	X	X
Obesity	X	X	X	X
Peripheral arterial and venous diseases	X	X	X	X

X identifies that either the disease or treatment of the disease has the potential to cause a delay or disruption in the identified phase of wound healing.

nation of increased bacterial burden, poor nutrition (deficiency in essential nutrients), repetitive trauma or injury (pressure, friction, or shear), exposure to moisture, the pathophysiology related to an underlying chronic disease, or, perhaps more often, the treatment or medications that an individual is receiving for the chronic disease (Kane).

Phase 1: Hemostasis

This phase occurs rapidly after injury. During *hemostasis*, platelets are recruited to the wound site to provide coagulation and form a blood clot to arrest bleeding and minimize blood loss. In addition, the platelets release platelet-derived growth factor (PDGF), which attracts neutrophils and fibroblasts to the site of injury (Kane, 2007; McNees, 2006; Moore, 2003). The formation of a provisional wound matrix is the final step in hemostasis. This matrix is strengthened by the synthesis of type III collagen by fibroblasts (Hartoch, McManus, Knapp, & Buettner, 2007). Once hemostasis is achieved, the process of wound healing moves to the next phase.

Phase 2: Inflammation

Inflammation is essential for wound repair and is a normal response to injury. It occurs quickly and is not in response to active infection. During the inflammation phase, keratinocytes, fibroblasts, endothelial cells, neutrophils, and macrophages arrive in the wound and assist in the production of *matrix metalloproteinases* (MMPs). MMPs remove debris and facilitate cell migration (Medina, Scott, Ghahary, & Tredget, 2005). These activities of cleansing and removing debris prepare the wound site for the next phase of healing (Kane, 2007; Moore, 2003). The inflammation phase begins immediately after the injury as a result of chemotaxis and lasts approximately three days (Colwell, 2005). An overabundance of MMPs can inhibit cell proliferation and angiogenesis because of the destruction of growth factors and matrix proteins that support cell migration and tissue integrity (Lobmann et al., 2002).

Phase 3: Proliferation and Granulation

The *proliferation and granulation* phase is important in building and strengthening the injured tissue (McNees, 2006). The wound contracts and fills with healthy replacement tissue and begins to close through the process of epithelialization (Colwell, 2005). Vascular endothelial growth factor and fibroblastic growth factor (FGF) stimulate *angiogenesis*, the formation of new blood vessels (Kane, 2007). Angiogenesis is an essential activity that provides oxygen and nutrients to the wound to promote healing (Angiogenesis Foundation, 2009). Proliferation of fibroblasts, whose primary function is collagen synthesis (Enoch & Price, 2004), begins the establishment of the foundation of the wound *extracellular matrix* (ECM) for granulation. This matrix supports re-epithelialization to build strength and wound integrity. The formation of connective tissue is generated by the synthesis and interactions of interleukin-1, tumor necrosis factor alpha (TNF-α), transforming growth factor beta (TGF-β), epidermal growth factor, PDGF, and nitric oxide (Kane). Phase III can take 3–24 days (Colwell, 2005).

Phase 4: Remodeling

The *remodeling* phase is a complex phase that can last from several months to several years (McNees, 2006). Remodeling of the wound is achieved by wound contraction brought about through the interaction of fibroblasts and the surrounding ECM (Grinnell, 1994) and is influenced by TGF-β, PDGF, and FGF (Slavin, 1996). The average wound contracts 0.6–0.75 mm per day toward its center four to five days after injury (Kane, 2007). Collagen is degraded by collagenase and other proteases in a delicate balance with collagen synthesis, whereas elastin is not synthesized in response to injury and therefore results in the lack of elasticity in scar tissue (Kane). At approximately four weeks, it is anticipated that the wound will reach 70% of the strength of undamaged tissue; however, it will never exceed 80% of the original tensile strength and therefore will always be at higher risk for breakdown (Madden & Peacock, 1968).

Impediments to Wound Healing

Regardless of the type of chronic disease an individual has, fundamental physiologic factors exist that will disrupt the phases of normal wound healing. Clinicians must consider the impediments that include hypoxia, infection, medications, injury, and malnutrition and their presence in chronic diseases (see Table 9-3) and organ failure.

Table 9-3. Chronic Diseases and Common Wound Healing Impediments					
Disease	Hypoxia	Infection	Medications	Injury	Malnutrition
Arthritis		X	X	X	
Cardiovascular disease	X		X	X	
Chronic kidney disease	X	X	X	X	X
Chronic pulmonary disease	X	X	X	X	X
Diabetes	X	X		X	
Obesity	X	X		X	X
Peripheral arterial and venous diseases	X		X	X	
X identifies that either the disease or treatment of the disease has the potential to contribute to common impediments of wound healing.					

Hypoxia

Oxygen is necessary for wound healing and is delivered to the tissue by way of hemoglobin and a patent vasculature. Several chronic illnesses can affect oxygen tissue perfusion, including cardiac and cardiovascular diseases, diabetes, peripheral arterial disease, chronic obstructive pulmonary disease (COPD), chronic kidney disease, and obesity. The result of inadequate tissue perfusion is tissue *ischemia*, which results in cell death as evidenced by necrotic tissue. Initially, hypoxia provides a significant stimulus for fibroblast proliferation and angiogenesis; however, wound healing will eventually deteriorate if hypoxia persists (Stadelmann, Digenis, & Tobin, 1998). The wound environment is dependent on oxygen for efficient leukocyte activity to suppress bacterial proliferation (Hunt, Hopf, & Hussain, 2000). A lack of oxygen also may contribute to the formation of a wound in individuals with arterial insufficiency, calcified vessels such as those found in patients with diabetes, or when tissue is exposed to external pressures that restrict the flow of oxygen. The relationship of soft tissue edema to impeded oxygen transfer to the tissue is not clear, but treatment such as compression stockings to reduce edema in patients with venous insufficiency and elevation of edematous extremities appear to be beneficial in the prevention and healing of an extremity wound (Hunt et al.).

Infection

Skin is the largest organ and has many functions, one of which is to cover and protect the body from organisms; hence, intact skin is the best defense against microorganisms. A number of chronic diseases predispose a patient to developing chronic wounds, such as diabetic foot ulcers and venous or arterial ulcers. Once the skin is broken, the first line of defense has been breached, and the opportunity arises for potential microorganism invasion. Whether this invasion develops into an infection is dependent on the following three major factors:

- The patient's ability to launch resistance against the various microorganisms
- The virulence of the organism
- The number of microorganisms present in the wound.

An imbalance in one or all of these factors can lead to infection (Landis, Ryan, Woo, & Sibbald, 2007; Stadelmann et al., 1998) and potentially to the death of the patient. This is of particular concern for many patients with cancer, especially if the patient receives systemic cytotoxic chemotherapy treatment, steroids, or radiation. All of these therapies can result in a dramatic imbalance of the normal bacterial flora and an opportunity to interfere with normal healing patterns.

Chronic disease can prevent patients from launching a satisfactory defense against this imbalance. Bacteria in a chronic wound can prolong the inflammatory phase with the persistent influx of neutrophils that release damaging substances such as free radicals, cytolytic enzymes, and inflammatory mediators (Landis et al., 2007). In addition, the overproduction of proteinases may occur and destroy growth factors, thus degrading the glycosaminoglycan matrix needed for wound healing (Stadelmann et al., 1998).

Medications

Individuals with a chronic disease rely on medications to control or treat their disease. Several classifications of medications interfere with wound healing. Among them are antineoplastic agents, steroids, and nonsteroidal anti-inflammatory drugs (NSAIDs) (Kane, 2007; Stotts, Wipke-Tevis, & Hopf, 2007). Systemic cancer treatment agents including traditional cytotoxic medications, molecular therapies that target the human epidermal growth factor receptors, and other biologic agents all affect wound healing (Stotts et al.).

Steroids are used for symptom management in many chronic illnesses, such as arthritis, COPD, and chronic kidney failure, as well as in many anticancer treatment protocols. The impact of these medications on wound healing begins in the inflammatory phase. The inflammatory phase is prolonged because of the decreased ability to mount an inflammatory response. In particular, steroids interfere with wound macrophages, angiogenesis, and fibrogenesis, in addition to inhibiting wound contraction (Stadelmann et al., 1998). These drugs reduce immunocompetent lymphocytes, decrease antibody production, and diminish antigen processing (Stotts et al., 2007). Signs and symptoms of inflammation are diminished when using steroids, particularly at the time of injury, because of their effect on the inflammatory phase (Ueno, Hunt, & Hopf, 2006).

NSAIDs such as acetylsalicylic acid (ASA) and phenylbutazones that are used for the management of pain and to complement other analgesics disrupt the normal healing process (Stotts et al., 2007). ASA also is used prophylactically in patients at risk for clot formation in conditions such as coronary artery disease to prevent platelet aggregation. Patients receiving these types of medications are at risk for prolonging the hemostasis phase as a result of impaired platelet function.

Injury

A break in the skin caused by unrelieved pressure, repeated shear, and friction may be associated with chronic disease and its association with immobility. Pressure ulcers are the result of unrelieved pressure, which causes tissue ischemia and necrosis. Pressure ulcers are classified into stages according to the depth of the tissue damage. For example, a stage 2 or partial-thickness pressure ulcer involves destruction of the epidermis and dermis resulting in ulceration (National Pressure Ulcer Advisory Panel, 2007). Moisture-related skin damage as a result of urinary and fecal incontinence exacerbates the effects of pressure and shear, as can excess wound drainage. Venous stasis ulcers are a result of peripheral artery disease and may contribute to the degradation of tissue at the wound edge. Diaphoresis and edema may cause skin to be fragile and easily injured.

People with diabetes may have varying degrees of neuropathy, particularly in the lower extremities, which results in a lack of normal protective sensation. The inability to detect pressure or pain may result in a wound caused by friction or pressure (Ueno et al., 2006). Examples include poorly fitting footwear or the presence of a foreign body in a shoe. Peripheral neuropathy can contribute to a much higher risk of heel ulcer development in patients with diabetes who are debilitated or confined to bed.

Malnutrition

An inadequate diet with vitamin deficiencies can lead to significant delays in wound healing. People with chronic diseases such as kidney disease or COPD may not ingest the required nutrients needed for wound healing. It is important to optimize, if not correct, nutritional deficits as early as possible in the wound healing process to avoid delays in healing. Bariatric patients also can have inadequate nutrition to promote wound healing because their diet may consist of foods that are high in calories but not necessarily nutritionally adequate (Mathison, 2003). For more information, see Chapter 13.

Organ Failure

In individuals with chronic illness, the internal organs lose their ability to function, mental and functional ability decline, and malnutrition occurs and results in fat and muscle wasting (Langemo & Brown, 2005). Progressive multisystem organ failure can be a consequence of chronic illness. The deleterious effects of body system organ failure are frequently evident in the skin, the largest organ of the body, when it is no longer supported by failing organs (Langemo & Brown). This deterioration of the skin is a result of hypoperfusion and presents as a pressure ulcer referred to as *skin failure* (Witkowski & Parish, 2000).

Skin failure in chronic illness occurs gradually over a period of time, usually in older adults with multiple comorbidities. In the final days and weeks of life, organ failure and the shunting of blood to vital organs can result in extensive and unusual presentations of skin failure (Langemo & Brown, 2005). Clinicians must initiate interventions to prevent skin failure; despite their best efforts, it may be difficult to decrease external skin damage, and wound healing may not be a reasonable goal. Discussions among the healthcare team, the patient, and family members regarding the patient's condition will identify and help to establish realistic treatment goals.

The Effects of Chronic Diseases on Wound Healing

Diabetes

The World Health Organization (WHO, 2008) estimated that 180 million people worldwide have diabetes. Diabetes occurs when the production of insulin from the pancreas is decreased (type 1 diabetes) or when the body is not able to effectively use the insulin it produces (type 2 diabetes). Type 2 diabetes comprises 90% of diabetes diagnoses and is largely the result of a lack of physical activity and increased body weight (WHO, 2008). The occurrence of diabetes is expected to rise rapidly in the future because of an increasing population of obese individuals and the reduced physical activity of the general population. The CDC (2009) estimated the total prevalence of diabetes to be 23.6 million in the United States. In 2007, the incidence of new cases of diabetes in people 20 years of age and older was 1.6 million (CDC, 2009). Diabetes varies from country to country, most likely based on the environment, genetics, and lifestyle, but also varies among ethnic populations within a country. In the United States, the estimated prevalence of diabetes in 2005 in people older than age 20 was 15.1% in Native Americans (American Indians and Alaska Natives), 13.3% in non-Hispanic blacks, 9.5% in Hispanic Americans, and 8.7% in non-Hispanic whites (CDC, 2008). Oncology clinicians need to know that approximately 15% of individuals with diabetes will develop a foot ulcer, and diabetes is the leading cause of nontraumatic lower extremity amputation in the United States (Powers, 2005). Risk factors for foot ulcers or amputation include (Powers)

- Diabetes for longer than 10 years
- Poor glycemic control
- Male gender
- Peripheral neuropathy
- Abnormal structure of foot (e.g., bony abnormalities, calluses, thickened nails)
- Peripheral arterial disease
- Tobacco use
- History of previous ulcer or amputation.

At the cellular level of wound healing, a number of deficiencies in patients with diabetes can be attributed to more than 100 known physiologic factors (Brem & Tomic-Canic, 2007). These physiologic factors involve

- Growth factor production
- Angiogenic response
- Keratinocyte and fibroblast migration and proliferation
- Epidermal barrier function
- Quantity of granulation tissue
- Collagen accumulation (Falanga, 2005)
- The balance between MMPs and the extracellular matrix (Lobmann et al., 2002)
- Macrophage function (Maruyama et al., 2007)
- Fewer epidermal nerves (Gibran et al., 2002).

All phases of wound healing are affected.

Over time, if diabetes is not well controlled, it can lead to damage to many of the key body organs and systems. Vascular complications include retinopathy, neuropathy, nephropathy, coronary artery disease, peripheral arterial disease, and cerebrovascular disease. Other nonvascular complications include gastroparesis, infections, and skin changes (Powers, 2005). People with diabetes are at risk not only for developing wounds such as thermal or traumatic foot injury because of peripheral neuropathy but also for infection and delay in wound healing (Hunt et al., 2000). Significant peripheral neuropathy can result in a *Charcot deformity*, described as acute bone destruction beneath the mid-foot in the area of the palmar arch (Steed, 2007). A greater frequency and severity of infection results because of incompletely defined abnormalities in cell-mediated immunity and phagocyte function associated with hyperglycemia, as well as diminished vascularization (Powers). Wound healing often becomes chronic in patients with diabetes when coupled with the inability to fight against infection and the inability of their bodies to mount an adequate inflammatory response (Brem & Tomic-Canic, 2007). Individuals with diabetes have an increased rate of colonization of *Staphylococcus aureus* in the skinfolds and nares, and such common infections are more frequent and severe. Increased colonization and growth of a variety of organisms (*Candida* and other fungal species) also are aided, in part, by hyperglycemia. Patients with diabetes tend to have a greater risk of postoperative wound infections (Powers).

Careful monitoring and control of blood glucose levels is essential in the successful management of diabetes and wound healing. Patients with vision impairment, decreased sensation, or limited physical mobility may not be aware of the development of a wound. Clinicians should regularly assess patients' skin integrity, evaluate their risk factors for skin breakdown, and plan appropriate interventions to avoid the development of a wound, especially in the lower extremities in order to avoid limb amputation.

Chronic Kidney Disease

In the United States, it is estimated that 20 million Americans (1 in 9 adults) have been diagnosed with chronic kidney disease (CKD) (National Kidney Foundation, 2007). The National Kidney Foundation (2007) estimated that 20 million more people are at increased risk for developing CKD during their lifetime. CKD is defined as having a glomerular filtration rate (GFR) of less than 60 ml/min/1.73 m^2 for more than three months, or kidney damage found either through imaging studies showing structural damage or chemistry abnormalities in urine or blood (National Kidney Foundation, 2002). Types I and II diabetes and hypertension are the most common causes of CKD, with hypertension being both a cause and a consequence of CKD (Skorecki, Green, & Brenner, 2005). Individuals with both CKD and hypertension are at greater risk for the development of cardiac disease (National Kidney Foundation, 2007). A family history of inheritable kidney disease, an episode of acute renal failure, autoimmune disease, older age, and indications of current kidney damage are additional risk factors (Skorecki et al.).

In CKD, a reduction of kidney mass (hypertrophy) occurs, causing both structural and functional hypertrophy of the nephrons. Vasoactive molecules, cytokines, and growth factors unsuccessfully attempt to mediate this hypertrophy, which was initially because of adaptive hyperfiltration and a subsequent increase in glomerular capillary pressure and flow (Skorecki et al., 2005). Kidney disease affects all organ systems. The result of untreated or inadequately treated kidney disease is *uremia*, a clinical and laboratory syndrome evident in the dysfunction of other organ systems, including renal excretory failure and a number of metabolic and endocrine functions supported by the kidney (Skorecki et al.). Individuals experience increased fatigue as a result of anemia, increasingly poor appetite, metabolic disorders associated with calcium and phosphorus metabolism, abnormalities in acid-base homeostasis, and hormonal abnormalities. A continued uremic state affects all activities of daily living and is fatal without dialysis (Skorecki et al.).

CKD can have a profound effect on the hematopoietic system. It significantly impairs the production of erythropoietin (Skorecki et al., 2005). Prolonged bleeding time, decreased activity of platelet factor III, abnormal platelet aggregation and adhesiveness, and impaired prothrombin consumption result in abnormal hemostasis (Skorecki et al.). Changes in the inflammatory response result in an increased susceptibility to infection with depressed neutrophils, leukopenia, decreased lymphocyte function, and decreased killer-cell activity (Colwell, 2005; Skorecki et al.). Individuals with CKD may experience peripheral neuropathy and bone pain—factors that may increase the incidence of skin injury, bone fractures, and incapacity, which ultimately increases the risk for development of pressure ulcers (Skorecki et al.). Some changes in skin are associated with the disease process that contributed to kidney failure or uremia (Headley & Wall, 2002). People with CKD experience degradation of collagen in the dermis and ecchymosis associated with platelet dysfunction, which results in changes in skin elasticity and pigmentation (Headley & Wall). Some skin manifestations are of little concern (e.g., pruritus), whereas others may be more indicative of the extent of the disease process. The extreme is *calciphylaxis*, a skin manifestation of CKD characterized by calcium deposits in the small vessels of the dermis that result in necrosis of skin and fat (Headley & Wall). It is a very painful, life-threatening condition and is a significant challenge for healthcare providers. The primary goal in this patient population is adequate pain management with dressing changes, rather than wound closure. Clinicians should be aware that injection puncture sites or inadvertent injury to the skin (skin tears) will probably develop into a calciphylatic lesion that is unlikely to heal. Patients with CKD also may become protein and energy malnourished, thereby affecting their ability to support wound healing in the proliferative phase (Colwell; National Kidney Foundation, 2007).

Cytokine elevation, interleukin-6 and TNF, and C-reactive protein in CKD are indications of inflammation and can result in atherogenesis, a risk for cardiovascular disease. The result is an accumulation of proinflammatory agents (Headley & Wall, 2002; Skorecki et al., 2005). Cardiovascular complications such as ischemic disease, congestive heart failure, and hypertension are present in 30%–45% of patients with CKD (Skorecki et al.). These complications precipitate hypoxia, delay wound healing, and increase the risk of further complications (Colwell, 2005). Blood flow to tissues is decreased in atherosclerotic disease associated with hypertension, resulting in poor tissue perfusion (Colwell; Skorecki et al.). Patients with both diabetes and CKD have impaired glucose metabolism, and elevation of insulin levels occurs because the kidneys, which normally contribute to insulin removal, are malfunctioning (Skorecki et al.). White blood cell phagocytic function, important in the inflammatory phase, is reduced in the presence of elevated blood glucose. Uncontrolled blood glucose levels can reduce collagen synthesis and deposition in the final stage of wound healing, resulting in weak wound tensile strength (Colwell). Clinicians must strive to minimize, manage, or eliminate the pathophysiologic factors of kidney disease and its associated comorbidities that alter the synchrony of normal wound healing to achieve wound closure.

Chronic Obstructive Pulmonary Disease

WHO (2007b) estimated that 210 million people have COPD. COPD is an inflammatory process affecting the tissue of the lung, which limits airflow (Agusti, 2001; Fiel, 2007). It is characterized by airway and systemic inflammation resulting from tobacco use, allergens, infections, airborne pollutants, and minerals (Agusti; Fiel). In some instances, no direct cause can be found. COPD is progressive and is not completely reversible (Fiel). In the past, the terms *emphysema* and *chronic bronchitis* were used to describe COPD, but these are no longer accepted (WHO, 2007b). According to WHO (2007b), 210 million people in the world have COPD, and more than 3 million people died of COPD in 2005. In the past, COPD was more common in men, but with increased use of tobacco among women, as well as other environmental factors, the disease now affects women and men almost equally. The death rate from COPD is expected to increase approximately 30% in the next 10 years unless tobacco use decreases and other environmental factors are altered (WHO, 2007b).

In the past, COPD was treated exclusively as a lung disease; however, current medical understanding recognizes COPD as a multisystem disease including pulmonary and systemic inflammatory disease with multiple comorbidities (Agusti, 2001; Fiel, 2007). For this reason, treatment is complex, and clinicians must consider all comorbid conditions. Bronchodilators, steroids, antibiotics, and mucolytics commonly are used to treat the symptoms of the disease, while long-term oxygen therapy is thought to be the only therapeutic measure that treats the entire body and improves survival rates (Agusti). If oxygen therapy is not optimized or if the individual is receiving steroids, there is a potential for poor wound healing. Additionally, individuals with COPD are at risk for decreased skeletal muscle mass related to an increased metabolic rate and the inability to respond to nutritional supplements. Agusti reported on a subset of patients with COPD who had an increase in the concentration of TNF-α in the blood plasma. TNF-α is a cytokine with a wide range of proinflammatory actions and is thought to contribute to the development of skeletal muscle wasting. The combination of steroid therapy, decreased muscle mass, nutritional imbalance, and decreased tolerance for exercise from muscle fatigue predisposes patients with COPD to delayed wound healing, skin tears, and pressure ulcers.

It is essential to optimize nutrition in patients with COPD to maintain an acceptable and stable weight needed to mitigate the pathophysiologic consequences of malnutrition such as reduced cell-mediated immune response and reduced protein synthesis (Schols, 2000) that delay wound healing. In addition, patients require education about the cutaneous effects of inhaled corticosteroids in order to avoid skin injury and subsequent delayed wound healing (Tashkin, Murray, Skeans, & Murray, 2004).

Arthritis

According to the Arthritis Foundation (2007), rheumatoid arthritis (RA) affects 1% of the U.S. population, or approximately 2.1 million individuals. RA is a chronic multisystem disease characterized by persistent inflammatory synovitis of peripheral joints for which the cause is unknown. It has been suggested that infection (viral or bacterial) is responsible for generating a chronic inflammatory response. The hallmark of the disease is synovial inflammation causing cartilage damage, bone erosions, and changes in joint integrity causing functional impairment (Lipsky, 2005). The cartilage damage initiates complement activation, which attracts leukocytes and stimulates the release of inflammatory mediators, which, in turn, exacerbates joint destruction ("Immune Disorders"; Lipsky). Lifestyle choices such as smoking are associated with the development of this disease (Lipsky). RA affects all races and affects women three times more than men in the early years; however, this gender difference decreases with age. Approximately 10% of individuals with RA will have an affected first-degree relative, indicating a genetic predisposition (Lipsky).

Clinical extra-articular manifestations of RA include vasculitis with its associated peripheral neuropathy, skin ulcerations, digital gangrene, dermal necrosis, visceral infarction with its multisystem complications, pleuropulmonary manifestations, rheumatoid nodules, and Felty syndrome, a combination of rheumatoid arthritis, enlarged spleen, decreased white blood cell count (MedlinePlus, 2008), which can potentially leave the individual at risk for infection related to the associated neutropenia ("Immune Disorders"; Lipsky, 2005). Within the next 25 years, an estimated one-quarter of the adult population will be diagnosed with arthritis, and 9.3% will experience activity limitations (CDC, 2007) as a result of joint deformity, muscle atrophy, and pain.

Physical deformity, activity limitations, and steroid therapy predispose patients with RA to skin breakdown. If injury occurs, common medications taken for the treatment of RA (steroids, anti-inflammatory, and antineoplastic agents) will inhibit normal wound healing. It is important for clinicians to assess patients' baseline activity level and consider the effects of medications.

Cardiac and Cardiovascular Diseases

The American Heart Association (AHA) reported a 37.1% prevalence rate of cardiovascular disease in the adult population based on 2005 statistics (AHA, 2008a). Cardiac and cardiovascular diseases can be classified as acute or chronic diseases depending on the duration and type of illness. An all-inclusive list of cardiac and cardiovascular diseases is extensive and beyond the scope of this discussion. This disease group includes coronary heart disease, cerebral vascular disease, rheumatic heart disease, and congenital heart disease (WHO, 2007a), systemic hypertension, hypertrophic cardiomyopathy, and mitral valve prolapse ("Approach to the Cardiac Patient," 2006).

AHA (2008a) estimated that 80,700,000 American adults (one in three) have one or more types of cardiovascular disease. Approximately 47% are estimated to be older than the age of 60. The National Center for Health Statistics (NCHS) estimated the prevalence of heart disease in the U.S. population to include American Indian/Alaska Natives, 16.2%; whites, 11.2%; blacks/African Americans, 10%; and Hispanics or Latinos, 7.6% (Pleis & Lethbridge-Cejku, 2007). The prevalence of hypertension is estimated to be 31.2% among blacks/African Americans and 25.7% among American Indian/Alaska Natives, is slightly lower in white populations (22.1%), and is lowest among Hispanics or Latinos (20.4%) (Pleis & Lethbridge-Cejku).

Any of these chronic diseases have the potential to alter the delivery of oxygen to tissues as a result of diminished pump function or poor circulation. An adequate blood flow to peripheral tissues is required to supply the necessary amount of oxygen for tissue viability and wound healing (Whitney, 1990), and this may be compromised to various degrees in these conditions. If tissue hypoxia persists, there is a risk of decreased collagen synthesis, decreased tensile strength, and reduced resistance to infection (Worley, 2004). Clinicians need to consider the comorbidities often present in patients with cardiac and cardiovascular diseases, such as diabetes, renal failure, COPD, and obesity.

Patients with cardiac and cardiovascular diseases frequently have additional factors that further alter wound healing, including advanced age, tobacco use, and immobility (Norris, Provo, & Stotts, 1990). Furthermore, the therapeutic treatments that patients receive to manage their cardiac disease, including NSAIDs, may disrupt wound healing and are important considerations for wound healing outcomes.

Vascular Diseases

Vascular diseases include a variety of diseases, with pathology affecting the peripheral arterial or venous vasculature. AHA (2008b) defined *peripheral vascular disease* (PVD) as a circulation disorder that narrows blood vessels, decreasing blood flow to the legs, arms, abdomen, or kidneys. Individuals with diabetes have a four- to fivefold increase in incidence of PVD. PVD is divided into two types. The first type involves structural damage to the blood vessel (i.e., peripheral arterial disease). The second type does not involve structural damage (i.e., Raynaud disease).

Peripheral arterial disease is a condition in which fatty deposits build along the inner lining of the arterial wall restricting blood flow. AHA (2008b) estimated that 8 million people are living with peripheral arterial disease. Initial symptoms can include cramping or fatigue of legs and buttocks during walking (intermittent claudication) that resolves when the activity is stopped.

Hypertension, hyperlipidemia, obesity, age, and smoking are factors that increase the risk of developing peripheral arterial disease (Mekkes, Loots, Van Der Wal, & Bos, 2003; Rubano & Kerstein, 1998).

Individuals with chronic disease of the peripheral vasculature are at risk for developing chronic leg ulcers. In this population, the pathophysiology of the leg ulcers may be related to valve incompetency resulting in venous hypertension, atherosclerosis resulting in ischemia, and diabetes (Mekkes et al., 2003; Sieggreen, 2005). Agren et al. (2000) reviewed the multifactorial pathogenesis of venous leg ulcers. They proposed that venous hypertension delays wound healing as it disturbs the microcirculation and changes the capillaries, resulting in a detrimental cascade with persistent levels of proinflammatory cytokines and proteases that prevents wound healing. As a result, fibroblasts do not respond normally to the growth factors. Optimal wound healing in patients with venous hypertension will not occur unless underlying pathology is resolved. Options to correct the pathology include surgical interventions to improve arterial flow by revascularization for ulcers with an arterial etiology, or for ulcers with venous etiology, medical interventions include compression treatment. It is essential that healthcare providers communicate the importance of compression therapy and support the patient's adherence to compression therapy, as it is thought to be the gold standard for venous ulcer wound healing. In this patient population, the healthcare provider also should consider other underlying comorbidities, including diabetes, hypertension, renal disease, and obesity, as causes for poor or delayed wound healing.

Obesity

WHO (2006) projected that by 2015, approximately 2.3 billion adults will be overweight and more than 700 million will be obese. NCHS (2006) reported that an estimated 66.3% of American adults are either overweight or obese. *Body mass index* (BMI) commonly is used to define overweight or obesity. BMI is expressed as weight/height squared (BMI = kg/m^2). A BMI of 25–29.9 is considered overweight, and a BMI of 30 or greater is defined as obesity among adults age 20 and older (NCHS, 2006). People who are overweight or obese frequently have comorbidities such as diabetes, venous stasis, osteoarthritis, cardiac, and pulmonary disease, which all can contribute to wound development and delayed wound healing (Norris et al., 1990). Obesity has been associated with several types of cancer, such as colorectal, prostate, breast, cervical, liver, and endometrial cancer (Khaodhiar, McCowen, & Blackburn, 1999). Obesity is a chronic health problem that can cause numerous skin complications, including the following (Hahler, 2006; Wright & Bauer, 2005):

- Candidiasis within skinfolds
- Skin irritation and dermatitis related to incontinence
- Moisture associated with the inability to perform personal hygiene
- Pressure ulcers
- Ulcers associated with venous insufficiency

- Cellulitis
- Lymphedema
- Surgical incision complications.

Preventing skin breakdown in obese patients can be a significant challenge as it relates to the patients' decreased mobility as a result of the underlying disease processes, lack of appropriately sized equipment, and the inability of staff to assist patients to mobilize (Mathison, 2003). In addition, it is not uncommon for bariatric patients to develop pressure ulcers in deep skinfolds, which can be difficult to heal because of the presence of excess adipose tissue and a warm, moist environment contributing to the possibility of bacterial imbalance. The blood supply in obese patients is limited in large areas of subcutaneous fat deposits, thereby causing less proportional blood supply and resulting in a higher risk of tissue hypoxia or ischemia (Norris et al., 1990), which may contribute to tissue injury and poor wound healing. After a surgical intervention, poor wound healing, dehiscence, and evisceration can occur in overweight patients because of increased tension on the edges of the fascia (Gallagher, 1997). Unfortunately, a diagnosis of extreme obesity increases the patient's risk of developing a variety of skin conditions causing a break in the skin integrity. The likelihood of multiple comorbidities associated with obesity places patients at increased risk for poor wound healing. Wound healing can be optimized in obese individuals by involving the entire interprofessional healthcare team in managing the plethora of intrinsic and extrinsic factors.

Conclusion

Several chronic diseases and their associated comorbidities and treatments negatively affect wound healing. Healing is a complex systemic response and requires an orderly process within an optimal environment to occur. Not all wounds will heal. Wound etiology, lifestyle choices, the physiologic impact of the treatments on patients with cancer, access to health care, psychological influences, and support systems will determine the success of healing a patient's wound.

References

Agren, M.S., Eaglstein, W.H., Ferguson, M.W., Harding, K.G., Moore, K., Saarialho-Kere, U.K., et al. (2000). Causes and effects of the chronic inflammation in venous leg ulcers. *Acta Dermato-Venereologica, Supplementum, 210*, 3–17.

Agusti, A.G.N. (2001). Systemic effects of chronic obstructive pulmonary disease. In D. Chadwick & J.A. Goode (Eds.), *Chronic obstructive pulmonary disease: Pathogenesis to treatment: Novartis Foundation Symposium, 234*, 242–254.

American Heart Association. (2008a). *Heart disease and stroke statistics—2008 update.* Dallas, TX: Author. Retrieved June 12, 2008, from http://www.americanheart.org/downloadable/heart/1200078608862HS_Stats%202008.final.pdf

American Heart Association. (2008b). *Peripheral artery disease (PAD)*. Retrieved June 12, 2008, from http://www.americanheart.org/presenter.jhtml?identifier=3020242

Angiogenesis Foundation. (2009). *Understanding angiogenesis*. Retrieved February 25, 2009, from http://www.angio.org/ua.php

Approach to the cardiac patient. (2006). In *Merck manual of diagnosis and therapy* (18th ed.). Retrieved February 25, 2008, from http://www.statref.com

Arthritis Foundation. (2007). *Disease center: Rheumatoid arthritis*. Retrieved November 25, 2007, from http://www.arthritis.org/disease-center.php?disease_id=31

Brem, H., & Tomic-Canic, M. (2007). Cellular and molecular basis of wound healing in diabetes. *Journal of Clinical Investigation, 117*(5), 1219–1222.

Centers for Disease Control and Prevention. (2007). *Arthritis: Arthritis related statistics*. Retrieved December 13, 2007, from http://www.cdc.gov/arthritis/data_statistics/arthritis_related_statistics.htm

Centers for Disease Control and Prevention. (2008). *Chronic disease prevention and health promotion: Featured items*. Retrieved June 12, 2008, from http://www.cdc.gov/nccdphp

Centers for Disease Control and Prevention. (2009). *Chronic disease prevention and health promotion: Diabetes successes and opportunities for population-based prevention and control*. Retrieved February 19, 2009, from http://www.cdc.gov/nccdphp/publications/aag/ddt.htm#aag

Colwell, J. (2005). The challenge of wound healing in patients with chronic kidney disease. *Nephrology Nursing Journal, 32*(1), 83–84.

Enoch, S., & Price, P. (2004). *Cellular, molecular and biochemical differences in the pathophysiology of healing between acute wounds, chronic wounds and wounds in the aged*. Retrieved October 25, 2007, from http://www.worldwidewounds.com/2004/august/Enoch/Pathophysiology-Of-Healing.html

Falanga, V. (2005). Wound healing and its impairment in the diabetic foot. *Lancet, 366*(9498), 1736–1743.

Fiel, S. (2007). COPD: A multisystem disease. In D.L. Kasper, E. Braunwald, A.S. Fauci, S.L. Hauser, D.L. Longo, J.L. Jameson, et al. (Eds.), *Harrison's principles of internal medicine* (16th ed.). New York: McGraw-Hill. Retrieved December 12, 2007, from https://www.accessmedicine.com/popup.a spx?aID=1001124

Gallagher, S. (1997). Morbid obesity: A chronic disease with impact on wounds and related problems. *Ostomy/Wound Management, 43*(5), 18–27.

Gibran, N., Jang, Y., Isik, F., Greenhalgh, D., Muffley, L., Underwood, R., et al. (2002). Diminished neuropeptide levels contribute to the impaired cutaneous healing response associated with diabetes mellitus. *Journal of Surgical Research, 108*(1), 122–128.

Grinnell, F. (1994). Fibroblasts, myofibroblasts, and wound contraction. *Journal of Cell Biology, 124*(4), 401–404.

Hahler, B. (2006). An overview of dermatological conditions commonly associated with the obese patient. *Ostomy/Wound Management, 52*(6). Retrieved December 11, 2007, from http://www.o-wm.com/article/5834

Hartoch, R.S., McManus, J.G., Knapp, S., & Buettner, M.F. (2007). Emergency management of chronic wounds. *Emergency Medicine Clinics of North America, 25*(1), 203–221.

Headley, C., & Wall, B. (2002). ESRD-associated cutaneous manifestations in a hemodialysis population. *Nephrology Nursing Journal, 29*(6), 525–541.

Hunt, T., Hopf, H., & Hussain, Z. (2000). Physiology of wound healing. *Advances in Skin and Wound Care, 13*(Suppl. 2), 6–11.

Immune disorders. (2006). In *Diseases: A nursing process approach to excellent care* (4th ed., pp. 411–486). Philadelphia: Lippincott Williams & Wilkins. Retrieved December 20, 2007, from http://ovidsp.ovid.com

Kane, D.P. (2007). Chronic wound healing and chronic wound management. In D.L. Krasner, G.T. Rodeheaver, & R.G. Sibbald (Eds.), *Chronic wound care: A clinical source book for healthcare professionals* (4th ed., pp. 11–24). Malvern, PA: HMP Communications.

Khaodhiar, L., McCowen, K., & Blackburn, G. (1999). Obesity and its comorbid conditions. *Clinical Cornerstone, 2*(3), 17–31, 54–60.

Landis, S., Ryan, S., Woo, K., & Sibbald, R.G. (2007). Infections in chronic wounds. In D.L. Krasner, G.T. Rodeheaver, & R.G. Sibbald (Eds.), *Chronic wound care: A clinical source book for healthcare professionals* (4th ed., pp. 299–321). Malvern, PA: HMP Communications.

Langemo, D., & Brown, G. (2005). Skin fails too: Acute, chronic, and end-stage skin failure. *Advances in Skin and Wound Care, 19*(4), 206–211.

Lipsky, P. (2005). Rheumatoid arthritis. In D.L. Kasper, E. Braunwald, A.S. Fauci, S.L. Hauser, D.L. Longo, J.L. Jameson, et al. (Eds.), *Harrison's principles of internal medicine* (16th ed.). New York: McGraw-Hill. Retrieved December 14, 2007, from http://www.accessmedicine.com/content.aspx?aID=94386

Lobmann, R., Ambrosch, A., Schultz, G., Waldmann, K., Schiweck, S., & Lehnert, H. (2002). Expression of matrix-metalloproteinases and their inhibitors in the wounds of diabetic and non-diabetic patients. *Diabetologia, 45*(7), 1011–1016.

Madden, J., & Peacock, E. (1968). Studies on biology and collagen during wound healing: Rate of collagen synthesis and deposition in cutaneous wounds of the rat. *Surgery, 64*(1), 288–294.

Maruyama, K., Asai, J., Ii, M., Thorne, T., Losordo, D., & D'Amore, P. (2007). Decreased macrophage number and activation lead to reduced lymphatic vessel formation and contribute to impaired diabetic wound healing. *American Journal of Pathology, 170*(4), 1178–1191.

Mathison, C. (2003). Skin and wound care challenges in the hospitalized morbidly obese patient. *Journal of Wound, Ostomy, and Continence Nursing, 30*(6), 78–83.

McNees, P. (2006). Skin and wound assessment and care in oncology. *Seminars in Oncology Nursing, 22*(3), 130–143.

MedicineNet.com. (2004). Definition of chronic disease. Retrieved November 25, 2007, from http://www.medterms.com/script/main/art.asp?articlekey=33490

Medina, A., Scott, P., Ghahary, A., & Tredget, E. (2005). Pathophysiology of chronic non-healing. *Journal of Burn Care and Rehabilitation, 26*(4), 306–319.

MedlinePlus. (2008). *Medical encyclopedia: Felty syndrome.* Retrieved February 19, 2009, from http://www.nlm.nih.gov/medlineplus/ency/article/000445.htm#Definition

Mekkes, J.R., Loots, M.A., Van Der Wal, A.D., & Bos, J.D. (2003). Causes, investigation and treatment of leg ulceration. *British Journal of Dermatology, 148*(3), 388–401.

Moore, K. (2003). Compromised wound healing: A scientific approach to treatment. *British Journal of Community Nursing, 8*(6), 274–278.

National Center for Health Statistics. (2006). *Health and stats: Prevalence of overweight and obesity among adults: United States, 2003–2004.* Retrieved February 23, 2009 http://www.cdc.gov/nchs/products/pubs/pubd/hestats/overweight/overwght_adult_03.htm

National Kidney Foundation. (2002). K/DOQI clinical practice guidelines for chronic kidney disease: Evaluation, classification, and stratification. *American Journal of Kidney Diseases, 39*(2, Suppl. 1), S46–S75.

National Kidney Foundation. (2007). *The facts about chronic disease (CKD).* Retrieved November 25, 2007, from http://www.kidney.org/kidneydisease/ckd/index.cfm#facts

National Pressure Ulcer Advisory Panel. (2007). *Updated staging system.* Retrieved December 18, 2007, from http://www.npuap.org/pr2.htm

Norris, S.O., Provo, B., & Stotts, N. (1990). Physiology of wound healing and risk factors that impede the healing process. *AACN Clinical Issues in Critical Care Nursing, 1*(3), 545–552.

Pleis, J.R., & Lethbridge-Cejku, M. (2007). Summary health statistics for U.S. adults: National Health Interview Survey, 2006. National Center for Health Statistics. *Vital and Health Statistics, 10*(235). Retrieved June 12, 2008, from http://www.cdc.gov/nchs/data/series/sr_10/sr10_235.pdf

Powers, A.C. (2005). Diabetes mellitus. In D.L. Kasper, E. Braunwald, A.S. Fauci, S.L. Hauser, D.L. Longo, J.L. Jameson, et al. (Eds.), *Harrison's principles of internal medicine* (16th ed.).

New York: McGraw-Hill. Retrieved December 8, 2007, from http://www.accessmedicine.com/content.aspx?aID=98925

Rubano, J., & Kerstein, M. (1998). Arterial insufficiency and vasculitis. *Journal of Wound, Ostomy, and Continence Nursing, 25*(3), 147–157.

Schols, A. (2000). Nutrition in chronic obstructive pulmonary disease. *Current Opinion in Pulmonary Medicine, 6*(2), 110–115.

Sieggreen, M. (2005). Lower extremity arterial and venous ulcers. *Nursing Clinics of North America, 40*(2), 391–410.

Skorecki, K., Green, J., & Brenner, B. (2005). Chronic renal failure. In D.L. Kasper, E. Braunwald, A.S. Fauci, S.L. Hauser, D.L. Longo, J.L. Jameson, et al. (Eds.), *Harrison's principles of internal medicine* (16th ed.). New York: McGraw-Hill. Retrieved December 14, 2007, from http://www.accessmedicine.com/content.aspx?aID=87373

Slavin, J. (1996). The role of cytokines in wound healing. *Journal of Pathology, 178*(1), 5–10.

Stadelmann, W., Digenis, A., & Tobin, G. (1998). Impediments to wound healing. *American Journal of Surgery, 176*(Suppl. 2A), 39S–47S.

Steed, D. (2007). Wounds in people with diabetes: Assessment, classification, and management. In D.L. Krasner, G.T. Rodeheaver, & R.G. Sibbald (Eds.), *Chronic wound care: A clinical source book for healthcare professionals* (4th ed., pp. 537–542). Malvern, PA: HMP Communications.

Stotts, N.A., Wipke-Tevis, D., & Hopf, H. (2007). Cofactors in impaired wound healing. In D.L. Krasner, G.T. Rodeheaver, & R.G. Sibbald (Eds.), *Chronic wound care: A clinical source book for healthcare professionals* (4th ed., pp. 215–220). Malvern, PA: HMP Communications.

Tashkin, D., Murray, H., Skeans, M., & Murray, R. (2004). Skin manifestations of inhaled corticosteroids in COPD patients: Results from lung health study II. *Chest, 126*(4), 1123–1133.

Ueno, C., Hunt, T., & Hopf, H. (2006). Using physiology to improve surgical wound outcomes. *Plastic and Reconstructive Surgery, 117*(Suppl. 7S), 59S–71S.

Whitney, J. (1990). The influence of tissue oxygen and perfusion on wound healing. *AACN Clinical Issues in Critical Care Nursing, 1*(3), 578–584.

Witkowski, J.A., & Parish, L.C. (2000). The decubitus ulcer: Skin failure and destructive behavior. *International Journal of Dermatology, 39*(12), 894–896.

World Health Organization. (2006). *Media centre: Fact sheet: Obesity and overweight.* Retrieved November 25, 2007, from http://www.who.int/mediacentre/factsheets/fs311/en/index.html

World Health Organization. (2007a). *Media centre: Fact sheet: Cardiovascular diseases.* Retrieved November 25, 2007, from http://www.who.int/mediacentre/factsheets/fs317/en/index.html

World Health Organization. (2007b). *Media centre: Fact sheet: Chronic obstructive pulmonary disease (COPD).* Retrieved November 25, 2007, from http://www.who.int/mediacentre/factsheets/fs315/en/index.html

World Health Organization. (2008). *Media centre: Fact sheet: Diabetes.* Retrieved February 23, 2009, from http://www.who.int/mediacentre/factsheets/fs312/en/index.html

Worley, C. (2004). Why won't this wound heal? Factors affecting wound repair. *Dermatology Nursing, 16*(4), 360–361.

Wright, K., & Bauer, C. (2005). Meeting bariatric patient care needs. Procedures and protocol development. *Journal of Wound, Ostomy, and Continence Nursing, 32*(6), 402–405.

CHAPTER 10

Impact of Systemic and Infectious Skin Disease During Cancer Treatment

Barbara Holmes Gobel, RN, MS, AOCN®,
and Anna Liza Rodriguez, RN, MSN, MHA, OCN®

Introduction

The skin is the largest human body organ and is the body's first line of defense against infection. In addition to protection, the skin provides sensation (pain and other stimuli) and temperature control (Elias, Feingold, & Fluhr, 2003; Wenger, 2003). A compromise in skin integrity, particularly in patients with cancer who are undergoing cancer treatment, can lead to an increased risk of wounds and problems with wound healing (Morris et al., 2003). Patients with cancer may undergo a variety of treatment modalities including surgical intervention, radiation therapy, and chemotherapy that have the potential to affect skin integrity. Surgical interventions may lead to both acute and chronic wounds depending on the ability of the body to heal postoperatively. Radiation therapy may lead to delayed wound healing as a result of interruption of mitosis in the basal membrane, which can lead to thinning or fibrosis of the epidermal layer of the skin (Goldberg & McGinn-Byer, 2000). Chemotherapy can cause neutropenia and thrombocytopenia, which decrease the availability of cells such as neutrophils and platelets that are needed for skin repair (Gerlach, 2005). An added stress to wound healing in patients with cancer is the problem of malnutrition, which is the most common comorbid condition in this population (Hayden, 2004). Malnutrition and inadequate wound healing have been found to be closely associated, particularly the protein-calorie malnutrition that is seen in patients undergoing chemotherapy and radiation therapy (Stillman, 2008).

A variety of skin disorders may affect patients with cancer, but in general, most skin disorders are not specific to patients with cancer. The skin disorders that will be reviewed in this chapter include psoriasis, herpes/varicella, sclero-derma, vitiligo, candidiasis, and mycobacterium. Skin disorders such as her-pes/varicella and candidiasis occur more commonly in patients with cancer.

Psoriasis

Psoriasis is an immune-mediated papulosquamous skin disease character-ized by well-demarcated, erythematous, scaly plaques on the scalp, extensor aspects of elbows and knees, and the sacral area. Psoriasis is estimated to af-fect more than 2 million people in the United States and up to 2% of the population worldwide (Stern, 1997). Histologic examination of lesions re-veals hyperkeratosis, hyperplasia of the epidermis, inflammatory cell infil-tration of leukocytes into the dermis and epidermis, and dilation of dermal capillaries. Several clinical variants of the disease exist, including (MacDon-ald & Burden, 2007)
- Chronic plaque psoriasis
- Guttate psoriasis
- Pustular psoriasis
- Flexural psoriasis
- Erythrodermic psoriasis.

Descriptions of psoriasis vary for each subcategory (see Table 10-1). *Chron-ic plaque psoriasis* is the most common presentation and is characterized by thick, scaly plaques affecting the scalp and extensor aspects of the limbs and trunk. *Guttate psoriasis* is a self-limiting, acute form of the disease affecting chil-dren and adolescents, often following a streptococcal throat infection (ton-sillitis or pharyngitis), and is characterized by small, scaly lesions less than 1 cm in diameter erupting on the trunk (Griffiths & Barker, 2007; MacDonald & Burden, 2007). *Generalized pustular psoriasis* presents as small monomorphic sterile pustules on painful inflamed skin precipitated by infection and abrupt withdrawal of systemic or strong topical corticosteroids (Griffiths & Barker).

Table 10-1. Clinical Variants of Psoriasis	
Type of Psoriasis	**Description**
Chronic plaque psoriasis	Thick, scaly plaques on the scalp and extensor aspects of limbs and trunk
Guttate psoriasis	Small, scaly lesions on the trunk
Pustular psoriasis	Small pustules on painful, inflamed skin
Flexural psoriasis	Shiny, erythematous plaques on the groin, axillae, and sub-mammary areas
Erythrodermic psoriasis	Widespread erythema

Flexural psoriasis presents as shiny erythematous plaques in the axillae, groin, and submammary areas and typically is devoid of scales. *Erythrodermic psoriasis* is the most serious, life-threatening form of the disease manifested by widespread erythema, which can lead to hypothermia, hypoalbuminemia, and cardiac failure (Griffiths & Barker; MacDonald & Burden).

Immunologic studies identify T cells as the driving force for inducing and maintaining the phenotypic changes in psoriasis; thus, emerging treatments for the disease, particularly biologic agents, are targeted to interfere with T-cell activation (Winterfield, Menter, Gordon, & Gottlieb, 2005). The trigger to T-cell activation in psoriasis remains unknown (MacDonald & Burden, 2007). The severity of psoriasis is the result of various factors such as ultraviolet (UV) exposure, streptococcal throat infections, alcohol, and physical and psychological stress (MacDonald & Burden). Population studies confirm genetic predisposition to psoriasis.

In patients with cancer, skin side effects take place more commonly in patients with incidental skin disorders such as psoriasis. Tomlinson (2001) presented a case study of a patient with breast cancer with a psoriasis flare in the irradiated chest wall six weeks after the completion of radiotherapy following mastectomy (total dose of 46 gray [Gy] in 20 fractions [2.3 Gy/fraction]). However, a study by Ben-Yosef, Soyfer, and Vexler (2005) demonstrated that using a daily radiotherapy dose of ≤ 2 Gy causes neither exacerbation nor development of psoriatic lesions. Feliu et al. (1997) reported a case of a 63-year-old patient with small cell lung cancer and psoriasis, with the psoriasis worsening during therapy with granulocyte–colony-stimulating factor (G-CSF). The coincidental worsening of psoriasis with G-CSF therapy and improvement after discontinuance of G-CSF suggests a causal role; however, the role of G-CSF in the pathogenesis of psoriasis has not been established (Feliu et al.).

Another case report by Adkins et al. (2000) demonstrated resolution of a patient's long-standing, extensive, refractory psoriasis following allogeneic bone marrow transplantation for chronic myeloid leukemia. A similar case report by Kojima et al. (2003) discussed complete remission of psoriasis following reduced-intensity stem cell transplantation from a human leukocyte antigen–identical sibling in a patient with acute myeloid leukemia. These case reports highlight the promising application of stem cell transplantation for autoimmune disorders such as psoriasis.

The optimal management of psoriasis begins with identification of the extent and severity of cutaneous disease, including comorbidities. In a flare of psoriasis, a cause should be sought, such as stress, trauma, infection, a new drug, or recent alcohol binge. Various strategies for the treatment of psoriasis exist, including topical, systemic, and biologic treatments. Topical treatment regimens include vitamin D, corticosteroids, coal tar, and dithranol (MacDonald & Burden, 2007). For patients with widespread disease or for those who do not respond to topical managements, ultraviolet B (UVB) and psoralen plus ultraviolet A (PUVA) treatments are viable options. The most common first-line systemic medications for severe psoriasis over the past several decades include methotrexate, acitretin, and cyclosporine (MacDonald & Burden). Second-line systemic treatments for severe psoriasis include hydroxycarbamide, azathioprine, leflunomide, and mycophenolate mofetil (MacDonald & Burden). Current biologic treatments for psoriasis include T-cell targeted agents such as efaluzimab and alefacept, and tumor necrosis factor-alpha antagonists such as infliximab, etanercept, and adalimumab.

Scleroderma

Systemic sclerosis (SSc or *scleroderma*) is a heterogeneous condition characterized by the deposition of excess collagen in skin and internal organs such as the lung, heart, kidney, gastrointestinal tract, and peripheral nervous system (Binks et al., 2001; Generini, Fiori, Pignone, Cerinic, & Cagnoni, 1999). Scleroderma has a reported incidence rate of about 19.3 cases per million per year from 1989 to 1991 (Mendoza & Derk, 2007). Scleroderma is derived from the words *skleros* (hard) and *derma* (skin) ("Scleroderma," 2009), aptly describing the characteristic skin hardening and thickening. The distinct underlying pathophysiologic processes in SSc include (Charles, Clements, & Furst, 2006; Hinchcliff & Varga, 2007)
- Small-vessel vasculopathy
- Inflammation or autoimmunity
- Excessive collagen production and deposition
- Fibrosis manifesting as Raynaud phenomenon
- Autoantibody production
- Varying degrees of skin thickening and internal organ dysfunction.

The immunologic abnormalities in SSc consist of chronic mononuclear cell infiltration of affected tissues (mainly by CD4+ T lymphocytes and macrophages), dysregulation of lymphokine and growth factor production, and the production of autoantibodies (Zuber & Spertini, 2006). It is hypothesized that the production of transforming growth factor-beta and the production of collagen by fibroblasts link the various immunologic abnormalities and the fibrosis observed in SSc (Zuber & Spertini). Although the etiology of SSc is unknown, the following are some of the various factors identified as potential causative agents (Charles et al., 2006; Varga & Abraham, 2007).
- Drugs
- Viruses including human cytomegalovirus
- Exposures to organic solvents, vinyl chloride, and silica
- Genetic predisposition

SSc is classified into two distinct clinical subsets based on patterns of skin involvement: *diffuse cutaneous SSc* (rapidly progressive fibrosis of the skin) and *limited cutaneous SSc* (limited and slow-progressing skin and organ fibrosis). Skin thickening in diffuse cutaneous SSc presents proximal as well as distal to the elbows and knees with or without facial or truncal effects, whereas skin thickening in limited cutaneous SSc presents in areas solely distal to the elbows and knees with or without facial effects (Charles et al., 2006). Initial symptoms of systemic sclerosis include fatigue, dysphagia, Raynaud disease, musculoskeletal complaints, and gastrointestinal reflux; skin thickening, swelling, and puffiness on the fingers and hands are the most reliable clinical signs for disease diagnosis (Charles et al.).

Patients with SSc present with a wide spectrum of vascular, respiratory, gastrointestinal, and musculoskeletal symptoms over time. In some patients, Raynaud phenomenon may be the only clinical manifestation of SSc (Ostojic & Damjanov, 2006). Nail-fold capillaroscopy detects morphologic and functional microcirculation changes that are characteristic of SSc. Sclerosis of the skin is the major characteristic of the disease. The extent and severity of sclerosis related to the skin may be determined using the modified Rodnan skin thickness scoring scale (Ostojic & Damjanov) (see Table 10-2). Using the Rodnan score, the skin thickness in 17 body surface areas is clinically assessed and assigned a score (with a possible maximum score of 51).

Scleroderma has other organ manifestations. Esophageal involvement related to the disease often is manifested as heartburn, dysphagia, and reflux esophagitis and is detected by contrast esophagography. Interstitial lung involvement and pulmonary hypertension are established by contrast radiography (chest radiography or high-resolution computed tomography) and pulmonary function tests. Heart involvement is often secondary to repeated myocardial ischemia during attacks of Raynaud phenomenon, resulting in chronic cardiac failure, arrhythmias, and other conduction disturbances, and can be detected by standard echocardiogram. Associated pericarditis is detected by echocardiography (Ostojic & Damjanov, 2006). Renal involvement in SSc is defined by a 24-hour creatinine clearance of less than 70 ml/min, proteinuria, hematuria, and/or acute renal failure (Ostojic & Damjanov).

Limited literature is available addressing the impact of scleroderma on wound healing. Numerous reports, however, have described severe radiation-induced toxicity in patients with scleroderma. The radiation-related injury may extend beyond the radiation field when patients with cancer and scleroderma are treated, even with localized high-dose radiation therapy (40–70 Gy) resulting in death or severe fibrosis (Burt et al., 2004). Case reports document systemic symptom progression, extremely poor cosmetic result, and exaggerated cutaneous and fibrotic reaction in the irradiated areas of patients with stable SSc with limited skin involvement following radiation therapy for cancer (Abu-Shakra & Lee, 1993; Robertson, Clarke, Pevzner, & Matter, 1991; Varga, Haustein, Creech, Dwyer, & Jimenez, 1991).

Treatment options for SSc involve management of organ-specific complications: angiotensin-converting enzyme inhibitors and endothelin-1 receptor antagonists effectively manage the acute renal failure and pulmonary arterial hypertension symptoms related to scleroderma (Hinchcliff & Varga, 2007). Oral and IV cyclophosphamide has been shown to induce improvements in dyspnea, forced vital capacity, and skin thickening (Hinchcliff & Varga). Smoking cessation and avoidance of cold exposure reduce the risks as-

Table 10-2. Modified Rodnan Skin Thickness Scoring Scale		
Grade	**Description**	**Definition**
0	Normal	Normal skin
1	Mild thickness	Skin thickened
2	Moderate thickness	Thickened skin unable to pinch
3	Severe thickness	Thickened skin unable to move
Maximum Score = 51		
Modified Rodnan Skin Surface Areas		
Site	**Skin Area**	**Number of Skin Areas to Assess**
Central	Face	1
	Anterior chest	1
	Abdomen	1
Bilateral	Fingers	2
	Dorsum of hands	2
	Forearms	2
	Upper arms	2
	Thighs	2
	Lower legs	2
	Dorsum of feet	2
Total Area Assessed		**17**

Note. Based on information from Clements et al., 2000; Silman, 1995.

sociated with Raynaud phenomenon. Gastroesophageal reflux disease symptoms can be managed by elevating the head of the bed during meals and offering patients small, frequent meals. Treatment for skin sclerosis related to scleroderma includes *phototherapy* (Sunderkotter, Kuhn, Hunzelmann, & Beissert, 2006). Phototherapy using UV irradiation is widely used as treatment for various dermatologic conditions. UV irradiation suppresses cellular immunity and has an antifibrotic effect accounting for its therapeutic effects in SSc (Sunderkotter et al.). During the past decade, hematopoietic stem cell transplantation (HSCT) using a cyclophosphamide and antithymocyte globulin regimen has emerged as a novel treatment for SSc. The aim for HSCT is to reset the deregulated immune system of patients (Van Laar & Tyndall, 2006) generating a new antigen-naïve immune system (Burt et al., 2004). A study by Burt et al. (2003) demonstrated rapid subjective and objective skin flexibility in patients with scleroderma following a dose-escalated cyclophosphamide conditioning regimen and HSCT.

Herpes Simplex and Varicella Zoster

Herpes simplex viruses types 1 and 2 (HSV1 and HSV2) and varicella zoster virus (VZV) belong to the *Herpesviridae* family of DNA viruses. These viruses share the following clinical features (Steiner, Kennedy, & Pachner, 2007).

1. The primary infection involves the mucocutaneous surfaces, which serve as the portal of entry of the viral particles into the peripheral nervous system.
2. The infection usually occurs within the same cutaneous distribution.
3. Under normal immunocompetent conditions, the reactivated infection usually does not spread beyond the anatomic distribution and vicinity of a single dorsal root ganglion.
4. Infection reactivation can occur at any time in the patient's life.

HSV, contracted via mucosal surfaces of damaged skin, generally is asymptomatic. HSV can recur multiple times during a person's lifetime but decreases in relation to age. The cutaneous distribution of lesions usually is local. HSV is not typically a disorder of immunocompromised hosts (Steiner et al., 2007).

VZV causes *varicella* (chicken pox) and *herpes zoster*. Varicella represents the primary infection in immunocompromised individuals. The highest incidence of varicella usually is in children ages 1–9; however, the infection can occur in older, immunocompromised, and pregnant adults. Varicella usually results in mild to moderate illness but is more severe in immunocompetent patients. Patients with lymphoproliferative malignancies and solid tumors are predisposed to developing disseminated varicella (Arvin, 1996). In bone marrow transplant recipients, varicella is of particular concern (Arvin). Clinical manifestations of varicella include prodromal symptoms including fever, malaise, headache, and abdominal pain 24–48 hours before the first lesions appear (Arvin). Systemic symptoms include fatigue and anorexia. The cutaneous lesions of varicella are erythematous macules evolving to small, painful, fluid-filled vesicles, often involving the scalp, face, trunk, and mucous membranes. The lesions crust and heal as new epithelial cells form at the base of the lesion. More serious complications of the disease include central nervous system involvement, pneumonia, secondary bacterial infection, and even death (Heininger & Seward, 2006). Secondary bacterial superinfection is a complication of varicella presenting as bullous progression or cellulitis surrounding the lesions and is treated with antibiotic therapy. Antiviral therapy with acyclovir prevents progressive varicella and visceral dissemination (Arvin).

Herpes zoster (shingles) results from the reactivation of VZV and mainly affects older or immunocompromised individuals, particularly bone marrow transplant recipients and HIV seropositive patients (Steiner et al., 2007). More than 300,000 cases of herpes zoster a year are treated in the United States (Gilden, Kleinschmidt-DeMasters, LaGuardia, Mahalingam, & Cohrs, 2000). Malignancies, particularly lymphomas, and conditions associated with immunosuppression such as AIDS, radiation therapy, bone marrow transplantation, and use of immunosuppressive agents (chemotherapy and corticosteroid use) are predisposing factors and triggers for the appearance of herpes zoster (Kleinschmidt-DeMasters & Gilden, 2001; Stankus, Dlugopolski, & Packer, 2000; Steiner et al.).

Herpes zoster presents as vesicular eruptions distributed unilaterally within a dermatome (see Figure 10-1) and usually involves cutaneous sites, particularly on the face and the thorax, where the highest burden of lesions was

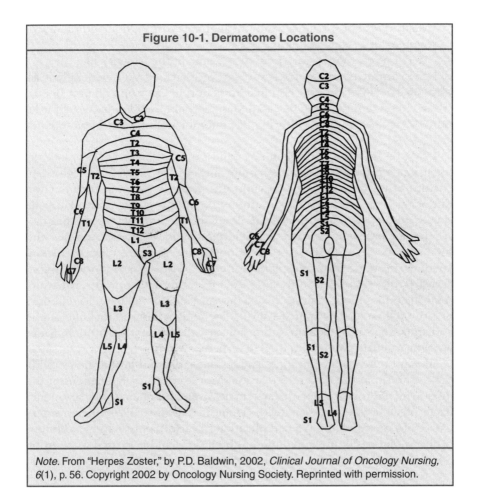

Figure 10-1. Dermatome Locations

Note. From "Herpes Zoster," by P.D. Baldwin, 2002, *Clinical Journal of Oncology Nursing, 6*(1), p. 56. Copyright 2002 by Oncology Nursing Society. Reprinted with permission.

present during varicella (Steiner et al., 2007). The vesicles are clear, become turbid, and crust within 5–10 days. Pain, itching, and paresthesia usually precede the vesicular eruptions, although the pain and itching are usual concomitants of the vesicular eruptions and can persist for several months after the rash resolves to become a self-limited postherpetic neuralgia (Stankus et al., 2000; Steiner et al.).

The diagnosis of herpes zoster is established using direct immunofluorescence assay and polymerase chain reaction (PCR). In immunocompetent patients, the treatment for herpes zoster is orally administered acyclovir (800 mg 5 times/day for 7–10 days), valacyclovir (1,000 mg every 8 hours for 7 days), or famciclovir (500 mg every 8 hours for 7 days) (Steiner et al., 2007), with doses adjusted accordingly for renal insufficiency. IV acyclovir is recommended for immunocompromised patients. Treatment for herpes simplex is continued until all lesions resolve (Steiner et al.). For pain control, low-dose narcotics, tricyclic antidepressants, or anticonvulsants may be administered. Topical capsaicin, lidocaine patches, and nerve blocks can also be used (Stankus et al., 2000).

Vitiligo

Vitiligo is a disorder of melanin pigmentation and is an example of a melanocytopenic disorder in which melanocytes (the site of melanin formation) are absent. Vitiligo is a specific acquired disorder that is often inherited (Ortonne, Bahadoran, Fitzpatrick, Mosher, & Hori, 2003). The disorder is characterized by well-circumscribed milky-white cutaneous macules in which identifiable melanocytes are absent, resulting in a lightening of the skin. Several types of vitiligo have been distinguished based on the distribution of the lesions. *Focal vitiligo* involves one or more maculae in one area. *Segmental vitiligo* is characterized by one or more maculae in a quasi-dermatomal pattern. The depigmentation does not cross the midline and affects one segment of the integument (Mollet, Ongenae, & Naeyaert, 2007). *Generalized vitiligo* is the most common type and is characterized by a few to widespread macules, either involving the distal extremities and face (*acrofacial vitiligo*) or by scattered macules over the entire body with a symmetrical distribution pattern (*vitiligo vulgaris*) (Han & Nordlund, 2000). Individuals with vitiligo carry a risk for ocular abnormalities, particularly iritis (Han & Nordlund).

The worldwide incidence of vitiligo is estimated at approximately 0.5%–1% (Njoo & Westerhof, 2001; Sehgal & Srivastava, 2007). Vitiligo affects all races, although it is more common in darker skin types (Ortonne et al., 2003). It is a skin disorder that affects both sexes equally and may develop at any age. Vitiligo has an unpredictable but often progressive course.

The etiology of vitiligo is not well understood, but it appears to involve a genetic predisposition and a number of potential precipitating factors. Multiple theories on the pathogenesis of vitiligo exist based on the mechanisms for the destruction of melanocytes, as there are no melanocytes in the evolved white macules (Ortonne et al., 2003). Individuals with vitiligo often list stressful life events, crises, or illnesses as the onset of their disorder. In some individuals, the onset of vitiligo follows trauma or a physical injury, such as a cut or an abrasion. This is known as the *Koebner phenomenon,* in which the vitiligo is congruent with a site of injury (Han & Nordlund, 2000). Case reports over the years have described patients with vitiligo who developed the Koebner phenomenon in the treated area following radiotherapy for carcinoma of the breast (Koo, Suh, & Hann, 1996; Levine & Ribeiro, 1994).

Diagnosis of vitiligo is largely a clinical diagnosis. Generally, melanocytes are completely absent in the chalk-white macules. Skin biopsies may be done, but they cannot distinguish vitiligo from chemical leukoderma or a number of other hypomelanotic disorders (Ortonne et al., 2003).

No definitive cure is available for vitiligo. The primary goal of treatment for vitiligo is to achieve repigmentation in the lesions and to stabilize the depigmenting process (Matz & Tur, 2007). Repigmentation of the lesions leads to improved cosmetic appearance and greater skin tolerance for sunburns. Individuals should be taught to use a sunscreen with sun protection factor (SPF) of 30 or higher to offer protection from sunburn and to attenuate the tanning of normally pigmented skin, which minimizes the contrast between vitiligo macules and normal skin. Cosmetics offer many patients an acceptable alternative to more aggressive therapies. Cosmetics may include dyes, self-tanning preparations, or conventional makeup. Many cosmetics can be custom mixed to match individual skin colors (Ortonne et al., 2003).

Few randomized controlled trials (RCTs) have been conducted to study the effects of various treatment modalities on vitiligo. Overall, therapies tend to be the most effective on the face and neck, whereas the acral areas are least responsive (Forschner, Buchholtz, & Stockfleth, 2007). Conservative therapies include photochemotherapy, phototherapy with UVB radiation, systemic steroids, and pseudocatalase. Newer therapeutic options include treatment with topical immunomodulators (tacrolimus, pimecrolimus) and analogs of vitamin D_3. Surgical options include excimer laser and surgery/transplantation.

Topical glucocorticoids have historically been used and have been found to be the most effective treatment for limited vitiligo. Hydrocortisone may be used for isolated macules, but highly potent glucocorticoids (e.g., clobetasol) have shown treatment success. In an RCT comparing topical clobetasol to tacrolimus, clobetasol was found to be more effective in restoring skin color in children with vitiligo, although tacrolimus was almost as effective and does not carry the same side effects as glucocorticoids (Lepe et al., 2003). Unfortunately, topical glucocorticoids have significant side effects, such as cutaneous atrophy and capillary fragility. Clobetasol also has been found to be superior to calcipotriol (a topical vitamin D_3 analog) in a prospective open study (Chiaverini, Passeron, & Ortonne, 2002).

Focal and segmental types of vitiligo have shown the best response to the use of photochemotherapy using photosensitizers (psoralen or khellin). One study demonstrated similar treatment results with the use of topical khellin and UVA therapy and systemic PUVA (Valkova, Trashlieva, & Christova, 2004). Two RCTs demonstrated that when PUVA was combined with calcipotriol, the response was more rapid and repigmentation was strong (Ermis, Alpsoy, Cetin, & Yilmaz, 2001; Parsad, Saini, & Verma, 1998).

Narrow-band and broad-band UVB therapy have been found to be beneficial for the treatment of segmental or generalized vitiligo, with narrow-band UVB showing more effectiveness (Hartmann, Lurz, Hamm, Brocker, & Hofmann, 2005). No controlled studies are available comparing surgical techniques for the management of vitiligo. Surgery generally is used for segmental vitiligo that has been stable for approximately two years. A variety of skin-grafting techniques are used to provide for direct repigmentation (Pianigiani, Andreassi, & Andreassi, 2005).

Mycobacterium

Mycobacteria are nonsporulating, nonmotile rods that are acid-fast and weakly gram-positive. Mycobacteria are the organisms responsible for tuberculosis (TB), including TB of the skin. The skin manifestations of TB are caused by *Mycobacterium (M.) tuberculosis, M. bovis*, and an attenuated strain of *M. bovis* of the bacillus Calmette-Guérin (Tappeiner & Wolff, 2003). Skin disease can occur as a result of either exogenous infection or endogenous spread (Barbagallo, Tager, Ingleton, Hirsch, & Weinberg, 2002). Cutaneous TB is relatively rare, with a reported incidence of 1%–4.4% of all cases of TB (Saral, Coskun, Ozturk, Bulut, & Cobanoglu, 2005). A wide range of skin manifestations are caused by TB, and these manifestations led to the development of a subclassification system. Of the various disease forms of TB of the skin, two forms will be covered in this chapter because of their potential occurrence in immunocompromised individuals.

Metastatic tuberculous abscess (tuberculous gumma) is caused by hematogenous spread of mycobacteria from a tuberculosis focus. This spread of the bacteria generally occurs in immunodeficient or severely immunosuppressed individuals. The spread of the bacteria leads to single or multiple subcutaneous lesions or abscesses, which generally are nontender and fluctuant. The lesions typically are found on the trunk and extremities. The lesions may invade the overlying skin and form ulcers and fistulas. Along with the clinical manifestations seen with metastatic tuberculous abscess, diagnosis is accomplished via culture, acid-fast bacilli stains, which usually reveal significant amount of mycobacteria, and PCR. The PCR does not diagnose mycobacterial disease, but it helps to identify the organism (Tappeiner & Wolff, 2003).

Acute miliary TB of the skin (tuberculosis cutis miliaris disseminata) is a very rare skin manifestation of fulminating miliary tuberculosis that is caused by hematogenous spread of mycobacteria. The disease may follow immunosuppressive infections and HIV (del Giudice et al., 2000). Lesions may occur anywhere on the body, particularly on the trunk. The lesions appear as minute erythematous macules or papules, as well as purpuric lesions. Mycobacteria are present both in and around blood vessels. Diagnosis is done via the same methods as with metastatic tuberculous abscesses. Prognosis related to this condition is poor (del Giudice et al.).

Treatment of skin TB follows the same guidelines as for treatment of TB of any other organ. A full antituberculosis regimen is indicated, even in localized forms of TB. First-line therapies include isoniazid, ethambutol, rifampin, and aminoglycosides. For patients with drug-resistant disease, second-line drugs include pyrazinamide, ethionamide, viomycin, kanamycin, capreomycin, and cycloserine (Tappeiner & Wolff, 2003). The mainstay of antituberculosis therapy is isoniazid, as it is both tuberculostatic and tuberculocidal. The drug penetrates into all body fluids and tissues. Patients generally are treated with multidrug regimens, as the goal of therapy is to cure the disease as rapidly as possible to prevent resistant strains of organisms.

Skin infections with atypical mycobacteria also exist. An atypical mycobacterial skin disease that may occur in individuals who are immunosuppressed is *M. kansaii*. This nontuberculous infection occurs in adults with AIDS and in patients receiving immunosuppression for renal transplantations and is associated with immunosuppressive diseases such as Hodgkin disease or hairy cell leukemia (Marras, Morris, Gonzalez, & Daley, 2004; Rose et al., 1997; Tappeiner & Wolff, 2003). *M. kansaii* usually is acquired from the environment. It has been found in tap water and in wild and domestic animals. It is an exogenous organism that generally is transmitted via an external wound.

Skin lesions related to *M. kansaii* in immunosuppressed patients are the result of the disseminated aspect of the organism. These lesions demonstrate as cellulitis and abscesses rather than granulomatous lesions. Progression of disease is slow, and chronic, persistent lesions can occur. The diagnosis is made by the isolation of the *M. kansaii* organism in bacterial culture.

M. kansaii is treated with antituberculosis drugs and multidrug regimens (Marras et al., 2004). Surgical excision is used for isolated skin lesions.

Candidiasis

Candidiasis is a diverse group of yeast infections generally caused by *Candida albicans*. The skin, nails, mucous membranes, and gastrointestinal tract typically are infected by these organisms, but they also may infect internal organs. The incidence of sepsis caused by fungal organisms, including candidiasis, increased 207% between 1979 and 2000 (Zaoutis et al., 2005). Factors related to this increase include the increase in intensive chemotherapy regimens leading to more immunosuppressed patients, allogeneic stem cell transplantation, prolonged stays in intensive care units, the increased use of vascular access devices, and the use of parenteral nutrition (Zaoutis et al.).

Candida albicans colonizes the mucous membranes of warm-blooded animals. The oral mucosa and vaginal mucosa are often colonized, yet the yeast is rarely isolated from normal human skin (Farah, Ashman, & Challacombe, 2000). Risk factors in the development of *Candida* infection (local and systemic) include (Klenk, Martin, & Heffernan, 2003)

- AIDS
- Trauma
- Local occlusion of the skin
- Generalized malnutrition
- Malignancy (especially hematologic and thymoma)
- Indwelling vascular access devices
- A variety of medications (such as glucocorticoids and antibiotics).

Candidal infection is aided by adherence of the organism to epithelial cells with subsequent invasion into the tissues (Staib, Kretschmar, Nichterlein, Kohler, & Morschhauser, 2000). Well-established investigations in human cutaneous candidiasis identified that cutaneous inoculation of *Candida albicans* could only develop into disease if the site of inoculation was occluded (Rebora, Marples, & Kligman, 1973).

Disseminated candidiasis is increasing in incidence as more patients are undergoing allogeneic stem cell transplantation and other organ transplantation and patients with hematologic diseases are being treated with highly immunosuppressive medications (Zaoutis et al., 2005). The organisms responsible for these disseminated infections include *Candida (C.) albicans, C. tropicalis, C. lusitaniae, C. krusei,* and *C. parapsilosis* (Lewis & Klepser, 1999). The hematogenous spread of these organisms occurs when patients have breaks in their skin, as with mucositis related to chemotherapy or infections related to central vascular access devices. Skin lesions may occur in some patients with disseminated infection. Skin lesions generally occur on the trunk and extremities and appear as 0.5–1 cm erythematous papulonodules. Skin lesions may be associated with fever and myalgias (Kressel, Szewczyk, & Tuazon, 1978). The management of disseminated candidiasis includes the early use of amphotericin B, including the lipid-based formulations (Klenk et al., 2003).

The *Candida* species is responsible for a significant number of oral infections in patients with cancer, including 50% of oral infections in patients with leukemia who are receiving chemotherapy and two-thirds of patients receiving antineoplastic therapy for solid tumors (Soysa, Samaranayake, & Ellepola, 2004). *Acute pseudomembranous candidiasis* (thrush) is the most common form of oral candidiasis and can occur as a result of cancer treatment such as chemotherapy and radiation therapy. Other predisposing factors for oral thrush include diabetes mellitus, antibiotic use, systemic steroids, and cell-mediated immunodeficiency such as HIV and AIDS. Oral candidiasis can lead to a number of negative consequences for patients with cancer, including poor nutrition, pain and discomfort, delays in drug administration, prolonged hospitalizations, and in some patients, the potential for life-threatening infections (septicemia and bacteremia).

Oral candidiasis appears as discrete white patches that may become confluent on the tongue, palate, gingivae, and buccal mucosa. Scraping of the patches produces a brightly erythematous surface underneath. Another manifestation of oral candidiasis seen in patients receiving radiation therapy to the
head and neck area is a black hairy tongue. The radiation therapy causes an
alteration in the normal flora of the tongue with fungi and bacteria. The surface of the tongue cannot undergo normal desquamation as the filiform pa-
pillae hypertrophy from the overgrowth (Klenk et al., 2003). Treatment of a
black hairy tongue consists of physical debridement and good oral hygiene
(McNally & Langlais, 1996).

A thorough oral assessment is critical to the prevention and treatment of
oral mucositis and oral candidiasis. The oral assessment is an ongoing process
that guides the development of a dynamic plan of care (Eilers & Epstein, 2004;
Jaroneski, 2006). Regular assessments of the oral cavity can provide for early
detection and intervention that may prevent problems such as pain and systemic infections (Eilers & Million, 2007). A number of valid and reliable oral
assessment instruments are available that can provide critical information to
guide nursing interventions. Instrument selection is guided by the purpose
of data collection (e.g., research or clinical). The Oncology Nursing Society
provides a comprehensive list of tools to measure mucositis on its outcomes
Web site (www.ons.org/outcomes/measures/mucositis.shtml). Some of the
well-established tools include the following.
- Oral Assessment Guide (Eilers, Berger, & Peterson, 1988)
- Oral Mucosa Rating Scale (Kolbinson, Schubert, & Flournoy, 1988)
- Oral Mucositis Index (McGuire et al., 2002; Schubert, Williams, Lloid, Donaldson, & Chapko, 1992)
- Oral Mucositis Assessment Scale (Sonis et al., 1999)
- Common Toxicity Criteria used by the World Health Organization (1979)
  and the National Cancer Institute Cancer Therapy Evaluation Program
  (2009)

Oral care protocols are recommended by the Multinational Association of
Supportive Care in Cancer/International Society for Oral Oncology (2005)
and other consensus groups, as these protocols may reduce the severity of mucositis from chemotherapy and radiation therapy (McGuire, Correa, Johnson,
& Wienandts, 2006; Rubenstein et al., 2004). The protocols should include
regular cleansing of the teeth (with a soft toothbrush) and mucosal tissues
and consultation with dental professionals, as well as education for staff and
patients. Although these recommendations are made for the prevention and
management of oral mucositis, it is prudent to encourage these practices for
the prevention and management of oral candidiasis because they often occur simultaneously in patients with cancer.

Strong evidence from RCTs has shown that antifungal drugs absorbed
(fluconazole, ketoconazole, and itraconazole) or partially absorbed (micon-
azole and clotrimazole) from the gastrointestinal tract prevent oral candidiasis in patients receiving treatment for cancer (Clarkson, Worthington, &

Eden, 2007). Evidence also supports that these drugs work significantly better at preventing oral candidiasis than drugs not absorbed (amphotericin B, nystatin, chlorhexidine, nystatin plus chlorhexidine, thymostimulin, amphotericin B plus nystatin, polyenes, natamycin, and norfloxacin plus amphotericin B) from the gastrointestinal tract (Clarkson et al.). Issues that are identified by the authors of the systematic review regarding prophylactic treatment of oral candidiasis that require further evidence include implications of drug toxicity, development of microbial drug resistance, and the cost of treatment (Clarkson et al.).

The evidence regarding treatment of oral candidiasis is not as strong. In a systematic review by Worthington, Clarkson, and Eden (2007) of interventions for treating oral candidiasis in patients with cancer who were receiving treatment, the authors found that trials are insufficient to make strong recommendations. They reported on one trial that found ketoconazole to be effective in treating oral candidiasis. Ketoconazole has a risk of hepatotoxicity with prolonged use; thus, it is advised that the potential benefit of use of this drug be weighed against the risk of liver damage (Worthington et al.). In practice, topical antifungal agents generally are used as first-line treatment for uncomplicated candidiasis. Commonly used drugs include nystatin suspension, clotrimazole troches, gentian violet, and chlorhexidine rinses (Klenk et al., 2003). Systematic reviews have shown that not only does chlorhexidine not prevent oral candidiasis, but may even make it worse because of debridement of good epithelial cells; therefore, it is not recommended in practice (Rubenstein et al., 2004). Good oral hygiene using a soft toothbrush that is replaced regularly is an essential component of treatment of oral candidiasis (Cheng, Molassiotis, Chang, Wai, & Cheung, 2001; McGuire et al., 2006). If a person with oral candidiasis wears dentures, the dentures are to be removed and soaked in 0.1% hypochlorite solution to eliminate *Candida* (Farah et al., 2000).

Conclusion

No risk for the development of cancer has been established in patients with documented skin diseases that are discussed in this chapter (psoriasis, systemic sclerosis, herpes simplex virus, varicella zoster virus, vitiligo, mycobacterium, and candidiasis). However, some evidence has shown (albeit some with case reports) that when a patient has an established skin disease, the symptoms of the skin disease may be exacerbated when a person is receiving cancer treatment. As noted in Table 10-3, which provides an overview of the skin diseases discussed in this chapter, evidence supports that the symptoms of psoriasis and systemic sclerosis can be exacerbated during radiation therapy treatment. The use of radiation therapy (in patients with breast cancer) also has been noted in a few case reports to be associated with depigmentation of the treated skin in patients with vitiligo.

Table 10-3. Summary of Skin Diseases and Nursing Implications

Skin Disease/Description	Issues	Nursing Implications
Psoriasis An immune-mediated papulosquamous skin disease characterized by well-demarcated, erythematous, scaly plaques on the scalp, extensor aspects of elbows and knees, and the sacral area	Evidence suggests that the symptoms of psoriasis may worsen during radiation therapy. In addition to other well-established treatments for psoriasis, some evidence has shown that stem cell transplantation may be of benefit to patients with refractory psoriasis.	Patients with cancer may experience exacerbation of preexisting skin disorders, including psoriasis, during the treatment of their cancer.
Systemic sclerosis (SSc or scleroderma) A heterogeneous condition characterized by the deposition of excess collagen in skin and internal organs, such as the lung, heart, kidney, gastrointestinal tract, and peripheral nervous system (Binks et al., 2001; Generini et al., 1999)	Numerous reports exist of severe radiation-induced skin toxicity in patients with scleroderma. Stem cell transplantation has emerged as a novel treatment for the management of scleroderma.	Patients with scleroderma may have significant organ dysfunction caused by the disease. Patients with scleroderma who are receiving radiation therapy may experience increased skin toxicity.
Herpes simplex virus and varicella zoster virus These viruses belong to the *Herpesviridae* family of DNA viruses. The primary infection of these viruses involves the mucocutaneous surfaces of the body.	Varicella represents the primary herpes infection in immunocompromised individuals. Patients with lymphoproliferative malignancies and solid tumors are predisposed to developing disseminated varicella (Arvin, 1996). Serious complications of varicella include central nervous system involvement, pneumonia, secondary bacterial infection, and even death (Heininger & Seward, 2006).	Varicella zoster virus can be severe in immunocompromised patients. Clinical manifestations of varicella zoster, including fever, malaise, headache, and abdominal pain, can occur up to 24–48 hours before any lesions appear on the body (Arvin, 1996). Patients with disseminated varicella zoster virus should be placed in respiratory isolation.

(Continued on next page)

Table 10-3. Summary of Skin Diseases and Nursing Implications *(Continued)*

Skin Disease/Description	Issues	Nursing Implications
Vitiligo A disorder of melanin pigmentation and an example of a melanocytopenic disorder in which melanocytes are absent. This condition is characterized by well-circumscribed milky-white cutaneous macules in which melanocytes are absent, resulting in a lightening of the skin.	A few case reports exist of patients with vitiligo who developed depigmentation of the treated skin area following radiotherapy for carcinoma of the breast (Koebner phenomenon). Generalized vitiligo is the most common type and is characterized by a few to widespread macules.	Patients with vitiligo should be taught to use sunscreen with a sun protection factor greater than 30 to offer protection from sunburn. In addition to other more aggressive therapies, many cosmetics can help to minimize skin color changes. Many cosmetics can be custom mixed to match individual skin colors (Ortonne et al., 2003).
Mycobacterium Mycobacteria are nonsporulating, nonmotile rods that are acid-fast and weakly gram-positive.	Mycobacteria are the organisms responsible for tuberculosis, including tuberculosis of the skin. Although uncommon, *metastatic tuberculous abscess* and *acute miliary tuberculosis of the skin* are two types of tuberculosis of the skin that may occur in patients who are immunosuppressed. Treatment of skin tuberculosis follows the same guidelines as treatment of tuberculosis of any other organ.	Metastatic tuberculous abscesses generally occur in immunodeficient or severely immunosuppressed individuals and are caused by a hematogenous spread of mycobacteria from a tuberculosis focus in the body. Acute miliary tuberculosis of the skin may follow immunosuppressive infections and HIV.

(Continued on next page)

Table 10-3. Summary of Skin Diseases and Nursing Implications *(Continued)*		
Skin Disease/Description	**Issues**	**Nursing Implications**
Candidiasis Candidiasis is a diverse group of yeast infections generally caused by *Candida albicans*. The skin, nails, mucous membranes, and gastrointestinal tract typically are infected by these organisms, but they also may infect internal organs.	Risk factors in the development of *Candida* infection (local and systemic) include AIDS, trauma, local occlusion of the skin, generalized malnutrition, malignancy (especially hematologic and thymoma), indwelling vascular access devices, and a variety of medications (such as glucocorticoids and antibiotics) (Klenk et al., 2003). Disseminated candidiasis is increasing in incidence as more patients are being treated with immunosuppressive medications.	Thorough oral assessment is critical to the prevention and successful treatment of oral mucositis and oral candidiasis. Strong evidence from randomized controlled trials supports that antifungal drugs absorbed (fluconazole, ketoconazole, and itraconazole) or partially absorbed (miconazole and clotrimazole) from the gastrointestinal tract prevent oral candidiasis in patients receiving treatment for cancer (Clarkson et al., 2007).

Immunosuppression related to cancer and cancer treatment is an established risk factor in the development of a variety of infections that are manifested as skin disorders, including herpes simplex, varicella zoster, mycobacterium, and candidiasis. These skin diseases can be severe in immunocompromised patients. Ongoing skin assessments by the nurse are critical in patients with cancer. While patients with cancer may experience a number of skin alterations related to their cancer or cancer therapy, including rashes related to medication therapy, skin diseases or infections manifested in the skin may be exacerbated by the cancer or cancer treatment.

References

Abu-Shakra, M., & Lee, P. (1993). Exaggerated fibrosis in patients with systemic sclerosis (scleroderma) following radiation therapy. *Journal of Rheumatology, 20*(9), 1601–1603.

Adkins, D.R., Abidi, M.H., Brown, R.A., Khoury, H., Goodnough, L.T., Vij, R., et al. (2000). Resolution of psoriasis after allogeneic bone marrow transplantation for chronic myelogenous leukemia: Late complications of therapy. *Bone Marrow Transplantation, 26*(11), 1239–1241.

Arvin, A.M. (1996). Varicella-zoster virus. *Clinical Microbiology Reviews, 9*(3), 361–381.

Barbagallo, J., Tager, P., Ingleton, R., Hirsch, R.J., & Weinberg, J.M. (2002). Cutaneous tuberculosis: Diagnosis and treatment. *American Journal of Clinical Dermatology, 3*(5), 319–328.

Ben-Yosef, R., Soyfer, V., & Vexler, A. (2005). Radiation therapy in cancer patients with psoriasis. The fractionated daily dose and the Koebner phenomenon. *Radiotherapy and Oncology, 74*(1), 21–23.

Binks, M., Passweg, J.R., Furst, D., McSweeney, P., Sullivan, K., Besenthal, C., et al. (2001). Phase I/II trial of autologous stem cell transplantation in systemic sclerosis: Procedure related mortality and impact on skin disease. *Annals of the Rheumatic Diseases, 60*(6), 577–584.

Burt, R.K., Kallunian, K., Patel, D., Thomas, J., Yeager, A., Traynor, A., et al. (2004). The rationale behind autologous autoimmune hematopoietic stem cell transplant conditioning regimens: Concerns over the use of total-body irradiation in systemic sclerosis. *Bone Marrow Transplantation, 34*(9), 745–751.

Burt, R.K., Oyama, Y., Traynor, A., Quigley, K., Brush, M., Rodriguez, J., et al. (2003). Hematopoietic stem cell transplantation for systemic sclerosis with rapid improvement in skin scores: Is neoangiogenesis occurring? *Bone Marrow Transplantation, 32*(Supp. 1), S65–S67.

Charles, C., Clements, P., & Furst, D.E. (2006). Systemic sclerosis: Hypothesis-driven treatment strategies. *Lancet, 367*(9523), 1683–1691.

Cheng, K.K., Molassiotis, A., Chang, A.M, Wai, W.C., & Cheung, S.S. (2001). Evaluation of an oral care protocol intervention in the prevention of chemotherapy-induced oral mucositis in pediatric cancer patients. *European Journal of Cancer, 37*(16), 2056–2063.

Chiaverini, C., Passeron, T., & Ortonne, J.P. (2002). Treatment of vitiligo by topical calcipotriol. *Journal of the European Academy of Dermatology and Venereology, 16*(2), 137–138.

Clarkson, J.E., Worthington, H.V., & Eden, T.O.B. (2007). Interventions for preventing oral candidiasis for patients with cancer receiving treatment. *Cochrane Database of Systematic Reviews 2007*, Issue 1. Art. No.: CD003807. DOI: 10.1002/14651858.CD003807.pub3.

Clements, P.J., Hurwitz, E.L., Wong, W.K., Seibold, J.R., Mayes, M., White, B., et al. (2000). Skin thickness score as a predictor and correlate of outcome in systemic sclerosis. *Arthritis and Rheumatism, 43*(11), 2445–2454.

del Giudice, P., Bernard, E., Perrin, C., Bernardin, G., Fouche, R., Boissy, C., et al. (2000). Unusual cutaneous manifestations of miliary tuberculosis. *Clinical Infectious Diseases, 30*(1), 201–204.

Eilers, J., Berger, A.M., & Peterson, M.C. (1988). Development, testing, and application of the oral assessment guide. *Oncology Nursing Forum, 15*(3), 325–330.

Eilers, J., & Epstein, J.B. (2004). Assessment and measurement of oral mucositis. *Seminars in Oncology Nursing, 20*(1), 22–29.

Eilers, J., & Million, R. (2007). Prevention and management of oral mucositis in patients with cancer. *Seminars in Oncology Nursing, 23*(3), 201–212.

Elias, P.M., Feingold, K.R., & Fluhr, J.W. (2003). Skin as an organ of protection. In I.M. Freedberg, A.Z. Eisen, K. Wolff, K.F. Austen, L.A. Goldsmith, & S.I. Katz (Eds.), *Fitzpatrick's dermatology in general medicine* (6th ed., pp. 107–118). New York: McGraw-Hill.

Ermis, O., Alpsoy, E., Cetin, L., & Yilmaz, E. (2001). Is the efficacy of psoralen plus ultraviolet A therapy for vitiligo enhanced by concurrent topical calcipotriol? A placebo controlled double-blind study. *British Journal of Dermatology, 145*(3), 472–475.

Farah, C.S., Ashman, R., & Challacombe, S.J. (2000). Oral candidosis. *Clinics in Dermatology, 18*(5), 553–562.

Feliu, J., Diaz, R., Contreras, F., Casado, M., Espinosa, E., & Baron, M.G. (1997). Worsening psoriasis after treatment with G-CSF in a patient with small-cell lung cancer. *Journal of the National Cancer Institute, 89*(17), 1315–1316.

Forschner, T., Buchholtz, S., & Stockfleth, E. (2007). Current state of vitiligo therapy-evidence-based analysis of the literature. *Journal of German Society of Dermatology, 5*(6), 467–475.

Generini, S., Fiori, G., Pignone, A.M., Cerinic, M.M., & Cagnoni, M. (1999). Systemic sclerosis: A clinical overview. *Advances in Experimental Medicine and Biology, 455*, 73–83.

Gerlach, M. (2005). Wound care issues in patients with cancer. *Nursing Clinics of North America, 40*(2), 295–323.

Gilden, D.H., Kleinschmidt-DeMasters, B.K., LaGuardia, J.J., Mahalingam, R., & Cohrs, R.J. (2000). Neurologic complications of the reactivation of varicella-zoster virus. *New England Journal of Medicine, 342*(9), 635–645.

Goldberg, M.T., & McGinn-Byer, P. (2000). Oncology-related skin damage. In R.A. Bryant (Ed.), *Acute and chronic wounds: Nursing management* (2nd ed., pp. 367–386). St. Louis, MO: Mosby.

Griffiths, C.E.M., & Barker, J.N. (2007). Pathogenesis and clinical features of psoriasis. *Lancet, 370*(9583), 263–271.

Han, S.K., & Nordlund, J.J. (2000). Definition of vitiligo. In S.K. Han & J.J. Nordlund (Eds.), *Vitiligo* (p. 3). London: Blackwell Science.

Hartmann, A., Lurz, C., Hamm, H., Brocker, E.B., & Hofmann, U.B. (2005). Narrowband UVB311 nm vs. broadband UVB therapy in combination with topical calcipotriol vs. placebo in vitiligo. *International Journal of Dermatology, 44*(9), 736–742.

Hayden, B.K. (2004). Skin ulcerations. In C.H. Yarbro, M.H. Frogge, & M. Goodman (Eds.), *Cancer symptom management* (3rd ed., pp. 293–318). Sudbury, MA: Jones and Bartlett.

Heininger, U., & Seward, J.F. (2006). Varicella. *Lancet, 368*(9544), 1365–1376.

Hinchcliff, M., & Varga, J. (2007). Substantial progress has been made in treatments for organ-specific problems—Managing systemic sclerosis and its complications. *Journal of Musculoskeletal Medicine, 24*(10), 411–421.

Jaroneski, L.A. (2006). The importance of assessment rating scales for chemotherapy-induced oral mucositis. *Oncology Nursing Forum, 33*(6), 1085–1093.

Kleinschmidt-DeMasters, B.K., & Gilden, D.H. (2001). Varicella-zoster virus infections of the nervous system: Clinical and pathologic correlates. *Archives of Pathology and Laboratory Medicine, 125*(6), 770–780.

Klenk, A.S., Martin, A.G., & Heffernan, M.P. (2003). Yeast infections: Candidiasis, pityriasis (tinea) versicolor. In I.M. Freedberg, A.Z. Eisen, K. Wolff, K.F. Austen, L.A. Goldsmith, & S.I. Katz (Eds.), *Fitzpatrick's dermatology in general medicine* (6th ed., pp. 2006–2018). New York: McGraw-Hill.

Kojima, R., Kami, M., Kim, S.W., Murashige, N., Kishi, Y., Hori, A., et al. (2003). Induction of graft-versus-autoimmune (GVA) disease effect against refractory psoriasis by complete donor-type chimerism and graft-versus-host disease after allogeneic hematopoietic stem cell transplantation. *Bone Marrow Transplantation, 32*(4), 439–442.

Kolbinson, D.A., Schubert, M.M., & Flournoy, N. (1988). Early oral changes following bone marrow transplantation. *Oral Surgery, 66*(1), 130–138.

Koo, S.W., Suh, C.O., & Hann, S.K. (1996). Vitiligo following radiotherapy for carcinoma of the breast. *British Journal of Dermatology, 135*(5), 852–853.

Kressel, B., Szewczyk, C., & Tuazon, C.U. (1978). Early clinical recognition of disseminated candidiasis by muscle and skin biopsy. *Archives of Internal Medicine, 138*(3), 429–433.

Lepe, V., Moncada, B., Castanedo-Cazares, J.P., Torres-Alvarez, M.B., Ortiz, C.A., & Torres-Rubalcava, A.B. (2003). A double-blind randomized trial of 0.1% tacrolimus vs. 0.05% clobetasol for the treatment of childhood vitiligo. *Archives of Dermatology, 139*(5), 581–585.

Levine, E.L., & Ribeiro, G.G. (1994). Vitiligo and radiotherapy: The Koebner phenomenon demonstrated in patients with vitiligo undergoing radiotherapy for carcinoma of the breast. *Clinical Oncology, 6*(2), 133–134.

Lewis, R.E., & Klepser, M.E. (1999). The changing face of nosocomial candidemia: Epidemiology, resistance, and drug therapy. *American Journal of Health-System Pharmacy, 56*(6), 525–530.

MacDonald, A., & Burden, A.D. (2007). Psoriasis: Advances in pathophysiology and management. *Post Graduate Medicine Journal, 83*(985), 690–697.

Marras, T.K., Morris, A., Gonzalez, L.C., & Daley, C.L. (2004). Mortality prediction in pulmonary *Mycobacterium kansaii* infection and human immunodeficiency virus. *American Journal of Respiratory and Critical Care Medicine, 170*(7), 793–798.

Matz, H., & Tur, E. (2007). Vitiligo. *Current Problems in Dermatology, 35,* 78–102.

McGuire, D.B., Correa, M., Johnson, J., & Wienandts, P. (2006). The role of basic oral care and good clinical practice principles in the management of oral mucositis. *Supportive Care in Cancer, 14*(6), 541–547.

McGuire, D.B., Peterson, D.E., Muller, S., Owen, D.C., Slemmons, M.F., & Schubert, M.M. (2002). The 20 item oral mucositis index: Reliability and validity in bone marrow and stem cell transplant patients. *Cancer Investigation, 20*(7–8), 893–903.

McNally, M.A., & Langlais, R.P. (1996). Conditions peculiar to the tongue. *Dermatology Clinics, 14*(2), 257.

Mendoza, F., & Derk, C.T. (2007). Systemic sclerosis mortality in the United States: 1999–2002 implications for patient care. *Journal of Clinical Rheumatology, 13*(4), 187–192.

Mollet, I., Ongenae, K., & Naeyaert, J.M. (2007). Origin, clinical presentation, and diagnosis of hypomelanotic skin disorders. *Dermatologic Clinics, 25*(3), 363–371.

Morris, C.D., Sepkowitz, K., Fonshell, C., Margetson, N., Eagan, J., Miransky, J., et al. (2003). Prospective identification of risk factors for wound infection after lower extremity oncologic surgery. *Annals of Surgical Oncology, 10*(7), 778–782.

Multinational Association of Supportive Care in Cancer/International Society for Oral Oncology. (2005). *Summary of evidence-based clinical practice guidelines for care of patients with oral and gastrointestinal mucositis (2005 update).* Retrieved January 20, 2007, from http://www.mascc.org/media/Resource_centers/Guidelines_mucositis.doc

National Cancer Institute Cancer Therapy Evaluation Program. (2009). *Common terminology criteria for adverse events* (version 4.0). Bethesda, MD: National Cancer Institute. Retrieved July 28, 2009, from http://ctep.cancer.gov/protocolDevelopment/electronic_applications/docs/ctcaev4.pdf

Njoo, M.D., & Westerhof, W. (2001). Vitiligo: Pathogenesis and treatment. *American Journal of Clinical Dermatology, 2*(3), 167–181.

Ortonne, J.P., Bahadoran, P., Fitzpatrick, T.B., Mosher, D.B., & Hori, Y. (2003). Hypomelanoses and hypermelanoses. In I.M. Freedberg, A.Z. Eisen, K. Wolff, K.F. Austen, L.A. Goldsmith, & S.I. Katz (Eds.), *Fitzpatrick's dermatology in general medicine* (6th ed., pp. 836–881). New York: McGraw-Hill.

Ostojic, P., & Damjanov, N. (2006). Different clinical features in patients with limited and diffuse cutaneous systemic sclerosis. *Clinical Rheumatology, 25*(4), 453–457.

Parsad, D., Saini, R., & Verma, N. (1998). Combination of PUVAsol and topical calcipotriol in vitiligo. *Dermatology, 197*(2), 167–170.

Pianigiani, E., Andreassi, A., & Andreassi, L. (2005). Autografts and cultured epidermis in the treatment of vitiligo. *Clinics in Dermatology, 23*(2), 424–429.

Rebora, A., Marples, R.R., & Kligman, A.M. (1973). Experimental infection with Candida albicans. *Archives of Dermatology, 108*(1), 69–73.

Robertson, J.M., Clarke, D.H., Pevzner, M.M., & Matter, R.C. (1991). Breast conservation therapy. Severe breast fibrosis after radiation therapy in patients with collagen vascular disease. *Cancer, 68*(3), 502–508.

Rose, C., Auxenfants, E., Noel, M.P., Mahieu, M., Demory, J.L., Croxo, C., et al. (1997). Tuberculosis, mycobacterium infection and hairy cell leukemia. *Presse Medicale, 26*(3), 110–114.

Rubenstein, E.B., Peterson, D.E., Schubert, M., Keefe, D., McGuire, D., Epstein, J., et al. (2004). Clinical practice guidelines for the prevention and treatment of cancer therapy-induced oral and gastrointestinal mucositis. *Cancer, 100*(Suppl. 9), 2026–2046.

Saral, Y., Coskun, B.K., Ozturk, P., Bulut, Y., & Cobanoglu, B. (2005). Multiple metastatic tuberculosis abscesses in a patient with Pott disease and lung tuberculosis: A case report. *Journal of Cutaneous Pathology, 32*(9), 629–633.

Schubert, M.M., Williams, B.B., Lloid, M.E., Donaldson, G., & Chapko, M.K. (1992). Clinical assessment scale for the rating of oral mucosal changes associated with bone marrow transplantation. Development of an oral mucositis index. *Cancer, 69*(10), 2469–2477.

Scleroderma. (2009). *Online etymology dictionary.* Retrieved February 22, 2009, from http://www.etymonline.com/index.php?term=scleroderma

Sehgal, V.N., & Srivastava, G. (2007). Vitiligo: Compendium of clinico-epidemiological features. *Indian Journal of Dermatology, Venereology and Leprology, 73*(3), 149–156.

Silman, A.J. (1995). Scleroderma. *Baillière's Clinical Rheumatology, 9*(3), 471–482.

Sonis, S.T., Eilers, J.G., Epstein, J.B., LeVeque, F.G., Liggett, W.H., Jr., Mulahga, M.T., et al. (1999). Validation of a new scoring system for the assessment of clinical trial research of oral mucositis induced by radiation or chemotherapy. Mucositis Study Group. *Cancer, 85*(10), 2103–2113.

Soysa, N.S., Samaranayake, L.P., & Ellepola, A.N. (2004). Cytotoxic drugs, radiotherapy and oral candidiasis. *Oral Oncology, 40*(10), 971–978.

Staib, P., Kretschmar, M., Nichterlein, T., Kohler, G., & Morschhauser, J. (2000). Expression of virulence genes in Candida albicans. *Advances in Experimental Medicine and Biology, 485*, 167–176.

Stankus, S.J., Dlugopolski, M., & Packer, D. (2000). Management of herpes zoster (shingles) and postherpetic neuralgia. *American Family Physician, 61*(8). Retrieved January 14, 2007, from http://www.aafp.org.ezproxy.galter.northwestern.edu/afp/20000415/2437.html

Steiner, I., Kennedy, P.G.E., & Pachner, A.R. (2007). The neurotropic herpes viruses: Herpes simplex and varicella-zoster. *Lancet Neurology, 6*(11), 1015–1028.

Stern, R.S. (1997). Psoriasis. *Lancet, 350*(9074), 349–353.

Stillman, R.M. (2008). *Wound care: Treatment.* Retrieved February 25, 2009, from http://emedicine.medscape.com/article/194018-treatment

Sunderkotter, C., Kuhn, A., Hunzelmann, N., & Beissert, S. (2006). Phototherapy: A promising treatment option for skin sclerosis in scleroderma? *Rheumatology, 45*(Suppl. 3), iii52–iii54.

Tappeiner, G., & Wolff, K. (2003). Tuberculosis and other mycobacterial infections. In I.M. Freedberg, A.Z. Eisen, K. Wolff, K.F. Austen, L.A. Goldsmith, & S.I. Katz (Eds.), *Fitzpatrick's dermatology in general medicine* (6th ed., pp. 1933–1950). New York: McGraw-Hill.

Tomlinson, M.J. (2001). Psoriasis and radiotherapy. *Clinical Oncology, 13*(2), 145–147.

Valkova, S., Trashlieva, M., & Christova, P. (2004). Treatment of vitiligo with local khellin and UVA: Comparison with systemic PUVA. *Clinical and Experimental Dermatology, 29*(2), 180–184.

Van Laar, J.M., & Tyndall, A. (2006). Adult stem cells in the treatment of autoimmune diseases. *Rheumatology, 45*(10), 1187–1193.

Varga, J., & Abraham, D. (2007). Systemic sclerosis: A prototypic multisystem fibrotic disorder. *Journal of Clinical Investigation, 117*(3), 557–567.

Varga, J., Haustein, U.F., Creech, R.H., Dwyer, J.P., & Jimenez, S.A. (1991). Exaggerated radiation-induced fibrosis in patients with systemic sclerosis. *JAMA, 265*(24), 3292–3295.

Wenger, C.B. (2003). Thermoregulation. In I.M. Freedberg, A.Z. Eisen, K. Wolff, K.F. Austen, L.A. Goldsmith, & S.I. Katz (Eds.), *Fitzpatrick's dermatology in general medicine* (6th ed., pp. 119–127). New York: McGraw-Hill.

Winterfield, L.S., Menter, A., Gordon, K., & Gottlieb, A. (2005). Psoriasis treatment: Current and emerging directed therapies. *Annals of the Rheumatic Diseases, 64*(Suppl. 2), ii87–ii90.

World Health Organization. (1979). *Handbook for reporting results of cancer treatment.* Geneva, Switzerland: Author.

Worthington, H.V., Clarkson, J.E., & Eden, O.B. (2007). Interventions for treating oral candidiasis for patients with cancer receiving treatment. *Cochrane Database of Systematic Reviews 2007*, Issue 2. Art. No.: CD001972. DOI: 10.1002/14651858.CD001972.pub3.

Zaoutis, T.E., Argon, J., Chu, J., Berlin, J.A., Walsh, T.J., & Feudtner, C. (2005). The epidemiology and attributable outcomes of candidemia in adults and children hospitalized in the United States: A propensity analysis. *Clinical Infectious Diseases, 41*(9), 1232–1239.

Zuber, J.P., & Spertini, F. (2006). Immunological basis of systemic sclerosis. *Rheumatology, 45*(Suppl. 3), iii23–iii25.

CHAPTER 11

Skin and Wound Pain: Assessment and Management

Dorothy B. Doughty, MN, RN, CWOCN, FAAN

Introduction

Pain is extremely common among patients with altered skin and tissue integrity, regardless of the etiology of the skin and tissue damage. Studies of pain in patients with chronic wounds reveal that 60%–90% of these individuals report pain, and pain is the wound-related factor with the greatest negative impact on quality of life (Coulling, 2007; Fleck, 2007; Krasner, Shapshak, & Hopf, 2007; Rastinehad, 2006; Szor & Bourguignon, 1999). These studies also found that skin and wound pain was not an area of focus for clinicians, who were more concerned with wound management and wound healing. In fact, one study of patients with pressure ulcers found that only 6% received analgesics for their pain (Szor & Bourguignon). The data regarding skin and wound pain have tremendous relevance to the oncology patient population because the therapies designed to eradicate or control the cancer also can cause significant skin and tissue damage—and resulting pain. Pain management is a key element of care for any patient with cancer, and oncology nurses are the primary "drivers" of programs to ensure that pain is routinely assessed and effectively managed. However, management of cancer-related pain does not necessarily provide relief of wound-based pain, and unrelieved skin and wound pain has an adverse effect on quality of life; if severe, it may even result in treatment dropout. Thus, knowledgeable assessment and management of skin and wound pain is a key skill in the oncology nurse's armamentarium. This chapter will address the pathology, assessment, and management of skin and wound pain.

Types of Pain

Effective management of wound-related pain is dependent on accurate assessment of the type of pain. Two classification systems are of particular benefit in assessing and managing wound-related pain: pathophysiology of the pain and occurrence and duration of the pain (Dallam, Barkauskas, Ayello, & Baranoski, 2004; Krasner et al., 2007).

Classification Based on Pathophysiology

From a pathophysiologic perspective, pain can be classified as either nociceptive or neuropathic, and nociceptive pain can be further classified as either somatic or visceral. *Nociceptive* pain is caused by tissue damage or inflammation, which causes release of substances (such as histamine, prostaglandins, and substance P) that stimulate the afferent nerve receptors, specifically the A-delta and C fibers. These activated nerve fibers transmit the pain message along the spinal cord to the brain, where it is processed and recognized as pain (Dallam et al., 2004; Krasner et al., 2007; McNaughton & Nimmo, 2004; Popescu & Salcido, 2004). The severity of the pain is determined partly by the intensity of the tissue damage or inflammation but is modulated considerably by other factors, such as the patient's sociocultural background, emotional status, level of anxiety, and beliefs regarding the cause of the pain (Briggs & Torra i Bou, 2002; Jones, 2004; McNaughton & Nimmo). Nociceptive pain originating from the skin, soft tissue, muscle, connective tissue, or bone is further classified as *somatic* pain. It typically is well localized and usually is described as sharp, throbbing, or aching. Skin and wound pain caused by chemotherapy or radiation therapy generally is somatic in nature. Nociceptive pain caused by inflammation of an internal organ is known as *visceral* pain; in contrast to somatic pain, visceral pain usually is poorly localized, more likely to be described as cramping, and more likely to be associated with autonomic symptoms such as nausea, vomiting, and diaphoresis (Krasner et al.). Nociceptive pain generally is time-limited, meaning that once the pathologic process has been effectively treated and resolved, the pain subsides. Nociceptive pain typically responds well to local measures to address the etiologic factors as well as to anti-inflammatory agents and opioid analgesics (American Medical Association [AMA], 2007; Dallam et al.; Krasner et al.).

Neuropathic pain differs considerably from nociceptive pain. Nociceptive pain is a response to local tissue damage or inflammation, whereas *neuropathic pain* is caused by damage to some component of the nervous system itself, which results in abnormal processing of stimuli and spontaneous generation of pain signals independent of any tissue trauma. One potential etiologic factor for neuropathic pain is persistent, poorly managed nociceptive pain; the prolonged activation of the nerve fibers is thought to cause morphologic changes that result in neuropathic pain. Neuropathic pain usually is described as burning, tingling, lancinating, or "electric shock" in nature and frequently is complicated by hyperalgesia and allodynia. *Hyperalgesia* is the state in which any touch is perceived as painful (because of abnormal processing of tactile stimuli), and *allodynia* refers to a severely exaggerated response to minor discomfort; for example, slow and careful removal of tape or an adhesive dressing may be perceived as acutely and severely painful. Unlike nociceptive pain, neuropathic pain responds poorly to anti-inflammatory agents and opioids. Topical anesthetics, tricyclic antidepressants, and anticonvulsants represent primary treatment options (AMA, 2007; Dallam et al., 2004; Krasner et al., 2007; Wulf & Baron, 2002).

Classification Based on Occurrence and Duration

Another approach to classification of wound pain is based on the occurrence and duration of the pain. Within this classification system, pain may be classified as either acute or persistent. *Acute pain* is elicited by manipulation of the wound such as with dressing changes or the application of topical agents. This type of pain usually is very responsive to simple measures such as premedication, the use of atraumatic wound care products, and gentle technique. In contrast, *persistent pain* is wound-related pain that persists even when the wound is not being disturbed or manipulated. This type of pain is obviously more difficult to manage and is not controlled by modifications in wound-care techniques. It requires around-the-clock analgesics along with adjuvant therapies such as relaxation therapy and possibly electrical stimulation (Dallam et al., 2004; Krasner, 2001; Krasner et al., 2007).

Pain Assessment

Strategies for effective pain management differ based on the type of pain (nociceptive versus neuropathic) and on the occurrence and duration of pain (acute versus persistent); thus, thorough assessment of the patient's pain is the first step in formulating an appropriate management plan (Young, 2007). Factors to be included in assessment of wound-related pain are highlighted in Table 11-1; the most critical elements include the following.

Description of Pain

Obtaining an accurate description of the pain is essential, because analgesics that are effective for nociceptive pain are typically ineffective for neuropathic pain. If patients have a difficult time describing the pain, they can be asked whether the pain is "aching or throbbing" in nature or whether it is more of a "burning, tingling, electric-shock" type sensation. In addition, oncology nurses should assess for any evidence of hyperalgesia or allodynia (e.g., wincing in response to light touch, or reporting severe pain with dressing removal). Finally, nurses should be aware that patients may have both nocice-

Table 11-1. Key Parameters in Assessment of Wound-Related Pain	
Assessment Parameter	**Descriptors**
Type of pain	Nociceptive (aching or throbbing pain) versus neuropathic (burning or lancinating pain) versus mixed
Occurrence	Persistent versus episodic (associated with wound care) versus persistent pain worsened by wound care
Severity (validated severity scale)	Numeric Pain Intensity Scale, Visual Analog Scale, Faces Pain Rating Scale, Pain Assessment in Advanced Dementia (PAINAD) Scale
Exacerbating and relieving factors	Factors increasing severity of pain or alleviating the pain
Impact on quality of life	Lifestyle changes caused by wound pain
Pain management goals	Established by patient; basis for determining efficacy of the pain management program
Relevant history	Past history of painful conditions, use of analgesics, drug or alcohol abuse

ptive and neuropathic pain occurring simultaneously; specifically, patients may describe "burning, throbbing" pain that is worsened by dressing changes and also may exhibit allodynia (AMA, 2007; Dallam et al., 2004; Krasner et al., 2007; McNaughton & Nimmo, 2004).

Occurrence

Another critical factor to be included in pain assessment is determination of when the pain occurs and whether it is acute, persistent, or both. Specifically, nurses need to determine which of the following scenarios best reflects the patient's wound-related pain: pain that primarily occurs during wound care or dressing changes, pain that is persistent but is worsened by wound care or dressing changes, or pain that is persistent and unaffected by wound care or dressing changes. Good questions to ask include the following (Krasner et al., 2007):
- Do you have pain related to wound care or dressing changes?
- Do you have pain that is constant/persistent (i.e., that extends beyond dressing changes and interferes with sleep and other activities of daily living)?
- If so, does the pain get worse during wound care?

Severity

It is important to determine the severity of the pain using a validated scale. This provides baseline data against which subsequent ratings can be compared and allows nurses and patients to more objectively evaluate the effectiveness of the current pain management program. In evaluating pain severity, it is critical to recognize that a patient's "self-report" is the single most reliable indicator of the pain's severity, duration, and impact so long as the patient is cognitively intact. Secondly, patients should be asked to self-report their pain using a validated scale that provides a quantifiable measure of severity. Several validated scales are available that are easy to use with cognitively intact adults and older children. These include the Numeric Pain Intensity Scale (NPIS), the Visual Analog Scale (VAS), and the Faces Pain Rating Scale (FPRS) (Bergstrom et al., 1994; Dallam et al., 2004; Krasner et al., 2007; McNaughton & Nimmo, 2004).

The NPIS is sometimes considered the "gold standard." In the Oncology Nursing Society (ONS) Patient Outcomes Survey conducted in October 2004, 83.4% of the 1,327 respondents reported that they utilized the NPIS (ONS, 2004). The NPIS is appropriate for children older than age seven and can be administered verbally or using a visual scale. The visual scale consists of a 10 cm line, with 0 at one end representing no pain and 10 at the other end representing the worst possible pain. The visual scale includes additional descriptors (2 represents mild pain; 4–6 represents moderate pain; and 8 represents severe pain). The VAS is similar to the NPIS except it has no numbers; instead, there is a 10 cm line with the indicators "no pain" and "pain as bad as it could possibly be" on the two ends of the straight line. The scale is explained to patients, and they are asked to indicate the point on the line that most accurately reflects the severity of their pain. The FPRS is the preferred tool for use with children ages 3 or older and also has been used effectively with patients for whom English is a second language and for adults with some degree of cognitive impairment. The FPRS consists of six faces ranging from a smiling face (no pain) to a frowning face (worst pain) (Dallam et al., 2004; Wong, Hockenberry-Eaton, Wilson, Winkelstein, & Schwartz, 2001).

Given that self-report is the most accurate indicator of pain severity, it is obviously difficult to accurately assess for presence and severity of pain when the patient is cognitively impaired or unable to communicate using a pain scale. An established tool for assessing pain severity among these patients is known as the Pain Assessment in Advanced Dementia (PAINAD) Scale. It consists of five indicators (breathing, negative vocalization, facial expression, body language, and consolability), each of which is rated on a scale of 0–2. In settings where this tool is not used, nurses should routinely assess for nonverbal indicators of pain such as grimacing, moaning, irritability, and withdrawal from touch (Krasner et al., 2007; Warden, Hurley, & Volicer, 2003).

Exacerbating and Relieving Factors

Nurses should ask patients about strategies and conditions that make the pain better or worse; relieving factors can then be incorporated into the management plan, while every effort should be made to avoid or compensate for exacerbating factors. For example, if wound care is a primary exacerbating factor, the management plan should include attention to selection of topical agents and dressings to eliminate or minimize the pain, as well as the possible need for premedication (Briggs & Torra i Bou, 2002; Krasner et al., 2007).

Impact on Quality of Life, and Pain Management Goals

Pain is the wound-related factor with the greatest negative impact on quality of life, and pain is an intensely individualized experience. Thus, only the patient can relate the impact of the pain in terms of ability to eat, sleep, carry out basic activities of daily living, and enjoy time with family and friends. Only patients can determine the level of pain that is "manageable and acceptable" for themselves, and it is critical to hear from the patients how the pain is affecting their lives. Phenomenologic studies addressing the impact of wound-related pain reported that healthcare providers frequently fail to "hear and acknowledge" the pain, and this lack of acknowledgment has a very negative impact on the patient (Rastinehad, 2006). If the patient reports significant pain but does not volunteer information about the impact, the oncology nurse should specifically ask about the patient's ability to sleep, eat, carry out critical activities, and interact with others. It is essential to ask the patient to establish a pain goal, to work aggressively toward reaching that goal, and to continually evaluate the effectiveness of the existing pain management program in light of that goal. A major goal of care for any patient with cancer is to optimize quality of life, and pain control is a critical element.

Relevant History

In addition to assessing the characteristics of the pain itself, the nurse should assess for prior painful conditions and episodes, past or present use of prescription analgesics, and any history of alcohol or drug abuse. Patients who have a history of alcohol or drug abuse and patients who have been taking opioid analgesics typically will require higher doses of medications to obtain comparable pain relief (Krasner et al., 2007).

Pain Management

Development of an effective pain management plan depends on accurate identification of the type of pain (nociceptive versus neuropathic versus mixed), the temporal features of the pain (acute pain related to dressing changes versus persistent pain versus persistent pain exacerbated by dressing changes), the severity of the pain in relation to the patient's established pain goal, and known exacerbating and relieving factors. The patient should be involved in the pain management plan, and the team should emphasize to the patient the importance of adequate pain relief, both in terms of wound healing and quality of life (Fleck, 2007; Krasner et al., 2007). Effective pain management strategies can be classified and selected based on the type of pain against which they are effective (i.e., acute pain related to wound care and dressing changes, persistent nociceptive pain, persistent neuropathic pain).

Management of Acute Pain

Shukla et al. (2005) conducted a descriptive study on wound-related pain and found that the most common type of wound-related pain was acute pain related to wound care; for many patients, dressing removal was the most painful specific aspect of wound care. These findings were echoed by an international survey of wound care providers, in which dressing removal and wound cleansing were reported as the most painful aspects of wound care (Moffatt, Franks, & Hollinworth, 2002; Shukla et al.). Fortunately, pain related to wound care is the easiest type of pain to manage. Effective strategies include general comfort measures and distraction, selection of wound care products and techniques that minimize or eliminate tissue trauma, and premedication with topical or systemic analgesics (Dallam et al., 2004; Krasner et al., 2007) .

General comfort measures: General comfort measures include temperature control, positioning for maximum comfort, creation of a soothing and relaxing environment to the extent possible (e.g., with music and lighting), and distraction during dressing removal and wound care. Distraction techniques can be as simple as talking with the patient during wound care or having the patient focus on deep breathing or imagery during dressing removal and wound cleansing. Another effective approach is to provide the patient with increased control. For example, many patients prefer to remove their own dressings; allowing them to do so reduces anxiety as well as discomfort and conveys to patients the nurse's concern for their comfort. Another patient-control strategy that helps to reduce anxiety is to allow patients to call "time out" at any point in the wound care process (Dallam et al., 2004; Krasner et al., 2007).

Product selection: Many modifications in dressing selection and wound care techniques can be used to minimize tissue trauma and the associated pain. These modifications fall into three major categories: product selection, modifications in wound care technique, and routine protection of the periwound skin. *Product selection* involves choice of a cleansing agent and a dressing or topical agent and possibly the selection of tape or an alternative product to secure the dressing. In selecting a cleanser, the guidelines are fairly simple: The cleansing agent should be noncytotoxic (and therefore nonirritating to the nerve receptors in the wound bed) and ideally should be close to body temperature (Jones, 2004). The best options typically are warm saline, tap water, or commercial wound cleansers. The following are key considerations in selecting dressings (Briggs & Torra i Bou, 2002; Dallam et al., 2004; Krasner et al., 2007):

- Effective control of exudate, because chronic wound exudate contains a high concentration of inflammatory mediators that can activate nociceptive nerve fibers and cause irritation of the periwound tissue

- Maintenance of a moist wound surface, because a layer of fluid at the wound surface bathes and protects the nerve fibers and also promotes the wound healing process
- Atraumatic removal (i.e., topical agents that do not stick to the wound bed and do not cause trauma with removal).

Good choices for dressing selection include gel dressings, absorptive dressings with silicone adhesive, and absorptive dressings with a nonadherent cover that does not stick to the wound. If the patient is at high risk for wound infection or has indicators of increased bioburden (such as increased exudate, increased pain, and deterioration in the wound surface), sustained-release silver dressings can be extremely helpful. Anecdotal reports suggest that silver dressings may help to reduce pain, probably because, in part, of their ability to reduce bacterial counts. Clearly, there is no one "best" dressing, as the optimal dressing for any wound must be selected based on the volume of exudate as well as the need for atraumatic removal. However, standard gauze dressings usually are *not* a good option because gauze sticks to the wound bed and causes trauma and pain with removal (Briggs & Torra i Bou, 2002; Ovington, 2001). If standard gauze dressings are the only dressings immediately available, a nonadherent contact layer such as Adaptic™ (Systagenix Wound Management) or Xeroform™ (Kendall Healthcare) gauze can be placed directly over the wound to provide protection of the wound surface and atraumatic removal. Appropriate dressings are highlighted in Table 11-2, along with indications and guidelines for use.

Although some of the recommended dressings include a silicone adhesive surface, some are nonadherent. When a nonadherent dressing is selected, the

Table 11-2. Pain-Reducing Dressings		
Category/Type of Dressing	Characteristics/Considerations	Examples
Silicone foam dressings	• Effectively manage moderate amounts of exudate • Maintain moist wound surface • Provide secure adhesion with atraumatic removal • Available with sustained-release silver	Mepilex®, Mepilex Ag (Mölnlycke Health Care)
Nonadherent foam dressings	• Effectively manage moderate amounts of exudate • Maintain moist wound surface • Provide atraumatic removal • Available with sustained-release silver • *Require securement with wrap gauze or tape*	PolyMem®, PolyMem Silver® (Ferris Mfg. Corp.) Allevyn™ (Smith & Nephew)

(Continued on next page)

Table 11-2. Pain-Reducing Dressings *(Continued)*

Category/Type of Dressing	Characteristics/Considerations	Examples
Amorphous gel dressings	• Maintain a moist wound surface • Appropriate only for wounds with minimal exudate • Available with sustained-release silver and with lidocaine • *Require secondary dressing and method of securement*	Curasol® (Health-point, Ltd.) SilvaSorb® Gel (Medline Industries, Inc.) Regenecare® (MPM Medical, Inc.)
Solid gel dressings (glycerine based or water based)	• Absorb small amounts of exudate • Maintain a moist wound surface • Provide atraumatic removal • *Require securement with wrap gauze or tape* • *Glycerine-based dressings are resistant to dehydration and do not cause maceration of intact skin.*	Glycerine-based: Derma-Gel™ (Medline Industries, Inc.) Water-based: Vigilon® (C.R. Bard, Inc.)
Gauze with nonadherent surface	• Effectively manages exudate • Provides a moist wound surface and atraumatic removal • Available in multiple sizes and shapes • *Requires securement with wrap gauze or tape*	Exu-Dry™ (Smith & Nephew) SofSorb® (DeRoyal Industries)
Contact layer dressings (used in conjunction with gauze secondary dressing)	• Provide nonadherent porous surface that protects wound bed while permitting exudate to pass through dressing for absorption by secondary dressing • *Require secondary dressing/method of securement*	Adaptic™ (Systagenix Wound Management) Xeroform™ (Kendall Healthcare)
Hydrofiber dressings	• Provide effective control of moderate amounts of exudate • Form solid gel that is soothing and maintains a moist wound surface • Available in flat and rope form • Available with sustained-release silver • *Require securement with wrap gauze or tape*	Aquacel®, Aquacel Ag (ConvaTec Inc.)
Sustained-release silver dressings	• Provides antimicrobial activity for up to seven days • Available in multiple forms: hydrofiber (for wet wounds), foam (for wet wounds), gel (for dry wounds), and contact layer (for wet or dry wounds)	SilvaSorb Algidex™ Ag (DeRoyal Industries)

Note. Based on information from Blackett, 2007; Dallam et al., 2004; Krasner et al., 2007; Maki & Clarey-Sanford, 2007.

final product decision involves the selection of a securement product that provides for atraumatic or minimally traumatic removal. When the wound is on the head, the neck, or an extremity, wrap gauze or stretch netting usually is the best option. For wounds on the trunk, it may be necessary to select one of the newer tapes with a fabric backing and less aggressive adhesive (e.g., Medipore™, 3M). If an adhesive agent *is* used to secure the dressing, it is helpful to use a petroleum-based adhesive removal product to ensure painless dressing removal (e.g., Uni-Solve™ [Smith & Nephew]). See Chapter 5 for more detailed information about dressings.

Modifications in wound care technique: In addition to selecting dressings and topical agents that are skin and wound "friendly," nurses need to practice and teach gentle wound care *technique*. For example, dressings should be removed slowly using a "press and peel" action as opposed to a "quick rip" approach, and wounds should be cleansed using gentle flushing and blotting as opposed to scrubbing.

Protection of periwound skin: Some of the pain related to wounds and wound care is caused by inflammation or trauma involving the periwound skin, which usually is caused either by removal of products with aggressive adhesive, or from exposure of the intact skin surrounding the wound to the inflammatory mediators in the wound exudate. Routine use of a skin "sealant" such as Skin-Prep™ (Smith & Nephew) is very helpful in providing protection of the periwound skin (Dallam et al., 2004). The copolymer sealant provides a plasticizing film on the periwound skin that serves as an artificial skin layer and helps to prevent epidermal stripping, and it also serves as a moisture barrier, thus protecting the periwound skin against the irritating effects of the exudate. If the wound is on the head, the neck, or an extremity and the dressing is being secured by wrap gauze, as opposed to an adhesive dressing, moisture barrier ointments such as petrolatum or dimethicone products can be used to protect the periwound skin from the exudate.

Premedication: Premedication is the third approach to prevention of acute pain related to wound care and dressing changes and may involve topical anesthetic agents, systemic analgesics, or combination therapy. Commonly used topical agents include lidocaine jelly (2% or 4%) or EMLA® (eutectic mixture of local anesthetics) cream (AstraZeneca Pharmaceuticals) applied immediately following dressing removal and prior to wound cleansing or manipulation (Dallam et al., 2004; Krasner et al., 2007). When using topical analgesics, it is critical to follow manufacturers' guidelines for use and to allow enough time for the medication to take effect before beginning any wound care; for example, EMLA cream should be covered with an occlusive plastic wrap and typically takes effect in about 20 minutes, although it sometimes takes longer (Evans & Gray, 2005). When systemic analgesics are used for premedication, the agent should be administered about 30 minutes to an hour before the wound care procedure. In an inpatient setting, the staff can premedicate the patient and then perform the dressing change once the patient reports good analgesic effect. In an outpatient setting, the patient should be counseled to take the medication before coming to the clinic. Oral transmucosal fentanyl citrate works extremely well for premedication because it takes effect in as little as 10 minutes (Dallam et al., 2004) (see Table 11-3). For very painful wounds or in situations where the patient is extremely anxious because of prior painful experiences, providing both systemic and topical premedication, in addition to general comfort measures and gentle wound care, may be beneficial.

Management of Persistent Nociceptive Pain

Persistent nociceptive pain cannot be managed simply with modifications in dressings, wound care techniques, and premedication; persistent pain re-

Table 11-3. Topical and Systemic Analgesics			
Category	Specific Drugs/ Agents	Usual Dosage	Characteristics/Considerations
Rapid-Acting			Typically used for prevention of acute episodic pain associated with wound care
• Topical	Lidocaine jelly/ solution	2%; 4%	Requires 10–20 minutes to take effect
	EMLA® cream (AstraZeneca Pharmaceuticals)	N/A	Should be applied to wound and covered with occlusive dressing; usually takes effect in 20 minutes
• Systemic	Oral transmucosal fentanyl	200–400 mcg	Onset < 10 minutes; duration 1–2 hours Potentiated by opioids, alcohol, central nervous system depressants Monitor respiratory function.
Sustained-Release			Required for relief of persistent pain
• Topical	Lidoderm® patch (5% lidocaine) (Endo Pharmaceuticals)	Applied for 12 out of 24 hours (up to 3 patches to involved area)	Applied to intact skin adjacent to affected area Effective for both nociceptive and neuropathic pain
	Regenecare® Gel (2% lidocaine) (MPM Medical, Inc.)	Applied 1–3 times/day	Provides a moist wound healing environment along with control of pain and itching

(Continued on next page)

Table 11-3. Topical and Systemic Analgesics *(Continued)*			
Category	**Specific Drugs/ Agents**	**Usual Dosage**	**Characteristics/Considerations**
• Systemic	Nonsteroidal anti-inflam-matory drugs (NSAIDs) (aspirin, ibuprofen, naproxen)	Aspirin: 325–1,000 mg every 4–6 hours Ibuprofen: 200–400 mg every 4–6 hours Naproxen: 500 mg as initial dose; then 250 mg every 6–8 hours	Provides local anti-inflammatory and central analgesic effects Does not cause sedation, tolerance, or dependence Should be taken with food or milk to reduce gastric irritation; if gastric irritation is a problem, consider use of a cyclooxygenase-2 inhibitor (e.g., celecoxib) Should be taken on schedule, not as needed
	Acetaminophen	325–650 mg every 4–6 hours	Used as alternative to NSAIDs for patients in whom gastric irritation a problem Must closely monitor total intake to prevent liver toxicity Should be taken on schedule, not as needed
	Mild opioids (codeine with or without acetaminophen, hydrocodone with acetaminophen, oxycodone with acetaminophen)	Codeine: 15–60 mg every 4–6 hrs Hydrocodone: 5–10 mg every 4– 6 hours Oxycodone: 10–30 mg every 4 hours	Used in combination with NSAIDs or acetaminophen for moderate pain (more effective for nociceptive pain than for neuropathic pain) Must monitor bowel function and initiate program to prevent or manage constipation Nausea and vomiting are common side effects; monitor and provide antiemetics as needed. May cause sedation, especially in combination with other central nervous system depressants

(Continued on next page)

Category	Specific Drugs/ Agents	Usual Dosage	Characteristics/Considerations
	Strong opioids (morphine, fentanyl, oxycodone)	Morphine (immediate release): 10–30 mg PO every 3–4 hours as initial dose Fentanyl transdermal: 25 mcg/hour as initial dose Oxycodone (immediate release): 10–30 mg every 4 hours	Used in combination with NSAIDs for moderate to severe pain (more effective for nociceptive pain) All available in sustained-release formulas as well as fast-acting; dose titrated to desired effect Nausea and constipation are common side effects; monitor and provide antiemetics and bowel program as needed.
	Anticonvulsants (gabapentin, pregabalin)	Gabapentin: 300–3,600 mg/day (dose titrated upward based on response) Pregabalin: 300–600 mg/day	Given for relief of neuropathic pain, either alone or in combination with NSAIDs and opioids Common side effects include dizziness and drowsiness, especially during initial therapy; patients should be counseled to avoid alcohol and to take at bedtime.
	Antidepressants (amitriptyline, desipramine)	Amitriptyline: 25–100 mg/day Desipramine: 75–300 mg/day	Help to relieve neuropathic pain by inhibiting reuptake of norepinephrine Common side effects include drowsiness and dry mouth; patients should be counseled to take at bedtime.

Table 11-3. Topical and Systemic Analgesics *(Continued)*

Note. Based on information from Evans & Gray, 2005; *Mosby's 2006 Drug Consult for Nurses*, 2006; Wong et al., 2007.

quires persistent therapy. This typically involves sustained-release topical analgesics or around-the-clock systemic analgesics, or some combination of these two approaches, in addition to general comfort measures and appropriate gentle wound care (Krasner et al., 2007; Senecal, 1999).

Sustained-release topical analgesics: The use of sustained-release topical analgesics is relatively new, and these agents represent one of the most important advances in topical wound care and pain management (see Table 11-3). For some patients, effective use of topical agents can eliminate the need for systemic analgesics, and for others, these agents can significantly reduce the required dose of systemic agents, thus effectively reducing the incidence of side effects related to the systemic medications. One of the most commonly used products at present is the Lidoderm® patch (Endo Pharmaceuticals). This adhesive patch, which provides sustained-release 5% lidocaine, is applied to intact skin *adjacent* to the wound or painful area for 12 out of 24 hours. Systemic absorption is minimal, so the product is considered safe for most individuals, although the prescribing provider should query the patient regarding use of any antiarrhythmic agents (Popescu & Salcido, 2004). Some concerns have been raised regarding the effects of lidocaine on wound healing; interestingly, early studies have suggested a positive impact, specifically an anti-inflammatory and possibly an antibacterial effect (Cassuto, Sinclair, & Bonderovic, 2006; Parr, Zoutman, & Davidson, 1999; Pecher, Bottiger, Graf, & Hollmann, 2004).

Dressings and wound care products are now emerging that provide sustained topical analgesia as well as support for moist wound healing. For example, Regenecare® (MPM Medical, Inc.) is an amorphous hydrogel that contains 2% lidocaine. It has been used for a number of painful wounds but specifically for the itching and painful skin rash associated with epidermal growth factor receptor inhibitors such as cetuximab, gefitinib, erlotinib, and panitumumab. In a pilot crossover study of patients with grade 2 skin rash, Wong et al. (2007) found significant reduction in self-reported levels of pain and itching. Another promising product, currently under investigation in Europe, is a foam dressing impregnated with ibuprofen (Biatain®-Ibu, Coloplast A/S). Initial studies include case reports, a randomized trial in which the impregnated foam was compared to local best practice, and a single-blinded crossover study in which the impregnated foam was compared to the same foam without the ibuprofen. In each of these studies, patients reported significant reduction in persistent pain, reduced pain with dressing changes, and improved quality of life (Hampton, 2007; Jorgensen, Friis, & Gottrup, 2006; Sibbald, Coutts, Fierheller, & Woo, 2007). A number of other dressings and wound care products currently are under investigation for their ability to provide sustained-release analgesia and a moist wound healing environment (Fleck, 2007; Popescu & Salcido, 2004). Thus, the future looks bright in terms of nurses' ability to simultaneously promote wound healing and patient comfort through appropriate product selection.

Systemic analgesics: While progress is occurring in the development of topical products for sustained analgesia, at present the primary intervention for management of persistent pain is administration of around-the-clock analgesics (see Table 11-3). In selecting and recommending specific medications for relief of persistent nociceptive pain, Senecal (1999) suggested a stepped approach that is modeled on the World Health Organization (WHO) pain management ladder (WHO, 1996). Specifically, he recommended nonsteroidal anti-inflammatory drugs (NSAIDs) as baseline therapy (with or without topical analgesic agents), with the addition of opioids as needed. In prescribing

opioids, he recommended beginning with a mild opioid and then replacing the mild opioid with a strong opioid if the mild opioid does not provide sufficient pain relief. Thus, management protocols would fall into three categories (Senecal):
- NSAIDs with or without topical agents
- NSAIDs (with or without topical agents) plus mild opioids
- NSAIDs (with or without topical agents) plus strong opioids.

NSAIDs with or without topical analgesics: NSAIDs are extremely appropriate baseline agents because they reduce pain through both local and central effects, can be used in conjunction with other agents, and do not produce sedation, tolerance, or dependence. Commonly used NSAIDs include acetylsalicylic acid (aspirin), ibuprofen, and naproxen. NSAIDs work partly by inhibiting the synthesis of inflammatory mediators such as prostaglandins, which reduces nociceptor activation, and partly by reducing the perception of pain at the central level (Krasner et al., 2007; McNaughton & Nimmo, 2004). The most common adverse effects include gastric irritation and bleeding because these agents inhibit the production of prostaglandin E_1, which protects the gastric mucosa and inhibits the production of prostaglandins involved in the inflammatory process. Counseling patients to take these drugs with food or milk can reduce the risk of gastric irritation. For patients at high risk for gastric irritation or patients who report gastric distress, alternative agents include acetaminophen or one of the cyclooxygenase-2 (COX-2) inhibitors (e.g., celecoxib). Acetaminophen does not affect prostaglandin synthesis, and COX-2 inhibitors block synthesis of the prostaglandins involved in inflammation but do not affect synthesis of prostaglandin E_1 (Krasner et al.; McNaughton & Nimmo). It is important to realize that excessive intake of acetaminophen can result in liver toxicity; therefore, close monitoring of total intake is critical (McNaughton & Nimmo). When educating patients regarding NSAIDs or alternative agents, nurses should emphasize the importance of taking the medication routinely as scheduled, as opposed to on an as-needed basis.

Mild opioids: Opioid analgesics relieve pain by binding to pain perception sites in the spinal cord and the brain and are extremely effective in relieving moderate to severe pain. Mild opioids are most effective for moderately severe pain (levels 4–6 on the NPIS), and they are the most appropriate next step for persistent nociceptive pain that is incompletely relieved by NSAIDs or acetaminophen (Dallam et al., 2004; Krasner et al., 2007; Senecal, 1999). Commonly used mild opioids include codeine with or without acetaminophen, hydrocodone with acetaminophen, and oxycodone with acetaminophen. Propoxyphene is used less commonly and should be avoided in older adults because of increased risk of central nervous system and cardiac toxicity (Dallam et al.). If the specific agent chosen for use is a combination product including acetaminophen, it is critical to ensure that the patient is not already taking acetaminophen. Patients who were prescribed acetaminophen as the baseline analgesic must be instructed to discontinue its use and to substitute the combination drug.

Strong opioids: Strong opioids are indicated when patients report severe persistent pain (level 7–10 on the NPIS) or when they report insufficient pain relief with mild opioids in combination with NSAIDs (Dallam et al., 2004; Senecal, 1999). If the patient has been on a mild opioid, that medication is discontinued; if the patient is on an NSAID, that medication is continued. Morphine, fentanyl, and oxycodone are the most commonly used strong opioids, and all are available in both short-acting and sustained-release compounds. The dose for any individual patient is titrated to the desired level of pain relief. The side effects of strong opioids are the same as those for mild opioids and are managed as described in the section on mild opioids (Dallam et al.; Krasner et al., 2007).

Patient education regarding opioids: Common side effects of opioid analgesics include nausea and constipation. Patients should be prescribed antiemetics for as-needed use and should be placed on a constipation-prevention program (Dallam et al., 2004; Krasner et al., 2007; McNaughton & Nimmo, 2004). Critical elements of a constipation prevention program include

• Adequate fluid intake (about 2,000 ml/day for the average adult)
• Adequate fiber intake (ideally about 30 g of fiber/day for adults)
• Stool softeners as needed.

Inulin (e.g., Fibersure™, Procter & Gamble) and guar gum (e.g., Benefiber®, Novartis AG) are excellent choices for fiber supplementation because they are nongelling and tasteless and can therefore be added to any food or fluid. However, many options are now available for fiber supplementation (including fiber-supplemented water, chewable fiber tablets, fiber wafers, and fiber capsules, in addition to the classic fiber powders that are mixed in water or other fluid), and nurses should assist patients in identifying a supplement they find acceptable. Patients should be instructed to use over-the-counter laxatives (e.g., magnesium citrate, milk of magnesia, senna products, lactulose, or bisacodyl) as needed to ensure defecation occurs at least every two days.

In educating patients regarding effective and appropriate use of opioid analgesics, nurses need to emphasize the following key points (Krasner et al., 2007).

• The medication should be taken routinely as scheduled, not as needed.
• The dose of medication frequently needs to be adjusted to obtain the desired level of pain relief.
• The dose may need to be increased over time because of the development of tolerance.
• Addiction is very uncommon (< 0.1%), and unrelieved pain has a negative impact on wound healing and the overall ability to tolerate the cancer therapy, so it is very important to take the medication and to accurately report the level of pain relief.

Management of Neuropathic Pain

The pathology of neuropathic pain differs significantly from that of nociceptive pain, and neuropathic pain typically is incompletely relieved by NSAIDs and opioids. The cornerstones of management for neuropathic pain at present are local anesthetic agents and adjuvant systemic agents, such as anticonvulsants and antidepressants; these agents may be given either alone or in conjunction with opioids (Keskinbora, Pekel, & Aydinli, 2007; McNaughton & Nimmo, 2004; Wound, Ostomy, and Continence Nurses Society, 2004) (see Table 11-3). Research is ongoing into the specific pathologic processes involved in neuropathic pain, which will undoubtedly lead to additional options for management.

Anticonvulsants such as gabapentin and pregabalin address neuropathic pain by reducing chemicals in the brain that act as neurotransmitters for pain signals. Typically therapy is initially low-dose, with upward titration to provide the desired clinical effects. The initial dose of gabapentin usually is 300 mg/day, with upward titration to as much as 1,800 mg/day. With pregabalin, the initial dose is 50 mg three times daily (total daily dose of 150 mg), and the maximum dose is 100 mg three times daily (total daily dose of 300 mg). Common side effects include dizziness and drowsiness, especially during the initiation of therapy, so patients should be counseled to avoid alcohol, to take the drug at bedtime during initial therapy, and to modify activities such as driving until adaptation occurs (Krasner et al., 2007).

Antidepressants such as amitriptyline and desipramine act to block pain impulses by inhibiting the reuptake of norepinephrine, which explains their role in the management of neuropathic pain. The most common side effects are drowsiness and dry mouth. Taking the drug at bedtime may improve the quality of sleep and reduce daytime drowsiness. For many patients, the side effects gradually subside as they adjust to the drug (Krasner et al., 2007).

Other therapies that may be beneficial in the management of neuropathic pain include transcutaneous electrical nerve stimulation and nerve blocks. These therapies usually are provided by specialists in pain management. Referral to a pain specialist or pain center should be a high priority for any patients who report persistent unrelieved pain.

Conclusion

Pain is a common problem among patients with skin and soft tissue damage and has a very negative impact on quality of life. It can be classified as nociceptive, neuropathic, or mixed, and as acute (such as pain associated with wound care and dressing changes) or persistent. The nurse should assume that any patient with skin or soft tissue damage has pain and should routinely complete a pain assessment that focuses on the description of pain, pain severity (using a validated severity scale), occurrence, and exacerbating and relieving factors.

The most common type of wound-related pain is acute pain related to dressing changes. This type of pain can be effectively managed by use of general comfort measures such as temperature control, distraction, and patient-controlled wound care; gentle technique and selection of products and dressings that absorb exudate, maintain a moist wound surface, and provide atraumatic removal; and premedication with topical or systemic analgesics.

Persistent pain requires around-the-clock analgesia, which can be provided by sustained-release topical agents (such as lidocaine) as well as routine administration of NSAIDs. This regimen should include opioid analgesics as needed. Weak opioids such as hydrocodone usually are sufficient for patients with moderate pain, whereas patients with severe pain typically require morphine, fentanyl, or oxycodone.

Neuropathic pain typically responds best to adjuvant agents such as antidepressants or anticonvulsants, either as monotherapy or in combination with opioids. Patients with refractory pain should be referred to a pain specialist or pain center.

References

American Medical Association. (2007). *Pathophysiology of pain and pain assessment.* Retrieved November 20, 2007, from http://www.ama-cmeonline.com/pain_mgmt/printversion/ama_painmgmt_m1.pdf

Bergstrom, N., Allman, R., Alvarez, O., Bennett, M., Carlson, C., Frantz, R., et al. (1994). *Treatment of pressure ulcers* [Clinical Practice Guideline No. 15, AHCPR Pub No. 94-0622]. Rockville, MD: Agency for Health Care Policy and Research, U.S. Department of Health and Human Services.

Blackett, A. (2007). Case study: Managing painful wounds. *Oncology (Nurse Edition), 21*(8), 16–19.

Briggs, M., & Torra i Bou, J.E. (2002). Pain at wound dressing changes: A guide to management. In *European Wound Management Association position document: Pain at wound dressing changes* (pp. 12–17). London: Medical Education Partnership.

Cassuto, J., Sinclair, R., & Bonderovic, M. (2006). Anti-inflammatory properties of local anesthetics and their present and potential clinical implications. *Acta Anaesthesiologica Scandinavica, 50*(3), 265–282.

Coulling, S. (2007). Fundamentals of pain management in wound care. *British Journal of Nursing, 16*(11), S4–S12.

Dallam, L., Barkauskas, C., Ayello, A., & Baranoski, S. (2004). Pain management and wounds. In S. Baranoski & E. Ayello (Eds.), *Wound care essentials: Practice and principles* (pp. 217–238). Philadelphia: Lippincott Williams & Wilkins.

Evans, E., & Gray, M. (2005). Do topical analgesics reduce pain associated with wound dressing changes or debridement of chronic wounds? *Journal Wound, Ostomy, and Continence Nursing, 32*(5), 287–290.

Fleck, C. (2007). Managing wound pain: Today and in the future. *Advances in Skin and Wound Care, 20*(3), 138–145.

Hampton, S. (2007). Chronic pain in wounds: A report on 11 case studies. *Nursing Times, 103*(15), 48–50.

Jones, M.L. (2004) Minimizing pain at dressing changes. *Nursing Standard, 18*(24), 65–70.

Jorgensen, B., Friis, G.J., & Gottrup, F. (2006). Pain and quality of life for patients with venous leg ulcers: Proof of concept of the efficacy of Biatain-Ibu, a new pain reducing wound dressing. *Wound Repair and Regeneration, 14*(3), 233–239.

Keskinbora, K., Pekel, A., & Aydinli, I. (2007). Gabapentin and an opioid combination versus opioid alone for the management of neuropathic cancer pain: A randomized open trial. *Journal of Pain and Symptom Management, 34*(2), 183–189.

Krasner, D. (2001). Caring for the person experiencing chronic wound pain. In D. Krasner, G. Rodeheaver, & G. Sibbald (Eds.), *Chronic wound care: A clinical source book for healthcare professionals* (3rd ed., pp. 79–89). Wayne, PA: HMP Communications.

Krasner, D., Shapshak, D., & Hopf, H. (2007). Managing wound pain. In R. Bryant & D. Nix (Eds.), *Acute and chronic wounds: Current management concepts* (3rd ed., pp. 539–565). St. Louis, MO: Elsevier.

Maki, L., & Clarey-Sanford, C. (2007). Using slow-released silver hydrofiber dressings on a neck radiation burn. *Journal of Wound, Ostomy, and Continence Nursing, 34*(5), 542–545.

McNaughton, D., & Nimmo, S. (2004). Pain assessment and management. In M. Morison, L. Ovington, & K. Wilkie (Eds.), *Chronic wound care: A problem-based learning approach* (pp. 194–210). London: Elsevier Mosby.

Moffatt, C.J., Franks, P.J., & Hollinworth, H. (2002). Understanding wound pain and trauma: An international perspective. In *European Wound Management Association position document: Pain at wound dressing changes* (pp. 2–7). London: Medical Education Partnership.

Mosby's 2006 drug consult for nurses. (2006). St. Louis, MO: Elsevier Mosby.

Oncology Nurses Society. (2004). *ONS patient outcomes survey.* Retrieved December 30, 2007, from http://www.ons.org/outcomes/measures/survey.shtml

Ovington, L. (2001). Hanging wet-to-dry dressings out to dry. *Home Healthcare Nurse, 19*(8), 477–484.

Parr, A., Zoutman, D., & Davidson, J. (1999). Antimicrobial activity of lidocaine against bacteria associated with nosocomial wound infection. *Annals of Plastic Surgery, 43*(3), 239–245.

Pecher, S., Bottiger, B., Graf, F., & Hollmann, M. (2004). Alternative effects of local anesthetic agents. *Anaesthetist, 53*(4), 316–325.

Popescu, A., & Salcido, R. (2004). Wound pain: A challenge for the patient and the wound care specialist. *Advances in Skin and Wound Care, 17*(1), 14–20.

Rastinehad, D. (2006). Pressure ulcer pain. *Journal of Wound, Ostomy, and Continence Nursing, 33*(3), 252–257.

Senecal, S.J. (1999). Pain management of wound care. *Nursing Clinics of North America, 34*(4), 847–860.

Shukla, D., Tripathi, A., Agrawal, S., Ansari, M., Rastogi, A., & Shukla, V. (2005). Pain in acute and chronic wounds: A descriptive study. *Ostomy Wound/Management, 51*(11), 47–51.

Sibbald, R.G., Coutts, P., Fierheller, M., & Woo, K. (2007). A pilot (real-life) randomised clinical evaluation of a pain-relieving foam dressing: Ibuprofen-foam versus local best practice. *International Wound Journal, 4*(Suppl. 1), 16–23.

Szor, J.K., & Bourguignon, C. (1999). Description of pressure ulcer pain at rest and at dressing changes. *Journal of Wound, Ostomy, and Continence Nursing, 26*(3), 115–120.

Warden, V., Hurley, A.C., & Volicer, L. (2003). Development and psychometric evaluation of the Pain Assessment in Advanced Dementia (PAINAD) scale. *Journal of American Medical Directors Association, 4*(1), 9–15.

Wong, D., Hockenberry-Eaton, M., Wilson, D., Winkelstein, M., & Schwartz, P. (2001). *Wong's essentials of pediatric nursing* (6th ed.). St. Louis, MO: Mosby.

Wong, S., Osann, K.I., Lloyd, K.P., Vasko, C.M., Arcinas, R.L., & Mummaneni, M. (2007). A pilot crossover study to evaluate the use of Regenecare topical wound gel in patients with cutaneous toxicity caused by epidermal growth factor receptor (HER 1/EGFR) inhibitors. *Journal of Clinical Oncology, 2007 ASCO Annual Meeting Proceedings, 25*(Suppl. 18), Abstract 19643.

World Health Organization. (1996). *Cancer pain relief* (2nd ed.). Geneva, Switzerland: Author.

Wound, Ostomy, and Continence Nurses Society. (2004). *Guideline for management of wounds in patients with lower extremity neuropathic disease* [WOCN Clinical Practice Guidelines Series, No. 3]. Glenview, IL: Author.

Wulf, H., & Baron, R. (2002). The theory of pain. In *European Wound Management Association position document: Pain at wound dressing changes* (pp. 8–11). London: Medical Education Partnership.

Young T. (2007). Assessment of wound pain: Overview and a new initiative. *British Journal of Nursing, 16*(8), 456, 458, 460–461.

CHAPTER 12

Psychological Distress Related to Skin Problems in the Oncology Patient Population

Giselle J. Moore-Higgs, ARNP, PhD(c), AOCN®

Introduction

Distress is defined by the National Comprehensive Cancer Network (NCCN) as

> a multifactorial unpleasant emotional experience of a psychological (cognitive, behavioral, emotional), social, and/or spiritual nature that may interfere with the ability to cope effectively with cancer, its physical symptoms and its treatment. Distress extends along a continuum, ranging from common normal feelings of vulnerability, sadness, and fears, to problems that can become disabling, such as depression, anxiety, panic, social isolation, and existential and spiritual crisis. (NCCN, 2008, p. DIS-2)

According to NCCN (2008), the diagnosis and treatment of cancer creates some degree of distress for all patients at various stages of the disease. Recently, the Canadian Strategy for Cancer Control (Rebalance Focus Action Group, 2005) designated emotional distress as the sixth vital sign in order to highlight the importance of distress as a marker of well-being and its reduction as a target outcome measure (Bultz & Carlson, 2006).

Across the trajectory of the illness (from diagnosis to treatment, termination of treatment, survivorship, or recurrence and palliation), the incidence of emotional distress in North America has been reported to be 35%–45%

(Bultz & Carlson, 2005; Carlson & Bultz, 2003; Carlson et al., 2004; Zabora, Szoc, Curbow, Hooker, & Piantadosi, 2001). Furthermore, up to 58% of patients receiving palliative care have reported significant levels of emotional distress (Bultz & Carlson, 2005; Potash & Breitbart, 2002). High levels of fatigue (49%), pain (26%), anxiety (24%), and depression (24%), in addition to severe financial hardship and material challenges, were reported in large studies of patients in the United States and Canada (Bultz & Carlson, 2005; Carlson et al.; Zabora et al.).

Unfortunately, despite the documentation that distress occurs and the extensive research that has been conducted focusing on different interventions, the initial assessment of a patient's distress often is delayed or goes unnoticed by oncology professionals (McDonald et al., 1999; Sollner et al., 2001). At a minimum, psychosocial screening provides nurses with the opportunity to identify and predict individuals who are at greater risk for distress and are unlikely to cope with the many stressors accompanying a cancer diagnosis and its treatment. Several common reasons for delays in psychosocial screening are the patient's reluctance to report concerns, the healthcare provider's lack of self-confidence in exploring psychosocial concerns, and the limited time available for assessment during clinic visits (NCCN, 2008). However, the successful management of distress is incumbent upon early recognition and appropriate management.

A cancer diagnosis is devastating on its own, but the additional development of a malodorous fungating tumor or skin-related complication, such as chronic graft-versus-host disease, can be a constant reminder of the disease and its effect on a patient's life (Lazelle-Ali, 2007). It can result in great distress and significantly affect the individual's quality of life (Lazelle-Ali). Not only do the physical aspects of the wound or skin problem need to be addressed but also significant psychosocial issues. The individual may experience shame and embarrassment related to a changed body image, which may result in social isolation and depression (Lazelle-Ali). A review of the literature reveals limited clinical research on the impact of chronic wounds on individuals and their families, much less on chronic skin problems related to cancer and its treatment. This chapter will provide an overview of distress as it relates to malignant skin problems by assimilating data from the chronic wound literature and identifying areas in need of further nursing research.

Chronic Wounds

Individuals of all ages (from neonates to older adults) and from all cultural and socioeconomic backgrounds develop chronic wounds. This is particularly true for people living with advanced or end-stage chronic illnesses, including cancer. Even with the best clinical care, an acute wound can become chronic. In addition, many treatments for cancer can result in chronic skin conditions that need aggressive management. Although wound care has historically focused on treating the underlying disease and healing the wounds, healthcare professionals now recognize that chronic skin problems, particularly chronic wounds, can cause significant distress and have a negative influence on an individual's quality of life. These wounds often are considered prognostic for poor treatment outcomes and may indicate a nearing of the end of life. Because malignant wounds have a tendency to become chronic and nonhealing, individuals with these types of wounds may experience a number of distressing symptoms, including pain, odor, excessive exudate, bleeding, functional compromise, and complications requiring hospitalizations (e.g., infection and fistula formation), which require complex management by clinicians. In addition, individuals and their families may face the impact of a change in body image, changes in social roles and family finances, and possible end-of-life grief if the disease fails to respond to treatment or if the treatment is not tolerated. If the lesions progress, such as with erosions of tumors to the surface of the skin, related symptoms may aggravate the situation, such as pain from the pressure of the tumor on surrounding structures, irritation, recurrent infection, and swelling as a consequence of impaired capillary and lymphatic drainage.

Physical Manifestations

Wounds often create profound psychological stress and affect the quality of life of patients, caregivers, families, and friends. van Rijswijk (2001) proposed that the state of having a wound implied imperfection, resulting in physical and emotional vulnerability. Restrictions in activities of daily living, pain, edema, fatigue, and bulky dressings make simple tasks, such as changing clothes and bathing, frustrating or unachievable, and tasks such as housework, leisure activities, grocery shopping, or returning to work impossible. The presence of a chronic wound may produce an offensive and embarrassing odor and drainage, alter the patient's ability to shower or bathe, and decrease the opportunity or desire for intimacy. For example, exudate leakage, odor from moist desquamation, and altered modes of dress, such as wearing slacks to hide dressings, can undermine the individual's body image. As a result, individuals have difficulty maintaining dignity, feel unclean, and may harbor feelings of isolation and limit their social contact. Roe, Cullum, and Hamer (1995) observed increased anxiety and depression scores, lower life satisfaction, and decreased social contacts among patients with malodorous leg ulcers.

Individuals with chronic wounds also may adapt unnecessary avoidance tactics to minimize the risk of aggravating an existing ulcer or incurring another wound. In addition, they may experience a heightened concern and vigilance associated with trying to retain as much skin integrity as possible and to guard against further damage, infection, or the development of a new problem.

An acute or chronic wound also can affect the family and may produce a change in the family social system. The wound may alter an individual's mobility, self-esteem, and role in the family, thus resulting in an alteration in the family structure and role functions. The individual with a wound may create a financial hardship on the family by decreasing income or increasing expenditures related to the cost of care and supplies. Space for supplies may become an issue as boxes of wound care products and other supplies accumulate, and the family's schedule may have to revolve around wound care, medication, home nursing visits, and doctor or rehabilitation appointments.

Wound Pain

Pain is a particular problem in wound management, where it often is regarded as an inevitable aspect of wound care. Studies have found that patients consider wound pain to be one of the most difficult symptoms to cope with in relation to chronic wounds (Price et al., 2008). The distress caused by wound pain can affect an individual's desire for treatment and reduce compliance with the wound management regimens (Price et al., 2008). Patients may report minimal pain despite the presence of a large fungating wound when dressings are suitable and adequate cancer pain management is provided. The most painful malignant lesions tend to be shallow ulcerating malignant wounds that have the potential to spread through the lymphatics, denuding the overlying epithelium (Price et al., 2008).

Wound pain has a variety of causes. Generally, pain associated with dressing changes, wound cleansing, and debridement appear to be the most problematic. In a recent study, the wound itself was the most painful location, and more than a third of patients described pain with dressing changes most or all of the time (Price et al., 2008). The touching or handling of the wound caused the most pain, followed by cleansing and dressing removal (Price et al., 2008). Adherent or dried-out dressings are the most likely wound coverings to cause pain and trauma. The anticipation of pain with dressing changes can further add to an individual's distress.

Pain related to the wound should be handled as a main priority in chronic wound management, as it is key to reducing distress. Management of pain in chronic wounds depends on the proper assessment, reporting, and documentation of the patient's experience with wound-related pain. The assessment should be based on six critical dimensions of the pain experience: location, duration, intensity, quality, onset, and impact on activities of daily living (Price et al., 2007). The management focus should be on controlling the sources of pain, applying topical anesthetics as required or providing oral analgesics, and carefully selecting dressings that cover the wound and exposed nerve endings yet adhere as little as possible and leave a minimal amount of residue behind (Price et al., 2007). Involving the individual in both the preparation for the dressing change as well as the actual procedure also can improve patient satisfaction.

Unfortunately, such management may fail for several reasons: inappropriate or nonexistent pain assessment; insufficient prescribing of analgesia; and confusion about the appropriate use of dressing products to reduce wound pain. In addition, healthcare professionals often lack knowledge about pain and may hold inappropriate beliefs and attitudes, particularly related to opioid drugs. Social and emotional factors also can contribute to the pain experience. Emotional responses such as depression, anger, and frustration may be related to the degree of acceptance of the situation, a feeling of helplessness, poor self-image, or a sense of isolation from family and friends.

Depression

Depression can affect the course of the cancer, morbidity, hospital stays, treatment compliance and efficacy, and even prognosis (Reich, 2008). According to the *Diagnostic and Statistical Manual of Mental Disorders* (American Psychiatric Association, 2000), major depression is defined by persistent low mood, or anhedonia (pervasive loss of interest or pleasure), for two weeks or more and with at least four of the following symptoms:
• Sleep disruption (especially early-morning insomnia)
• Weight loss or change in appetite
• Psychomotor retardation or agitation
• Fatigue or loss of energy
• Feelings of worthlessness or excessive guilt
• Diminished ability to think or concentrate
• Recurrent thoughts of death or suicidal ideation.
Depressive disorders are syndromes, not diseases, and may include a variety of mood disturbances and clinical presentations (Pasquini & Biondi, 2007).

The reported prevalence of depression in patients with cancer varies widely depending on several factors considered in a particular study (Reich, 2008). Things to consider include the time and stage of the cancer, patient populations studied, social network and availability of support, and the diagnostic criteria and method of assessment used (e.g., self-reports, structured interviews) (Reich). Moreover, the prevalence of depression often is underestimated because many of its symptoms, such as fatigue, weight loss, loss of appetite, or sleep disruption, closely mirror the physiologic effects of cancer. Additionally, the use of certain treatments and medications for symptom management may prevent appropriate diagnosis (Pasquini & Biondi, 2007). The prevalence rate of depression for patients with solid tumors is reported to be 20%–50% (Pasquini & Biondi). Depression has been reported to occur in 5%– 26% of individuals with advanced disease and in 6.7%–17.8% of individuals with terminal illness (Miovic & Block, 2007).

Depression frequently is found in patients with acute or chronic wounds. A recent study in the United Kingdom found both depression (27%) and anxiety (26%) in 190 patients with chronic venous ulceration (Jones, Barr, Robinson, & Carlisle, 2006). Two symptoms that appeared to be associated with depression and anxiety were pain and odor. Other studies also have mentioned negative effects on mood and feelings. Feelings of regret, depression, loss of will power, loss of control, and feelings of helplessness and hopelessness have been reported (Charles, 1995; Douglas, 2001; Hyland, Ley, & Thomson, 1994). Such findings can be assimilated into patients with chronic malignant wounds, which only serves to compound the depression related to the diagnosis of cancer.

Psychological factors such as depression and anxiety also may have both a direct and indirect impact on wound healing through the impairment of immune function. Several mechanisms have been suggested, including disruption of the activity of macrophages and lymphocytes in the healing process, impairment of both cellular and humoral immunity, and a negative impact on the secretion of proinflammatory cytokines at an actual wound site. Further research is needed to confirm this relationship.

Unfortunately, few data from clinical trials are available on the effectiveness of treatment for depression among patients with cancer (Williams & Dale, 2006). Treatment usually is a combination of psychotherapy and pharmacologic therapy (Reich, 2008). Prescribing antidepressants to patients with cancer requires specific knowledge, experience, and caution. Practitioners must consider the anticholinergic side effects of tricyclic antidepressants, the proemetic effect of selective serotonin reuptake inhibitors and how they may affect the pharmacokinetics of other drugs, and the specific syndromes occurring with chemotherapy (Pasquini & Biondi, 2007; Richards, Umbreit, Fanucchi, Giblin, & Khuri, 2003). All medications should be prescribed based on the characteristics of the various drugs and the specific needs of the individual patient (Pasquini & Biondi). In terms of nonpharmacologic treatments, few studies have assessed their effectiveness in patients with cancer (Reich). Many of the results conflict because of the variety of techniques used and a lack of clearly defined procedures, thus making them difficult to reproduce (Pasquini & Biondi).

Assessment

The NCCN (2008) standards for managing distress recommend screening all patients for their levels of distress at their initial visit, at appropriate intervals, and as clinically indicated, especially with changes in disease status such as remission, recurrence, or progression. A number of identified risk factors may place an individual at increased risk of distress: younger age, female gender, living alone, having young children, patients with cumulative stress and past psychiatric treatment, and a history of alcohol or substance abuse. These factors should be assessed during the initial evaluation. Those with a history of psychiatric disorder or depression, substance abuse, cognitive impairment, severe comorbid illnesses, social problems, and communication barriers have greater risk for distress (NCCN).

NCCN (2008) and the American Psychosocial Oncology Society (2000) have both issued consensus panel statements in which they recommend the development of improved screening mechanisms to enhance the detection and management of emotional distress in patients with cancer. Included in these recommendations are the development and utilization of practical and efficient screening tools. Current techniques for psychosocial screening of patients with a new diagnosis of cancer range from structured interviews to self-report instruments. Brief and efficient methods that use self-report measures also tend to be cost-effective. A number of short methods are available to screen for distress in patients with cancer (NCCN). These include the distress thermometer (DT) (Roth et al., 1998), the Functional Assessment of Cancer Therapy–General (Cella et al., 1993), and the Brief Symptom Inventory (Derogatis & Melisaratos, 1983).

The DT (see Figure 12-1) is a one-item, self-reporting tool that is easy to administer, nonstigmatizing, and easy to score and interpret. The DT measures distress levels over the past week using a thermometer-like Likert scale with scores from 0 (no distress) to 10 (extreme distress) and a midpoint anchor labeled "moderate distress." The NCCN distress practice guidelines panel endorsed it for use in all oncology settings (NCCN, 2008).

Gessler et al. (2008) suggested an easy clinical approach to the interpretation of DT results. They use a "traffic light" system with three levels: green-light scores (DT = 0–4), yellow-light scores (DT = 5–6), and red-light scores (DT ≥ 7). A score of 0–4 would result in care as usual. A score of 5–6 would draw the attention of the clinical team, who could then monitor the patient more closely. A score higher than 7 would alert the clinician to discuss distress with the patient (Gessler et al.) and provide the opportunity to refer appropriately. Limitations of the DT include limited evidence of its ability to monitor change over time, limited evidence of its sensitivity to cross-cultural comparisons, and its stability and sensitivity to minor changes. However, the tool's quick and easy administration and transparency and acceptability to patients make it more likely to be used successfully in a busy clinical setting, where longer, more complex assessments are impossible. Furthermore, clinicians can use the problem checklist to identify sources of distress and then incorporate these into treatment. Another benefit is that use of the DT demonstrates the clinical team's concern for the patient as a whole (Gessler et al.).

Treatment

The NCCN (2008) guidelines on distress management provide a great resource for oncology healthcare teams in terms of management and referral options. A multidisciplinary approach is critical to a successful outcome. Patients with malignant wounds require not only individualized physical wound care but also emotional support that takes into account the nature of their un-

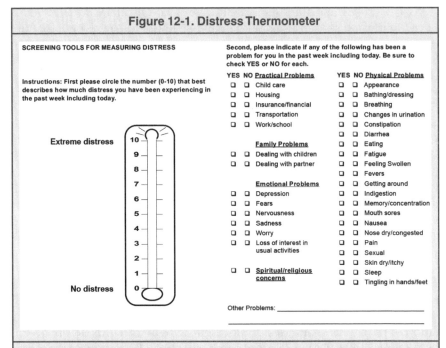

Figure 12-1. Distress Thermometer

SCREENING TOOLS FOR MEASURING DISTRESS

Instructions: First please circle the number (0-10) that best describes how much distress you have been experiencing in the past week including today.

Extreme distress 10

9
8
7
6
5
4
3
2
1
No distress 0

Second, please indicate if any of the following has been a problem for you in the past week including today. Be sure to check YES or NO for each.

YES NO **Practical Problems**
☐ ☐ Child care
☐ ☐ Housing
☐ ☐ Insurance/financial
☐ ☐ Transportation
☐ ☐ Work/school

Family Problems
☐ ☐ Dealing with children
☐ ☐ Dealing with partner

Emotional Problems
☐ ☐ Depression
☐ ☐ Fears
☐ ☐ Nervousness
☐ ☐ Sadness
☐ ☐ Worry
☐ ☐ Loss of interest in usual activities

☐ ☐ **Spiritual/religious concerns**

YES NO **Physical Problems**
☐ ☐ Appearance
☐ ☐ Bathing/dressing
☐ ☐ Breathing
☐ ☐ Changes in urination
☐ ☐ Constipation
☐ ☐ Diarrhea
☐ ☐ Eating
☐ ☐ Fatigue
☐ ☐ Feeling Swollen
☐ ☐ Fevers
☐ ☐ Getting around
☐ ☐ Indigestion
☐ ☐ Memory/concentration
☐ ☐ Mouth sores
☐ ☐ Nausea
☐ ☐ Nose dry/congested
☐ ☐ Pain
☐ ☐ Sexual
☐ ☐ Skin dry/itchy
☐ ☐ Sleep
☐ ☐ Tingling in hands/feet

Other Problems: _____
_____

Note. Reproduced with permission from *The NCCN 1.2008 Distress Management Clinical Practice Guidelines in Oncology.* © National Comprehensive Cancer Network, 2008. Available at http://www.nccn.org. Accessed March 27, 2008. To view the most recent and complete version of the guideline, go online to www.nccn.org.

These Guidelines are a work in progress that will be refined as often as new significant data becomes available.

The NCCN Guidelines are a statement of consensus of its authors regarding their views of currently accepted approaches to treatment. Any clinician seeking to apply or consult any NCCN guideline is expected to use independent medical judgment in the context of individual clinical circumstances to determine any patient's care or treatment. The National Comprehensive Cancer Network makes no warranties of any kind whatsoever regarding their content, use or application and disclaims any responsibility for their application or use in any way.

These Guidelines are copyrighted by the National Comprehensive Cancer Network. All rights reserved. These Guidelines and illustrations herein may not be reproduced in any form for any purpose without the express written permission of the NCCN.

derlying malignancy and its prognosis. In the clinical setting, healthcare providers need to be aware of the potential impact of the wound on the patient, the caregiver, and the family. Assessment of the family and its adaptation to the wound needs to be a component of the care plan. Providers should treat the patient in the context of his or her environment and not focus only on the outcome of care (wound healing), particularly in a patient with a poor overall cancer-related prognosis. A referral for counseling or psychiatric intervention may be necessary if the patient and/or family members appear distressed and unable to cope with the current situation.

Conclusion

Malignant wound–related distress still is poorly understood and not well described in the literature. It can have a significant impact on patients and families. Acute wounds that occur with oncology treatments deserve more attention and research. Although the chronic wound literature provides some data that can be assimilated, further research is needed into the impact of malignant wounds on individuals and their families. Specifically, research on the assessment and management of wound pain, effective wound dressings, and nonpharmaceutical options for distress is needed. In addition, the potential for family distress caused by these wounds grows, and further research into family coping mechanisms and other resources is needed.

References

American Psychiatric Association. (2000). *Diagnostic and statistical manual of mental disorders* (4th ed., text revision). Washington, DC: Author.

American Psychosocial Oncology Society. (2000). *APOS standards of care for the management of distress in patients with cancer.* Charlottesville, VA: Author.

Bultz, B.D., & Carlson, L.E. (2005). Emotional distress: The sixth vital sign in cancer care [Correspondence]. *Journal of Clinical Oncology, 23*(26), 6440–6441.

Bultz, B.D., & Carlson, L.E. (2006). Emotional distress: The sixth vital sign—future directions in cancer care. *Psycho-Oncology, 15*(2), 93–95.

Carlson, L.E., Angen, M., Cullum, J., Goodey, E., Koopmans, J., Lamont, L., et al. (2004). High levels of untreated distress and fatigue in cancer patients. *British Journal of Cancer, 90*(12), 2297–2304.

Carlson, L.E., & Bultz, B.D. (2003). Cancer distress screening: Needs, models and methods. *Journal of Psychosomatic Research, 55*(5), 403–409.

Cella, D.F., Tulsky, D.S., Gray, G., Sarafien, B., Linn, E., Bonomi, A., et al. (1993). The Functional Assessment of Cancer Therapy scale: Development and validation of the general measure. *Journal of Clinical Oncology, 11*(3), 570–579.

Charles, H. (1995). The impact of leg ulcers on patients' quality of life. *Professional Nurse, 10*(2), 571–573.

Derogatis, L.R., & Melisaratos, N. (1983). The Brief Symptom Inventory: An introductory report. *Psychological Medicine, 13*(3), 595–605.

Douglas, V. (2001). Living with a chronic leg ulcer: An insight into patients' experiences and feelings. *Journal of Wound Care, 10*(9), 355–360.

Gessler, S., Low, J., Daniells, E., Williams, R., Brough, V., Tookman, A., et al. (2008). Screening for distress in cancer patients: Is the distress thermometer a valid measure in the UK and does it measure change over time? A prospective validation study. *Psycho-Oncology, 17*(6), 538–547.

Hyland, M.E., Ley A., & Thomson, B. (1994). Quality of life of leg ulcer patients: Questionnaire and preliminary findings. *Journal of Wound Care, 3*(6), 294–298.

Jones, J., Barr, W., Robinson, J., & Carlisle, C. (2006). Depression in patients with chronic venous ulceration. *British Journal of Nursing, 15*(11), S17–S23.

Lazelle-Ali, C. (2007). Psychological and physical care of malodorous fungating wounds. *British Journal of Nursing, 16*(Suppl. 15), S16–S24.

McDonald, M.V., Passik, S.D., Dugan, W., Rosenfeld, B., Theobald, D.E., & Edgerton, S. (1999). Nurses' recognition of depression in their patients with cancer. *Oncology Nursing Forum, 26*(3), 593–599.

Miovic, M., & Block, S. (2007). Psychiatric disorders in advanced cancer. *Cancer, 110*(8), 1665–1676.

National Comprehensive Cancer Network. (2008). *NCCN Clinical Practice Guidelines in Oncology™: Distress management* [v.1.2008]. Fort Washington, PA: National Comprehensive Cancer Network. Retrieved March 13, 2008, from http://www.nccn.org/professionals/physician_gls/PDF/distress.pdf

Pasquini, M., & Biondi, M. (2007). Depression in cancer patients: A critical review. *Clinical Practice and Epidemiology in Mental Health, 3,* 2.

Potash, M., & Breitbart, W. (2002). Affective disorders in advanced cancer. *Hematology/Oncology Clinics of North America, 16*(3), 671–700.

Price, P., Fogh, K., Glynn, C., Krasner, D.L., Osterbrink, J., & Sibbald, R.G. (2007). Managing painful chronic wounds: The Wound Pain Management Model. *International Wound Journal, 4*(Suppl. 1), 4–15.

Price, P.E., Fagervik-Morton, H., Mudge, E.J., Beele, H., Ruiz, J.C., Nystrom, T.H., et al. (2008). Dressing-related pain in patients with chronic wounds: An international patient perspective. *International Wound Journal, 5*(2), 159–171.

Rebalance Focus Action Group. (2005). A position paper: Screening key indicators in cancer patients: Pain as a 5th vital sign and emotional distress as a 6th vital sign. *Canadian Strategy for Cancer Control Bulletin, 7*(Suppl. 4), 93–95.

Reich, M. (2008). Depression and cancer: Recent data on clinical issues, research challenges and treatment approaches. *Current Opinion in Oncology, 20*(4), 353–359.

Richards, S., Umbreit, J.N., Fanucchi, M.P., Giblin, J., & Khuri, F. (2003). Selective serotonin reuptake inhibitor-induced rhabdomyolysis associated with irinotecan. *Southern Medical Journal, 96*(10), 1031–1033.

Roe, B., Cullum, N., & Hamer, C. (1995). Patients' perceptions of chronic leg ulcers. In N. Cullum & B. Roe (Eds.), *Leg ulcers: Nursing management: A research-based guide* (pp. 125–134). Harrow, UK: Scutari Press.

Roth, A.J., Kornblith, A.B., Batel-Copel, L., Peabody, E., Scher, H.I., & Holland, J.C. (1998). Rapid screening for psychologic distress in men with prostate carcinoma. *Cancer, 82*(10), 1904–1908.

Sollner, W., DeVries, A., Steixner, E., Lukas, P., Sprinzl, G., Rumpold, G., et al. (2001). How successful are oncologists in identifying patient distress, perceived social support, and need for psychosocial counseling? *British Journal of Cancer, 84*(2), 179–185.

van Rijswijk, L. (2001). The language of wounds. In D. Krasner (Ed.), *Chronic wound care: A clinical sourcebook for health care professionals* (3rd ed., pp. 101–115). Wayne, PA: HMP Communications.

Williams, S., & Dale, J. (2006). The effectiveness of treatment for depression/depressive symptoms in adults with cancer: A systematic review. *British Journal of Cancer, 13*(3), 372–390.

Zabora, J., Szoc, K.B., Curbow, B., Hooker, C., & Piantadosi, S. (2001). The prevalence of psychological distress by cancer site. *Psycho-Oncology, 10*(1), 19–28.

CHAPTER 13

Nutrition Needs for Healing Skin

Tammy Fansabedian, BASc, RD, and Diane Candiotto, BASc, RD

Introduction

> "Healing is a matter of time, but it is sometimes also a matter of opportunity."
> —Hippocrates, Greek physician (460 BC–377 BC)

Healing is a body's natural response to wound or injury, and, given time, most wounds will eventually heal regardless of internal or external conditions. Optimal conditions, however, will facilitate and speed healing, and optimal nutrition provides a vital role in this process. Nutrition is fundamental for proper skin integrity as well as wound healing. A joint statement by the American Academy of Family Physicians, the American Dietetic Association, and the National Council on Aging emphasized the importance of nutrition in a patient's wound healing status: "Nutrition is one of the important vital signs, just as blood pressure or pulse. Well-nourished people tend to have shorter hospital stays, fewer complications and speedier wound healing after surgery" (as cited in Ayello, Thomas, & Litchford, 1999, p. 719).

Proper wound healing has three fundamental prerequisites: adequate tissue perfusion, oxygenation, and blood flow. Tissue perfusion may be seen as the most important step, as it allows for the delivery of nutrients and oxygen to the wound site (Leininger, 2002). The absence of adequate nutrients will inhibit healing. In well-nourished patients, the availability of nutrients creates *anabolism* leading to repair and eventual healing. When nutrients are lacking, tissue breakdown and *catabolism* occurs, perpetuating the cycle of inflammation and poor healing until the malnutrition can be corrected. Treatment for cancer, including surgery, chemotherapy, and radiation therapy, can have a significant impact on the delivery of nutrients both acutely and long term.

Wound healing is a multifactorial process, one that encompasses patient variables as well as location, severity, and etiology of the wound. In essence, the three stages of wound healing—inflammation (lasting four to six days), proliferation (lasting approximately two weeks), and maturation (lasting up to two years)—each rely upon different nutrients. The final stage, maturation, is where collagen stabilization takes place. Collagen increases the tensile strength of the wound and is essential for successful wound healing (Campos, Groth, & Branco, 2008).

Malnutrition

Malnutrition is widely implicated in delayed wound healing along with factors including infection, organ failure, and hypoxia (Albina, 1994; Johnson, 1993). Malnourished patients are at risk for postoperative complications such as sepsis, infection, and increased length of stay, as well as death (Dempsey, Mullen, & Buzby, 1988; Young, 1988). Patients who are well-nourished prior to sustaining a wound and have adequate nutrients throughout have the optimal conditions for healing. Malnutrition also has been implicated in a person's vulnerability to developing pressure ulcers (Albina).

The definition of *malnutrition* is beyond the scope of this chapter, as the interpretation of malnutrition can range a wide gamut from macronutrient to micronutrient intake and status. Hengstermann, Fischer, Steinhagen-Thiessen, and Schulz (2007) suggested that one of the confounding reasons for a lack of research into the area of nutrition and wound healing is the inability to unanimously define malnutrition. In its simplest terms, however, it can be seen as either an excess or insufficiency of nutrients. The consequences are grim because malnutrition can delay healing and decrease the tensile strength of a wound, as well as increase the possibility of infection (Hughes, 2003). Encouragingly, malnutrition is reversible, and wound healing can be corrected.

Several tools can help to define a patient's nutritional status. These include a Mini Nutritional Assessment® (MNA) (Société des Produits Nestlé S.A.) and body mass index (BMI). Hengstermann et al. (2007) studied 484 geriatric patients 48 hours after hospital admission. They found the prevalence of pressure ulcers was 16.7% among the overall study group and that the nutritional status, as reflected in the MNA, was significantly better in the patients without pressure ulcers ($p < 0.001$). The group also found that patients with pressure ulcers had significantly lower BMIs (22.8 ± 5.3 versus 24.8 ± 5.2 kg/m^2, $p = 0.003$). A patient's nutritional status prior to injury has been demonstrated to affect healing. When looking at patients undergoing elective gastrointestinal resection, a 50% less than normal intake coincided with a reduction in the amount of hydroxyproline, an indicator of collagen formation (Windsor, Knight, & Hill, 1988).

Nurses play a vital role in the initial nutritional screening of patients and are on the front lines in assessing wound healing. Simple tools to screen nutritional status should be included in routine practice. Weighing patients with wounds is one way nurses can assist registered dietitians in monitoring patients' nutrition status (Casey, 1998). Routine calorie counts can be effective; however, a recent study found a 20% overestimation of intake when nurses were asked to complete calorie counts (Ferguson, Cook, Rimmasch, Bender, & Voss, 2000). Dietitians should be notified when a patient appears to be at risk for malnutrition or if there are concerns about inadequate intake.

Energy Requirements

There is tremendous interest in research looking to the micronutrient level to determine how vitamins and minerals affect wound healing. From a macronutrient standpoint, however, total energy and protein must be met first and foremost to meet metabolic demands. In addition, adequate hydration must also be provided. Providing adequate energy in the form of kilocalories may be a challenge for several reasons. The presence of a wound puts a patient in a *hypermetabolic* state increasing the metabolic demand on the body as both inflammation and cellular activity in the wound increase energy demands (Casey, 2003). The process of wound healing is estimated to increase metabolic demand. The extent of the increased need depends on the size of the wound, the amount of wound exudate, and patient's pre-wound nutritional status (Collins, 1996). A hypermetabolic state, if left uncorrected, will lead to weight loss and, perhaps more importantly, muscle loss. The inflammatory response interferes with the patient's appetite (Fuhrman, 2003), thus making the act of nourishing injured patients even more of a challenge.

It is difficult to quantify exact energy requirements for optimal wound healing, and yet adequate energy intake is perhaps the primary nutritional indicator in wound healing. As outlined in the working definition of malnutrition, either excess or insufficient energy may exacerbate poor wound healing. An excess of energy may result in overweight or obesity, which may, in itself, deter proper wound healing. Adipose tissue can be poorly vascularized, potentially leading to decreased blood flow and delivery of nutrients to the wound site. Higher rates of wound dehiscence may be evident, as obesity can cause more of a surgical challenge because of an increased hematoma formation (Armstrong, 1998). Adjusted body weights often are used in calculating energy requirements for these patients. No known benefit exists to overfeeding a wound. In fact, overfeeding may increase metabolic stress, leading to increased carbon dioxide production, impaired respiration, and promotion of hyperglycemia (Leininger, 2002). Furthermore, excessive or rapid reestablishment of feeding in malnourished patients can put them at risk for *refeeding syndrome*, a metabolic disturbance characterized by a fluid and electrolyte imbalance.

Alternately, insufficient energy may result in catabolic conditions leading to muscle atrophy, less muscle function, and loss of adipose stores (Hughes, 2003). A loss of just 10% of usual body weight can increase an individual's potential for unhealed wounds as the process of anabolism competes with the wound for nutrients.

Optimal energy requirements for wound healing vary based on multiple factors including severity, type, and size of wound; nutritional status; disease state; age; sex; mobility; or activity. Levels range from 25–30 kcal/kg (Evans, Andrews, Chutka, Fleming, & Garness, 1995) up to 30–35 kcal/kg (Chernoff, 1996; Mathus-Vliegen, 2001; Thomas, 1997; Thompson & Fuhrman, 2005).

Protein Requirements

Protein is the only macronutrient that provides nitrogen, and nitrogen balance is crucial to healing. Protein is a substrate for energy and is needed for electrolyte and fluid balance as well as for the growth, maintenance, and structure of the skin. A protein-deficient diet may impede fibroblast proliferation, angiogenesis, and collagen synthesis (Worley, 2004). A lack of total dietary energy (kilocalories) or stored glycogen forces the body to turn to protein stores and skeletal muscle to fuel gluconeogenesis. To prevent protein catabolism, the provision of adequate energy is needed in the form of carbohydrates and fat to prevent the loss of structural or functional proteins. Protein deficiency appears to delay wound healing by prolonging the inflammatory phase and inhibiting fibroblast proliferation, collagen synthesis, and wound remodeling (Hughes, 2003). Depleted protein stores can decrease the tensile strength of the wound and slow the formation of connective tissue (Wallace, 1994).

Structural Proteins

Amino acids, the building blocks of proteins, are vital to cell division, scar tissue formation, and collagen synthesis (Casey, 1998). Protein is required for fibroblast production, angiogenesis, and collagen production—all important factors in the healing process. Collagen is the major extracellular protein, making up approximately 25% of dry body weight (Alberts et al., 1989). The main fiber in skin and scar tissue is type I collagen, which replaces type III during the granulation phase of healing. Collagen is remodeled during maturation, but the structure of a wound never regains the structure of normal skin, with a scar being approximately 70%–80% as strong as normal tissue (Casey). *Hydroxyproline*, an amino acid found in collagen, often is used as an indirect measure for wound healing progress. However, its validity as a useful marker has been questioned in the literature (Albina, 1994).

Serum albumin frequently is looked to as a marker of nutritional status, yet it is not reliable in times of injury, inflammation, or edema. Hypoalbuminemia can be more closely correlated with severity of illness rather than level of malnutrition. Prealbumin has a short half-life of approximately two days and a small body pool and perhaps is a better indicator of nutritional status than albumin (Scholl & Langkamp-Henken, 2001).

Dietary Protein

Inadequate dietary protein may delay wound healing and prolong the inflammatory phase. Ensuring adequate kilocalories is important in order to spare structural protein losses caused by hypermetabolism. Heavily exudating wounds can easily increase protein losses (Alexander, Spungen, Liu, Losada, & Bauman, 1995). That, coupled with inadequate dietary intake, can prolong the inflammatory response, leading to edema caused by hypoalbuminemia and resulting in impaired healing (Brylinsky, 1995). Adequate energy intake coupled with adequate protein is the optimal environment to promote positive nitrogen balance essential for wound healing (Scholl & Langkamp-Henken, 2001).

When energy intake is adequate but protein intake is low, *protein malnutrition* results. Plasma proteins decrease and can result in peripheral edema, which may affect tissue damage (Doweiko & Nompleggi, 1991; Mora, 1999). When energy and protein intake are both inadequate, *protein energy malnutrition* (PEM) results. Signs of PEM include unintentional weight loss and low body weight for height. Those at risk for PEM include older adults and hospitalized patients.

The recommended dietary allowance for protein in healthy adults is 0.8 g/kg/day. However, because of increased losses and needs, the recommended dietary allowance for adults is likely inadequate to put most patients with wounds into positive nitrogen balance (Thomas, 2001). Evidence suggests that higher protein intake helps to decrease the size of wounds (Breslow, Hallfrisch, Guy, Crawley, & Goldberg, 1993; Chernoff, Milton, & Lipschitz, 1990). The Agency for Healthcare Research and Quality (formerly the Agency for Health Care Policy and Research) has recommended 1.25–1.5 g/kg/day (Bergstrom et al., 1994). Other recommendations in the literature range from 1–2 g/kg/day as being sufficient to put a person into positive nitrogen balance (Bergstrom et al.; Mathus-Vliegen, 2001; Scholl & Langkamp-Henken, 2001). It is essential, however, to consider individual patient needs and comorbidities such as decreased renal and hepatic function, which warrant caution with excessive protein intake. In addition, increased protein without adequate fluid can compromise patient hydration status, especially in older adults (Ayello et al., 1999).

A study of participants with varying degrees of PEM illustrated that the people with higher degrees of PEM had significantly lower rates of healing than the nourished control subjects (Haydock & Hill, 1986). Several studies have suggested that protein is important in the healing of pressure ulcers (Breslow et al., 1993; Chernoff et al., 1990). Chernoff et al. suggested that higher protein intake aids in the healing of pressure ulcers despite the patient's nitrogen balance. Patients on enteral support were randomized to receive 17% (1.2 g/kg) versus 25% (1.8 g/kg) of total energy from protein. The higher protein group had a 73% improvement in healing versus 42% in the lower protein group, despite the fact that the group randomized to the higher protein level had ulcers with larger surface areas (Chernoff et al.). Breslow et al. evaluated patients with stage 2–4 pressure ulcers and found that those consuming a 24% protein diet healed at a greater rate than those consuming a standard 14% protein diet.

Hydration

In addition to energy and protein, fluid plays a vital role in wound healing. Water makes up a large portion of plasma, thus is essential in maintaining the blood volume needed to transport oxygen, nutrients, and growth factors to the wound tissue. Fluid maintains skin turgor and elasticity, whereas dehydrated skin is less elastic and prone to easier breakdown.

Dehydration and malnutrition often exist concurrently, and dehydration is a known risk factor for pressure ulcer formation and delayed wound healing. Fluid recommendations are estimated at 30–35 ml/kg or 1 ml/kcal provided, which is a minimum of 1,500 ml/day (American Dietetic Association & Dietitians of Canada, 2000). Needs may be higher if there is excessive loss from an open wound, diarrhea, or emesis. With fever, the recommendation is for a 12.5% increase of fluid with each degree above 37°C (American Dietetic Association & Dietitians of Canada). The drying effects of air-fluidized beds may, in themselves, be a risk factor for dehydration. As such, the recommendation is to add 10–15 ml/kg for patients on these beds (Ayello et al., 1999; Breslow, 1994; Leininger, 2002). Conversely, levels may need to be lowered if fluid restriction is medically warranted, as both edema and hypervolemia can adversely affect healing.

In monitoring fluids and assessing hydration status, daily intakes and outputs are invaluable, along with routine weights and physical examinations. Laboratory data including hemoglobin, hematocrit, the ratio of blood urea nitrogen to creatinine, chloride, and albumin, as well as urine-specific osmolalities, are helpful but might not always be specific or sensitive to wound status.

Fasting and Surgical Procedures

It has been suggested that current practice of keeping patients fasting for long periods of time before and after surgery may exacerbate poor healing (Field & Bjarnason, 2002; Ruberg, 1984). This would include prolonged nil-per-mouth orders before and after surgery and too slow of a progression back to a diet as tolerated. Some degree of fasting before surgery is necessary to prevent aspiration of gastric contents. In the literature, four to six hours fasting of food and two to four hours fasting of clear fluids prior to surgery is sufficient in patients with normal gastric emptying (Hung, 1992). However, prolonged fasting often is, unfortunately, the case. In a study by Windsor et al. (1988), the authors hypothesized that a patient's recent food intake is more important in the wound healing response than the patient's overall or prior nutritional status. They divided 83 patients awaiting gastrointestinal resection to receive adequate versus inadequate intake. A significant difference was found in the wound healing response, suggesting that maintaining adequate food intake up until the time of surgery is an important aspect of wound healing.

The fact that patients with a good nutritional intake prior to surgery have better wound healing than those with suboptimal intakes (Windsor et al., 1988) suggests that it may be to the patient's advantage to defer surgery, when possible, to optimize nutrition intake.

Nutrients Affecting Wound Healing

Amino Acids

Glutamine: Glutamine is a conditionally indispensable amino acid, meaning that although it is normally nonessential as it is synthesized in the body, it does become conditionally essential in times of stress or disease as levels are decreased. It is needed for DNA synthesis, cell growth, protein synthesis, and immunity (Barton, 1997; Brylinsky, 1995) and makes up the largest proportion of nitrogen in the body (Williams, Abumrad, & Barbul, 2002).

Glutamine may be the primary energy source for the cells of the gastrointestinal tract and immune system (Buchman, 2001; Food and Nutrition Board, 2005; Savy, 1999). The clinical significance of decreased cellular glutamine concentrations is unknown, and it has been debated whether supplementation is truly necessary (Buchman; Savy).

Glutamine may play an indirect role in wound healing, as it is used by inflammatory cells within the wound for proliferation and as a source of energy (Kadowaki & Kanazawa, 2003; Vinnars, Hammarvist, von der Decken, & Wernerman, 1990). Fibroblasts use glutamine as a fuel, as well as for protein and nucleic acid synthesis. Optimal functioning of these cells is paramount to the healing process; thus, glutamine often is discussed as a component in the process of tissue repair (MacKay & Miller, 2003). In addition, it has been shown to improve nitrogen balance after elective surgery (Wilmore, 2001).

In some clinical areas, supplemental glutamine has been shown to be effective; however, little evidence exists to suggest noticeable effects on wound healing (McCauley, Platell, Hall, & McCulloch, 1991; Ziegler et al., 1992). However indirectly, glutamine may improve gut permeability and protein synthesis and normalize serum protein levels, thus leading to decreased length of hospital stay (Flaring, Rooyackers, Wernerman, & Hammarqvist, 2003; Peng, Yan, You, Wang, & Wang, 2005; Zhou et al., 2003).

According to the Food and Nutrition Board (2005), many studies on glutamine supplementation in humans have been published, and very few, if any, adverse effects have been reported. Elevation of liver enzymes was a result of patients supplemented with glutamine via total parenteral nutrition, which resolved after treatment (Hornsby-Lewis et al., 1994).

The Food and Nutrition Board (2005) cautions that glutamine may have effects on tumorigenesis, which is of concern for patients with cancer. Glutamine is a fuel used by rapidly growing tumors (Kovacevic & Morris, 1972) and may reduce the body's own ability to use the amino acid (Chen, Espat, Bland, Copeland, & Souba, 1993; Chen et al., 1991; Klimberg & McClellan, 1996). The Food and Nutrition Board (2005) therefore cautions that although glutamine supplements may help to restore the body's glutamine pool, a possibility exists that it may fuel the cancer cells. In vivo studies on rats, however, did not show tumor growth (Klimberg et al., 1990), and several studies in rats showed that glutamine might even depress tumor growth (Fahr, Kornbluth, Blossom, Schaeffer, & Klimberg, 1994; Klimberg & McClellan).

Although data on glutamine are conflicting, maximum supplementation of 0.57 g/kg has been reported as safe in the literature (Ziegler et al., 1990). Because glutamine is metabolized to ammonia and glutamate, there is concern that it may exacerbate neurologic effects in people with neurologic and psychiatric diseases (Food and Nutrition Board, 2005).

Arginine: Similar to glutamine, arginine is conditionally indispensable, and dietary sources are only needed in times of stress. Arginine is important to cell function, particularly during inflammation and an immune response (Efron & Barbul, 1998). It is the most widely used amino acid to promote wound healing, and the literature suggests arginine supplementation may benefit wound healing irrespective of deficiency (Meyer, Muller, & Herndon, 1994; Wu, Meininger, Knabe, Bazer, & Rhoads, 2000).

The mechanism by which arginine may influence wound healing is unknown at this time, but the end products of arginine metabolism, including nitrous oxide, ornithine, and citrulline, all play important roles. Immune cells catabolize arginine to nitric oxide or ornithine (Scholl & Langkamp-Henken, 2001). Nitric oxide acts as a vasodilator and stimulates fibroblast and collagen synthesis, as well as mediating macrophage antibacterial function (Schaffer et al., 1997). Ornithine can either be converted to proline and eventually hydroxyproline, which assists in collagen synthesis, or may be converted to polyamines, which are needed in cell growth (Albina, Abate, & Mastrofrancesco, 1993; Langkamp-Henken, Johnson, Viar, Geller, & Kotb, 1998). Studies have shown that 8.5–25 g of arginine increased hydroxyproline and collagen deposition (Langkamp-Henken et al., 2000; Williams et al., 2002).

Arginine stimulates anabolism by affecting growth hormone, insulin-like growth factor (IGF-I), and insulin release (Albina et al., 1988; Witte & Barbul, 2002). Arginine increases the body's level of IGF-I, a hormone essential to wound healing. Furthermore, it works indirectly by stimulating levels of both insulin and prolactin, hormones also needed to stimulate healing (Albina, 1994).

Kirk et al. (1993) studied 30 healthy volunteers older than age 65 for a period of two weeks. Fifteen participants received 17 g of free arginine per day, whereas the control group received a placebo. The arginine group showed significantly higher protein and hydroxyproline content, greater lymphocyte responses, and elevated levels of IGF-I, leading the authors to conclude that arginine supplementation improved wound healing in this group (Kirk et al.). Barbul, Lazarou, Efron, Wasserkrug, and Efron (1990) found similar results. In their two-week study, 36 healthy volunteers were randomized into three groups receiving either 24.8 g of free arginine, 17 g of free arginine, or a placebo. Both of the arginine-supplemented groups demonstrated a significant enhancement in collagen and hydroxyproline deposition, as well as greater lymphocyte response. This study was not without side effects; one patient in the placebo group, three patients in the group receiving 17 g of free arginine, and six patients in the group receiving 24.8 g of free arginine reported bloating, mild anorexia, and diarrhea. Conversely, in a study by Hurson, Regan, Kirk, Wasserkrug, and Barbul (1995), 30 older adults receiving 17 g of free arginine per day for 14 days reported no adverse effects.

A randomized, double-blind study by Williams et al. (2002) illustrated that an oral supplement containing a mixture of arginine, glutamine, and beta-hydroxy beta-methylbutyrate (HMB) significantly enhanced collagen synthesis in healthy older adult volunteers by 67%. HMB is a metabolite of the amino acid leucine, and the supplement contained 3 g of this metabolite along with 14 g of arginine and 14 g of glutamine. It is important to note that although the supplement showed enhanced collagen synthesis, it did not seem to have an effect on total protein levels.

Two randomized controlled clinical trials (RCTs) examined postoperative patients with head and neck cancers. When enterally fed an arginine-enhanced formula versus an isocaloric, isonitrogenous formula, both groups showed significant improvement in plasma proteins and immune parameters but with no significant difference between the study and control groups (de Luis et al., 2005; de Luis, Izaola, Cuellar, Terroba, & Aller, 2004).

An RCT by de Luis, Aller, Izaola, Cuellar, and Terroba (2002) examined the impact of an arginine-enhanced formula in the same patient population. Outcome measures included plasma proteins, weight, postoperative infection rates, wound complications, mortality, and length of stay in hospital. The only significant difference found between the study and control groups was a lower incidence of postoperative fistula formation in the study group. Similarly, an RCT by de Luis et al. (2004) also demonstrated decreased postoperative fistula formation and shortened length of stay in the group receiving arginine-enhanced enteral formula arginine.

Gastrointestinal symptoms are a reported side effect of arginine supplementation. In one study of 21 healthy adults orally supplemented with arginine, a small percentage of the participants reported nausea and diarrhea (Barbul, Sisto, Wasserkrug, & Efron, 1981). These side effects were mediated by altering the individual doses without changing the total daily dose of supplement. In another study, postoperative patients receiving an enteral formula supplemented with arginine experienced statistically significant ($p = 0.05$) increases in diarrhea compared to the control group (de Luis et al., 2004). A similar study by de Luis et al. (2002) showed a higher incidence of diarrhea in the arginine group, although it was not statistically significant.

Arginine is the only precursor to nitric oxide, and there is controversy that excess production of nitric oxide can be detrimental. Excess nitric oxide may enhance a systemic inflammatory response (SIRS) in critically ill patients; therefore, arginine may be contraindicated in times of SIRS or sepsis (Suchner, Heyland, & Peter, 2002). In addition, hepatic, renal, and hydration status must be monitored regularly because of the high nitrogen load in large therapeutic doses.

The evidence is conflicting regarding arginine supplementation in the area of cancer research. Park et al. (1992) gave 30 g of oral arginine per day to 10 patients with breast cancer three days immediately prior to surgery. A control group that did not receive supplementation also was monitored. The daily median rate of tumor protein synthesis for individuals receiving arginine supplementation was more than double that found in the control group, leading the authors to indicate that large oral doses of arginine may stimulate tumor growth. The evidence from this study indicates that dietary supplementation with arginine is not advisable for patients with cancer. The Food and Nutrition Board (2005) suggested that only at-risk children with congenital defects affecting arginine metabolism take arginine supplementation.

Fatty Acids

Omega-3 and omega-6 are the body's two essential polyunsaturated fatty acids important to cell membrane integrity and function. The body cannot produce these fatty acids, so they must be supplied exogenously; however, a deficiency of either essential fatty acid is extremely rare in healthy people. Patients with fat malabsorption or those on total parenteral nutrition with insufficient lipids may be at risk. Symptoms include scaly skin, dermatitis, and delayed growth (Food and Nutrition Board, 2005). Both series of fatty acids are precursors to the *eicosanoids*, molecules that affect inflammation, immunity, and central nervous system signaling. Eicosanoids send the signal to initiate wound healing, although research has suggested that eicosanoids derived from the omega-3 series have less inflammatory and immunologic effect than those from the omega-6 series (Shepherd, 2002b).

The use of omega-3 fatty acids for their anti-inflammatory effects has received recent interest. Inflammation is helpful to wound healing because it promotes delivery of nutrients and removal of debris and bacteria from the wound site (Phillips, 2000). Prolonged inflammation, however, can be detrimental as cellular activity is compromised and the inflammatory process competes with the body for nutrients, suppressing the immune system (Cerra, 1991). Dietary manipulation of omega-3s may be beneficial to curb inflammation in a chronic wound with overactive macrophages (Cerra). Ruthig and Meckling-Gill (1999) suggested that providing omega-3 fatty acids may reduce the immunosuppressive effects of omega-6 fatty acids. Omega-3 supplementation has demonstrated benefits such as reduced infection rates postoperatively (Heller & Koch, 2000) and increased collagen synthesis (Hankenson, Watkins, Schoenlein, Allen, & Turek, 2000). However, the caveat for adverse effects on patients in the inflammatory phase of healing needs to be considered. A possible reduction in metabolic response can occur, although much of this information is garnered from animal studies (Fuhrman, 2003). Additional research on omega-3 supplementation is needed to verify or disprove current available information.

In general, a lack of consensus exists regarding the use of supplementation of omega-3 fats. Most of the research on wound healing and fat requirements is based on animal models, thus limiting application. However, it is generally accepted practice that high-dose supplements of omega-3 fatty acids can increase synthesis of prostaglandins and impair inflammatory response, leading to a wound with decreased strength (Lown, 1998). For this reason, supplemental omega-3 currently is not recommended for wound healing.

In addition, individuals taking oral hypoglycemic agents or anticoagulant medications should be cautioned with omega-3 supplementation because it may promote prolonged bleeding time (Food and Nutrition Board, 2005). Currently, insufficient evidence exists to recommend omega-3 supplementation in patients with cancer, as conclusive RCTs are lacking (Food and Nutrition Board, 2005).

Micronutrients

Healthcare professionals in the United States and Canada turn to the Food and Nutrition Board of the Institute of Medicine for recommendations on micronutrient intakes developed as part of the dietary reference intake (DRI) program. The *recommended dietary allowance* is the average daily nutrient intake via diet that is sufficient to meet the nutrient requirements of nearly all (97%–98%) healthy individuals according to age and gender. The *tolerable upper intake level* (UL) is the highest average daily nutrient intake level that may pose no risk of adverse health effects to almost all individuals in the general population. At intakes greater than the UL, the risk of adverse effects may increase. DRIs are based on healthy people and are not reflective of illness or disease state.

Micronutrient requirements and supplementation pose a nutritional challenge to practice in the care of patients with cancer who have wounds. Recommendations are not without controversy as there currently is no clear consensus in the scientific community. The following is a summary of the evidence on what is known about micronutrient needs and supplementation in the area of wound care.

Vitamin A: Vitamin A is a fat-soluble vitamin required for epithelial development; therefore, it is of great interest in wound healing. Vitamin A may function as an immunostimulant by increasing the quantity of monocytes and macrophages in the wound or by stabilizing the intracellular lysosomes of white blood cells (Barbul, Thysen, Rettura, Levenson, & Seifter, 1978; Ehrlich & Hunt, 1968). Vitamin A also may play a role by increasing collagen synthesis and epithelization stimulating fibroplasia (Connor, 1986; Demetriou, Levenson, Rettura, & Seifter, 1985). Thus, a vitamin A deficiency appears to impair healing, secondary to decreased collagen formation and increased vulnerability to infection.

It is suggested that vitamin A should only be supplemented if a deficiency is suspected, as in the case of fat malabsorption or if the serum retinol levels are low (American Dietetic Association & Morrison Health Care, Inc., 1997; Bergstrom et al., 1994). *Clinical deficiencies* are defined as serum retinol levels less than 0.35 mmol/L (Scholl & Langkamp-Henken, 2001); however, many factors may affect vitamin A status, and lab values should not be considered in isolation (Scholl & Langkamp-Henken).

Most of the research in vitamin A deficiency and wound healing has been garnered in animals. Levenson et al. (1984) suggested that supplemental vitamin A prevented impaired wound healing and reduced weight loss in wounded rats receiving radiation. Researchers found that the supplemental vitamin A was beneficial regardless of whether initiated before or after radiation and wounding. They also found that vitamin A worked to enhance early inflammatory phase wound healing by increasing the amount of monocytes and macrophages at the wound site, modulating collagenase activity, supporting epithelial cell differentiation, improving localization and stimulation of the immune response, and lessening the adverse reactions of radiation (Levenson et al.). It is questionable whether supplementation with vitamin A will actually improve wound healing in animals unless a deficiency state is present (Ehrlich & Hunt, 1968; Niu, Cushin, Reisner, Levenson, & Demetriou, 1987).

Corticosteroid use is implicated in delayed wound healing and increased risk of developing a wound-related infection (Ehrlich & Hunt, 1968; Hunt, Ehrlich, Garcia, & Dunphy, 1969; Phillips, Kim, Fonkalsrud, Zeng, & Dindat, 1992). Steroids are known to impair inflammation, fibroblast proliferation, collagen deposition, capillary regeneration, wound contraction, and epithelial migration (Levenson & Demetriou, 1992; Lown, 1998; Stadelmann, Digenis, & Tobin, 1998; Wicke et al., 2000). A recommended dose of vitamin A of 10,000–15,000 IU/day for up to seven days has been suggested for patients on steroids (Hadley & Fitzsimmons, 1990; Lown). Animal studies have shown that vitamin A may counter the anti-inflammatory action of steroids and help to increase the tensile strength of the wound (Ehrlich & Hunt; Petry, 1999; Phillips et al.). The level of supplementation currently recommended is not strongly justified, as most of the scientific data in vitamin A, wounds, and steroid treatment are from animal research (Scholl & Langkamp-Henken, 2001).

Supplementation with vitamin A should be administered cautiously. Because it is a fat-soluble vitamin that is stored in the liver, toxicity is a risk. Signs of toxicity include headache, vomiting, and bone and muscle pain (Ross, 1999). Supplementation may be contraindicated in individuals with existing liver disease or severe protein malnutrition, high alcohol intake, or hyperlipidemia (Food and Nutrition Board, 2001). Furthermore, in chronic renal failure, levels of vitamin A typically are high, leading to an increased risk of hypercalcemia secondary to the osteolytic action of retinoids on bone (Beijer & Planken, 2001; Doireau, Macher, Brun, Bernard, & Loirat, 1996; Weiland, Hendricks, Amat y Leon, Gutierrez, & Jones, 1971).

Vitamin C: Vitamin C is a water-soluble vitamin that acts as an antioxidant or free-radical scavenger. Its antioxidant properties have been demonstrated to lessen DNA damage (Food and Nutrition Board, 2000; Jacob, 1999). Humans lack long-term storage ability for vitamin C; therefore, daily intake is crucial in maintaining adequate levels, although deficiency does not appear to be an issue in the United States and Canada (Food and Nutrition Board, 2000). Vitamin C deficiency has been linked to poor healing (Crandon, Lund, & Dill, 1940). However, it is unknown whether patients without deficiency will benefit from supplementation. A serum level of 0.2 mg/dl is considered deficient (Jacob).

Early vitamin C deficiencies manifested as scurvy in 18th century sailors whose diets lacked sufficient fruits and vegetables. Body pools of 300 mg or less of vitamin C are associated with scurvy, and individuals most at risk for deficiency include individuals who smoke, people living with cancer or liver disease, and substance abusers (Hughes, 2003; Scholl & Langkamp-Henken, 2001). Older adults may be at risk for poor vitamin C status secondary to edentulous states (Shepherd, 2002a). Smokers have an increased requirement for vitamin C secondary to an increased metabolic turnover, necessitating approximately 35 mg/day more than nonsmokers to maintain body pools (Food and Nutrition Board, 2000).

In wounds, vitamin C plays a role in the synthesis of connective tissue and collagen. It acts as a cofactor with iron in the hydroxylation of proline and lysine needed in the synthesis and cross-linking of collagen—essential to the proliferation and remodeling phases of wound healing (Bailey, 1978). Deficiency can therefore compromise wound healing as it contributes to less mature and sufficiently cross-linked collagen fibers needed for tensile strength (Hughes, 2003). Deficiencies also may result in weakened capillaries because collagen is necessary for blood vessel synthesis (Scholl & Langkamp-Henken, 2001). In addition, vitamin C is essential to neutrophil function, which helps to prevent infection and plays a role in angiogenesis, helping to supply vital nutrients to the skin tissue (Levenson & Demetriou, 1992; Goetzl, Wasserman, Gigli, & Austen, 1974; Nicosia, Belser, Bonanno, & Diven, 1991). When vitamin C is deficient, abnormal changes occur in the intracellular matrix, leading to poor adhesion of endothelial cells (MacKay & Miller, 2003). Without adequate formation of collagen, wounds are more likely to dehisce (Scholl & Langkamp-Henken). The incidence of wound dehiscence in patients with depleted vitamin C was eight times as high compared those with normal levels (Zaloga, 1994).

Historically, supplementation with vitamin C for wound healing has its roots in World War II. British citizens had a limited supply of fresh foods and, thus, likely had low levels of vitamin C intake. With air strikes, surgery rates increased, and physicians initiated vitamin C supplementation of 1,000 mg three days before surgery and 100 mg after surgery for recovery. As a result, the incidence of nonhealing wounds dropped by 76% (Hunt, 1941).

An early prospective, double-blind clinical trial tested the effect of vitamin C on existing pressure ulcers. Twenty patients with pressure ulcers were randomized to receive either 500 mg of ascorbic acid twice daily or a placebo. The experimental group showed a better reduction in the area of their pressure ulcer at month one (84% mean reduction versus 43% mean reduction for placebo). However, in a study by ter Riet, Kessels, and Knipschild (1995), patients with pressure ulcers did not benefit any more with 500 mg twice a day than with 10 mg twice a day. The investigators found no statistical difference between the velocity of the wound closure or its global appearance (ter Riet et al.). Although no difference occurred in improvement of healing rates between 1,000 mg or 20 mg of vitamin C daily, a difference was seen between supplementation versus placebo. This could suggest, in accordance with the literature, that higher doses do not necessarily correlate with increased wound healing (Taylor, Rimmer, Day, Butcher, & Dymock, 1974).

Although supplementation has been shown to aid healing in deficient, stressed, or injured patients, it remains controversial as to whether supplementation can benefit those who are not deficient. In addition, although the amount of supplementation recommended in the literature ranges from 100–4,000 mg/day, little evidence indicates that supplementing greater than 1,000 mg/day promotes wound healing. Tissue saturation occurs at approximately 200 mg/day (Levine, Rumsey, Daruwala, Park, & Wang, 1999). Higher doses up to 300 mg may only be beneficial in cases of sepsis or critical illness (Williams, 2002). Levenson and Demetriou (1992) recommended 1,000–2,000 mg/day, as no adverse effects have been reported at these doses.

Excessive supplementation may have risks. There is some evidence of gastrointestinal distress including nausea, diarrhea, and cramping, as well as oxidative damage, with amounts of 3,000 mg or more (Food and Nutrition Board, 2000; Jacob, 1999; Vilter, 1980). Lastly, a few case reports exist of increased urinary oxalate secretion increasing risk of kidney stones in individuals taking more than 500 mg of vitamin C (Commission of the European Communities, 1993). However, a recent review article by Hathcock et al. (2005) concluded that vitamin C supplements of less than 2,000 mg/day are safe for most adults.

Vitamin E: Vitamin E is an essential, fat-soluble vitamin that acts as an antioxidant by inhibiting free-radical reactions (Food and Nutrition Board,

2000; MacKay & Miller, 2003). Vitamin E has eight naturally occurring forms, but only *alpha-tocopherol* is maintained in plasma (Food and Nutrition Board, 2000). Deficiencies of vitamin E are very rare but may be seen in patients with fat malabsorption, patients on very low-fat diets, individuals with genetic abnormalities of vitamin E metabolism, or people with protein-energy malnutrition (Food and Nutrition Board, 2000; Traber, 1999). There is no indication that vitamin E supplementation may help in wound healing, and in fact, it may adversely affect healing.

According to the Food and Nutrition Board (2000), vitamin E supplement use is high in the U.S. population. Vitamin E in amounts above the UL of 1,000 IU/day may impair wound healing in humans and has been shown to inhibit clot formation in animals (Ehrlich, Tarver, & Hunt, 1972; Greenwald, Sharzer, Padawer, Levenson, & Seifter, 1990; Havlik, 1997). Interestingly, a recent review by Hathcock et al. (2005) suggested that 1,600 IU/day may actually be safe for the general population, even though this amount is above the UL. Individuals who are deficient in vitamin K or on anticoagulant therapy should be monitored if on vitamin E supplements (Food and Nutrition Board, 2000).

Vitamin E has become a popular ingredient in skin care products for topical use. Although it enhances the immune response, its role in wound healing is controversial. Many of the recommendations about vitamin E supplementation historically have been anecdotal, as several trials did not detect any benefit in wound healing for surgical or pressure ulcers (Baumann & Spencer, 1999; Jenkins, Alexander, MacMillan, Waymack, & Kopcha, 1986). Fifty-seven patients with venous stasis ulcers of the leg received 400 mg/day of vitamin E orally and demonstrated no difference from the control group in either the frequency or rate of healing, or incidence of relapse (Lee, 1953). It has been suggested that perhaps the anti-inflammatory properties of vitamin E can inhibit collagen synthesis by decreasing tensile strength, adversely affecting healing in animal studies (Ehrlich et al., 1972; Greenwald et al., 1990; Havlik, 1997).

Vitamin K: Vitamin K is a fat-soluble vitamin that acts as a coenzyme for bone metabolism and is essential for blood clotting (Food and Nutrition Board, 2001). In addition, vitamin K acts as a cofactor for the synthesis of proteins, including prothrombin, involved in the wound healing process. Vitamin K has been shown to reduce the risk of infection and wound dehiscence (Cartwright, 2002). Deficiency of vitamin K is rare but is seen in cases of fat malabsorption or with medications affecting vitamin K metabolism. In cases of deficiency, excessive bleeding can occur at the site of the wound and may increase the risk of wound infections (Levenson & Demetriou, 1992; Lown, 1998). No UL has been set for vitamin K because data were insufficient, but no adverse effects have been reported in healthy individuals from food or supplements. Patients on anticoagulants should be cautioned against supplemental use of vitamin K because of its blood clotting action. In addition, elevated intakes of vitamin E may affect the action of vitamin K; however, the metabolic reason is unknown, and more research is needed (Food and Nutrition Board, 2000).

Iron: Iron is a component of proteins, enzymes, and hemoglobin, the latter of which transports oxygen in the body (Food and Nutrition Board, 2001). Susceptibility to deficiency includes patients with impaired iron absorption or individuals on a vegetarian diet. Calcium may inhibit the absorption of heme and non-heme iron (Food and Nutrition Board, 2001). Data have suggested that supplemental iron may inhibit zinc absorption unless consumed with food (Food and Nutrition Board, 2001).

Iron has implications for wound healing. It is a cofactor for the hydroxylation of lysine and proline, needed for synthesis of collagen (Lewis, 2002), and aids in reducing the risk of infection. Lack of iron can lead to iron deficiency and iron-deficiency anemia, which affect oxygen transport because oxygen delivery to the wound is proportional to the concentration of oxygen in the blood (Casey, 1998). Deficiency of iron can lead to reduced peripheral circulation to preserve oxygen delivery to organs, which can have implications for wounds in peripheral areas (Casey, 1998). However, the literature has shown that low hemoglobin may, in fact, not be as critical a factor in wound healing as long as cardiac output and tissue perfusion are maintained (Hunt & Hopf, 1997; Stadelmann et al., 1998).

Excess iron may promote growth of certain bacteria, and it has been postulated that *anemia of inflammation* (also referred to as *anemia of chronic disease*) may be the body's attempt to withhold iron from these microbes (Jurado, 1997). Routine iron supplementation therefore is not recommended for wound healing unless a deficiency is confirmed via laboratory indicators.

Zinc: Zinc is an essential trace mineral needed for cellular growth and replication and is required for enzymatic processes in macronutrient metabolism (Food and Nutrition Board, 2001). Zinc demands increase when cell division and protein needs increase (Casey, 1998; Chandra, 1984; Levenson & Demetriou, 1992). Low serum zinc levels have been associated with poor wound healing (Orgill & Demling, 1998; Scholl & Langkamp-Henken, 2001). Supplementation may help, but only in patients who are deficient.

Zinc deficiency is rare because the body tightly regulates serum zinc levels to 10–15 μmol/L. Stress, trauma, and infection, however, can cause decreases in serum zinc levels (Ehrlichman, Seckel, Bryan, & Moschella, 1991; Greaves & Skillen, 1970; Selmanpakoglu, Cetin, Sayal, & Isimer, 1994). For example, low serum zinc levels have been found in patients with chronic leg ulcers (Carlson, 1999) and spinal cord injuries (Cruse et al., 2000). In inflammatory conditions, serum zinc levels may not be reliable because zinc is more than 90% protein bound (Galloway, McMillan, & Sattar, 2000).

Zinc has received much attention in the area of wound care, perhaps secondary to its role in DNA synthesis, cell division, and protein synthesis—all necessary processes for tissue regeneration and repair (MacKay & Miller, 2003). Zinc demands are considered to be high in all stages of wound healing (Lansdown, 1996; MacKay & Miller); thus, deficiency can inhibit both protein and collagen formation (Fernandez-Madrid, Prasad, & Oberleas, 1973).

Two early studies showed positive results in the area of zinc supplementation. In 1967, a study of 20 men undergoing surgical removal of pilonidal sinuses received 220 mg zinc sulfate (50 mg elemental zinc) three times daily. It was found that they had a significantly faster healing rate than the control group (Pories, Henzel, Rob, & Strain, 1967). In a 1972 double-blind trial of 27 patients with chronic leg ulcers, 13 received 600 mg/day zinc sulfate and the remainder received a placebo. Only the patients with low serum zinc levels benefited from the supplemental zinc (Hallbrook & Lanner, 1972). Supplementation has been shown to promote wound healing in these early studies (Lansdown, 1996) but may be beneficial only in those who have proven deficiency (Hallbrook & Lanner; Levenson & Demetriou, 1992; MacKay & Miller, 2003; Weisman, 1980).

Not all studies, however, have shown improved healing with routine zinc supplementation. In a retrospective study, older, institutionalized patients who received 440 mg zinc showed no significant decrease in duration of wound healing compared to the control group (Haggard, Houston, Williford, Meserve, & Shewokis, 1999). A small, blinded, crossover design study did not show significant improvement in ulcer volume with supplementation of 220 mg zinc sulfate after 12 weeks (Norris & Reynolds, 1971).

Supplementation of 15–25 mg/day has been recommended for wound healing (American Dietetic Association & Morrison Health Care, Inc., 1997). Reasons for supplementation include increased losses from large skin wounds, as up to 20% of total-body zinc is found in the skin (Andrews & Gallagher-Allred, 1999). In addition, zinc is lost in times of skin cell turnover, and more zinc is excreted through the urine in times of starvation or trauma (Food and Nutrition Board, 2001).

If a zinc deficiency is suspected or increased losses are present, it is suggested that supplementation should be given for no longer than two to three weeks to minimize the risk of adverse affects (Lown, 1998).

Lown (1998) suggested high-dose supplements should be limited based on adverse clinical effects. High-dose intakes have been shown to cause gastrointestinal side effects including nausea and vomiting (Fosmire, 1990). Excess levels of 150 mg orally twice a day for six weeks were shown to impair neutrophil and lymphocyte function (Chandra, 1984). Decreased high-density lipoprotein (HDL) cholesterol and increased low-density lipoprotein cholesterol were adverse effects reported in a study of volunteers given 300 mg elemental zinc per day (Chandra). Similarly, reduced HDL was reported when subjects were given 160 mg of elemental zinc per day for six weeks (Fosmire).

Excess zinc may interfere with *lysyl oxidase*, an enzyme required for catalysis of collagen cross-linking needed for tensile strength. In this manner, excess zinc may actually exacerbate poor wound healing (Andrews & Gallagher-Allred, 1999).

Zinc supplementation may interfere with other nutrients, potentially contributing to a negative effect on wound healing. Copper status may be reduced with increased zinc intake. Intakes as low as 25 mg/day of zinc have been shown to have an effect on copper absorption and may lead to copper deficiency (Fosmire, 1990). Excess plasma zinc levels also may lead to a vitamin A deficiency (Lown, 1998; Sandstrom, 2001). Concurrent iron and zinc supplementation may decrease the absorption of zinc from the intestine (Casey, 1998). Calcium and phosphorus may decrease zinc absorption, but more evidence is needed in this area (Food and Nutrition Board, 1997).

Other nutrients: Meyer et al. (1994) suggested manganese, selenium, and silicon as other nutrients that may help the wound healing process when deficient. Manganese, along with copper, may be important to tissue regeneration (Lewis, 2002; Lown, 1998) Copper plays a role in bone formation and in maintaining the integrity of connective tissue, as well as in collagen synthesis (Lown). Thiamin, riboflavin, and pantothenic acid are needed for collagen production (Lewis; Lown). More research is needed to determine whether amounts greater than the recommended dietary allowance are necessary in wound healing.

Antioxidants and Radiation Therapy

The process of wound healing generates free radicals and thereby oxidative stress, which causes cellular damage, an impediment to wound healing (Gordillo & Sen, 2003). Dietary antioxidants (vitamins C, E, and carotenoids) historically have been used to suppress the oxidative process in general wound care management; however, supplementation in patients undergoing radiation or chemotherapy warrants caution.

Two hypotheses exist to antioxidant supplementation during cancer treatment. One maintains that high-dose antioxidants (vitamins C, E, and carotenoids) may enhance the effect of radiation and chemotherapy by increasing tumor response to treatment while decreasing some toxic effects of radiation on toxic cells (Prasad, Cole, Kumar, & Prasad, 2001). The opposing hypothesis (Salganik, 2001) is that high doses of antioxidants should not be taken during radiation therapy as they may protect cancer cells against radiation. Currently, some cancer centers do not recommend the use of large-dose antioxidant supplements during radiation therapy. Dietary sources present in a balanced diet are not of concern. More evidence is required to recommended changes to practice in the area of antioxidant supplementation.

Comorbidities

Diabetes Mellitus

Wound healing in patients with diabetes mellitus presents unique challenges. If blood glucose is not well controlled, the cell walls become rigid and blood flow is impaired through the vessels at the cell surface (Collins, 2003). In general, maintaining targeted blood sugar levels will often show improved wound healing (Bohannon & Jack, 1996; Gore et al., 2001). Patients with diabetes have decreased wound healing rates and develop chronic wounds secondary to neurologic and microvascular changes (Casey, 1998). A relationship exists between glycosylated hemoglobin and the tensile strength of wounds (Lewis, Biondo, & Page, 1994).

In RCTs by Van den Berghe et al. (2001, 2003), critically ill surgical patients whose blood glucose levels were maintained at 80–110 mg/dl had significantly reduced inflammation and infections. A smaller RCT by Grey and Perdrizet (2004) replicated the findings of reduced infectious rates. Furnary, Zerr, Grunkemeier, and Starr (1999) found that deep sternal wound infections following coronary artery bypass graft surgery were decreased when blood glucose was less than 200 mg/dl.

Monitoring blood glucose in patients with diabetes should be done regularly not only for wound healing but also to reduce other complications associated with prolonged hyperglycemia. Possible long-term complications of poorly managed diabetes include neuropathies, which can impair protective sensation against wounds. Tissue perfusion may be affected by vascular complications of unmanaged diabetes or cardiac or pulmonary conditions.

Another side effect of hyperglycemia is its interference in the transport of vitamin C into fibroblasts and leukocytes and subsequent decreased leukocyte chemotaxis. As glucose and vitamin C have similar structures, it has been suggested that they compete for membrane transport (Mann & Newton, 1975) in diabetic patients, thus inhibiting vitamin C entry into cells. With relation to leukocytes, hypergylcemia may affect early inflammatory response, thereby increasing the risk of infection and decreasing wound healing (Mann & Newton).

Chronic Renal Failure and Dialysis

Renal insufficiency should be considered when increasing protein needs secondary to wounds. According to the National Kidney Foundation Kidney Disease Outcomes Quality Initiative (2000), individuals with *chronic renal failure*, defined by a glomerular filtration rate of 25 ml/min or less, should receive 0.6–0.75 g/kg of protein. This range has been suggested in order to retard the progression of kidney disease by unduly taxing renal function (National Kidney Foundation). Once dialysis therapy is initiated, however, protein restriction is no longer applicable.

Patients with renal disease have a higher incidence of concurrent diabetes, which could have implications for wounds and wound healing. In addition, individuals undergoing dialysis have a higher risk of wounds secondary to decreased mobility and potential vascular disease. Nutrient supplementation in patients undergoing dialysis therapy requires modification when wound healing is needed. The final stage of wound healing, collagen remodeling and reepithelialization, is dependent on zinc, vitamin C, and protein intake (Winkler & Mandry, 1992). A thorough assessment of nutritional status and correction of nutritional deficits must be considered.

Energy and protein: Patients on dialysis have higher energy and protein requirements. Energy requirements may range from 30–35 kcal/kg depending on age; protein needs range from 1.2–1.3 grams of protein per kilogram of body weight depending on modality (hemodialysis versus peritoneal) (Kopple, 2001).

Zinc: Dialysis patients may consume inadequate amounts of zinc-rich protein foods, in part because of altered taste perceptions. Coupled with the difficulty in estimating losses in the dialysate and altered zinc stores, suboptimal zinc intake may be a factor for this population. Zinc supplementation therefore should be considered if deficiency is suspected.

Vitamin C: Additional vitamin C greater than what is delivered in a typical renal-formulated multivitamin should not be administered to renal patients. Vitamin C acts as an oxalate precursor and in the absence of renal function, oxalate cannot be excreted, increasing the risk of tissue calcification. In addition, if patients are on supplemental iron and erythropoietin, the antioxidant capability of vitamin C changes. Iron in the ferric form causes vitamin C to become a pro-oxidant and can penetrate ferritin, leading to losses of free iron in the blood (Herbert, Shaw, & Jayatileke, 1995). Doses of vitamin C of 300 mg or more given three times a week at the time of dialysis caused free iron from ferritin in recombinant human erythropoietin resistance (Gastaldelo, Vereerstraeten, Nzame-Nze, Vanherweghem, & Tielemans, 1995; Tarng & Huang, 1998). A renal-formulated multivitamin typically contains approximately 60–100 mg vitamin C and is appropriate to meet nutritional needs for dialysis patients with wounds (Elfert & Drees, 1999). Limiting vitamin C to a dose of 60–120 mg/day has been suggested in practice (Wiggins, 2004) because of increased risk of developing oxalates in bone and muscle (Wiggins, 1999).

Vitamin E: Vitamin E given in the dialysate or by the oral route may attenuate the pro-oxidant detriment when an individual receives iron (Roob et al., 2000). It has been suggested to limit vitamin E to 400 IU daily in dialysis patients (Roob et al.).

Vitamin A: It is not advisable to initiate vitamin A supplementation in dialysis patients. Retinol-binding protein cannot be degraded without adequate kidney function, and high levels of vitamin A can lead to hypercalcemia, bone loss, and osteolytic activity. Intake from foods, multiple micronutrient supplements, and oral supplements should not exceed 1,000 mcg/day (Chazot & Kopple, 2004).

Oral nutritional supplements containing arginine may contain up to 250 mg vitamin C and 1,000 IU of vitamin A, and thus should be considered in the patients' total intake with additional vitamin levels adjusted accordingly.

Conclusion

As suggested in the opening quotation, most wounds, given time, will heal. The objective of medical nutritional therapy, however, is to provide the optimal conditions for healing to occur. As with most interventions, nutrition therapy is most effective when initiated early and reassessed routinely by a registered dietitian. There has been much research as to the effect of micronutrients on healing status. The importance of micronutrients cannot be disputed, but the question still remains as to whether supplementation in nondeficient patients is appropriate. The challenge is that it is not always feasible to obtain accurate and timely lab values in clinical practice; therefore, supplements may be suggested based on suspicion of deficiency derived from clinical assessment versus a proven deficiency.

What cannot be disputed, however, is that the macronutrients, in particular overall kilocalories, protein, and fluid, will undoubtedly contribute to patients' overall nutritional status and ultimately to their ability to heal. Wound healing involves a combination of effective medical, nursing, and nutrition intervention and when applied correctly will contribute to patients' morbidity, well-being, and quality of life.

References

Alberts, B., Bray, D., Lewis, J., Raff, M., Roberts, K., & Watson, J.D. (1989). *Molecular biology of the cell* (2nd ed.). New York: Garland.

Albina, J.E. (1994). Nutrition and wound healing. *Journal of Parenteral and Enteral Nutrition, 18*(4), 367–376.

Albina, J.E., Abate, J.A., & Mastrofrancesco, B. (1993). Role of ornithine as a proline precursor in healing wounds. *Journal of Surgical Research, 55*(1), 97–102.

Albina, J.E., Mills, C.D., Barbul, A., Thirkill, C.E., Henry, W.L., Jr., Mastrofrancesco, B., et al. (1988). Arginine metabolism in wounds. *American Journal of Physiology, 254*(4), E459–E467.

Alexander, L.R., Spungen, A.M., Liu, M.H., Losada, M., & Bauman, W.A. (1995). Resting metabolic rate in subjects with paraplegia: The effect of pressure sores. *Archives of Physical Medicine and Rehabilitation, 76*(9), 819–822.

American Dietetic Association & Dietitians of Canada. (2000). *Manual of clinical dietetics* (6th ed.). Chicago: American Dietetic Association.

American Dietetic Association & Morrison Health Care, Inc. (1997). *Medical nutrition therapy across the continuum of care*. Chicago: American Dietetic Association.

Andrews, M., & Gallagher-Allred, C. (1999). The role of zinc in wound healing. *Advances in Wound Care, 12*(3), 137–138.

Armstrong, M. (1998). Obesity as an intrinsic factor affecting wound healing. *Journal of Wound Care, 7*(5), 220–221.

Ayello, E.A., Thomas, D.R., & Litchford, M.A. (1999). Nutritional aspects of wound healing. *Home Healthcare Nurse, 17*(11), 719–729.

Bailey, A.J. (1978). Collagen and elastic fibres. *Journal of Clinical Pathology, 21*(Suppl. 12), 49–58.

Barbul, A., Lazarou, S.A., Efron, D.T., Wasserkrug, H.L., & Efron, G. (1990). Arginine enhances wound healing and lymphocyte immune responses in humans. *Surgery, 108*(2), 331–336.

Barbul, A., Sisto, D.A., Wasserkrug, H.L., & Efron, G. (1981). Arginine stimulates lymphocyte immune response in healthy human beings. *Surgery, 90*(2), 244–251.

Barbul, A., Thysen, B., Rettura, G., Levenson, S.M., & Seifter, E. (1978). White cell involvement in the inflammatory, wound healing and immune actions of vitamin A. *Journal of Enteral and Parenteral Nutrition, 2*(2), 129–138.

Barton, R.G. (1997). Immune-enhancing enteral formulas: Are they beneficial in critically ill patients? *Nutrition in Clinical Practice, 12*(2), 51–62.

Baumann, L.S., & Spencer, J. (1999). The effects of topical vitamin E on the cosmetic appearance of scars. *Dermatologic Surgery, 25*(4), 311–315.

Beijer, C., & Planken, E.V. (2001). Hypercalcemia due to chronic vitamin A use by an elderly patient with renal insufficiency. *Nederlands Tijdschrift Voor Geneeskunde, 145*(2), 90–93.

Bergstrom, N., Allman, R.M., Alvarez, O.M., Bennett, M.A., Carlson, C.E., Frantz, R.A., et al. (1994). *Treatment of pressure ulcers* [Clinical Practice Guideline No. 15, AHCPR Publication No. 95-0652]. Rockville, MD: Agency for Health Care Policy and Research, Public Health Service, U.S. Department of Health and Human Services.

Bohannon, N., & Jack, D. (1996). Type II diabetes: Tips for managing your older patients. *Geriatrics, 51*(3), 28–35.

Breslow, R.A. (1994). Nutrition and air-fluidized beds: A literature review. *Advances in Wound Care, 7*(3), 57–62.

Breslow, R.A., Hallfrisch, J., Guy, D.G., Crawley, D., & Goldberg, A.P. (1993). The importance of dietary protein in healing pressure ulcers. *Journal of the American Geriatrics Society, 41*(4), 357–362.

Brylinsky, C.M. (1995). Nutrition and wound healing. *Ostomy/Wound Management, 41*(10), 14–26.

Buchman, A.L. (2001). Glutamine: Commercially essential or conditionally essential? A critical appraisal of the human data. *American Journal of Clinical Nutrition, 74*(1), 25–32.

Campos, A.C.L., Groth, A.K., & Branco, A.B. (2008). Assessment of nutritional aspects of wound healing. *Current Opinion in Clinical Nutrition and Metabolic Care, 11*(3), 281–288.

Carlson, G. (1999). The influence of nutrition and sepsis upon wound healing. *Journal of Wound Care, 8*(9), 471–474.

Cartwright, A. (2002). Nutritional assessment as part of wound management. *Nursing Times, 98*(44), 62–63.

Casey, G. (1998). The importance of nutrition in wound healing. *Nursing Standard, 7*(13), 51–56.

Casey, G. (2003). Nutritional support in wound healing. *Nursing Standard, 17*(23), 55–58.

Cerra, F.B. (1991). Nutrient modulation of inflammatory and immune function. *American Journal of Surgery, 161*(2), 230–234.

Chandra, R.K. (1984). Excessive intake of zinc impairs immune responses. *JAMA, 252*(11), 1443–1446.

Chazot, C., & Kopple, J. (2004). Vitamin metabolism and requirements in renal disease and renal failure. In J. Kopple & S.G. Massry (Eds.), *Nutritional management of renal disease* (pp. 315–356). Baltimore: Williams & Wilkins.

Chen, M.K., Espat, N.J., Bland, K.I., Copeland, E.M., III, & Souba, W.W. (1993). Influence of progressive tumor growth on glutamine metabolism in skeletal muscle and kidney. *Annals of Surgery, 217*(6), 655–667.

Chen, M.K., Salloum, R.M., Austgen, T.R., Bland, J.B., Bland, K.I., Copeland, E.M., III, et al. (1991). Tumor regulation of hepatic glutamine metabolism. *Journal of Parenteral and Enteral Nutrition, 15*(2), 159–164.

Chernoff, R. (1996). Policy: Nutrition standards for treatment of pressure ulcers. *Nutrition Reviews, 54*(1, Pt. 2), S43–S44.

Chernoff, R.S., Milton, K.Y., & Lipschitz, D.A. (1990). The effect of a very high-protein liquid formula (Replete®) on decubitus ulcer healing in long-term tube-fed institutionalized patients. *Journal of the American Dietetic Association, 90*(9), A-130–A-139.

Collins, C. (1996). Nutrition and wound healing. *Care of the Critically Ill, 12*(3), 87–90.

Collins, N. (2003). Diabetes, nutrition and wound healing. *Advances in Skin and Wound Care, 16*(6), 291–294.

Commission of the European Communities. (1993). *Nutrient and energy intakes for the European Community Reports of the Scientific Committee for Food.* Luxembourg: Commission of the European Communities.

Connor, M.J. (1986). Retinoid stimulation of epidermal differentiation in vivo. *Life Science, 38*(20), 1807–1812.

Crandon, J.H., Lund, C.C., & Dill, D.B. (1940). Experimental human scurvy. *New England Journal of Medicine, 223*(10), 353–369.

Cruse, J.M., Lewis, R.E., Roe, D.L., Dilioglou, S., Blaine, M.C., Wallace, W.F., et al. (2000). Facilitation of immune function, healing of pressure ulcers, and nutritional status in spinal cord injury patients. *Experimental and Molecular Pathology, 68*(1), 38–54.

de Luis, D.A., Aller, R., Izaola, O., Cuellar, L., & Terroba, M.C. (2002). Postsurgery enteral nutrition in head and neck cancer patients. *European Journal of Clinical Nutrition, 56*(11), 1126–1129.

de Luis, D.A., Arranz, M., Aller, R., Izaola, O., Cuellar, L., & Terroba, M.C. (2005). Immunoenhanced enteral nutrition, effect on inflammatory markers in head and neck cancer patients. *European Journal of Clinical Nutrition, 59*(1), 145–147.

de Luis, D.A., Izaola, O., Cuellar, L., Terroba, M.C., & Aller, R. (2004). Randomized clinical trial with an enteral arginine-enhanced formula in early postsurgical head and neck cancer patients. *European Journal of Clinical Nutrition, 58*(11), 1505–1508.

Demetriou, A.A., Levenson, S.M., Rettura, G., & Seifter, E. (1985). Vitamin A and retinoic acid: Induced fibroblast differentiation in vitro. *Surgery, 98*(5), 931–934.

Dempsey, D.T., Mullen, J.T., & Buzby, G.P. (1988). The link between nutritional status and clinical outcome: Can nutritional intervention modify it? *American Journal of Clinical Nutrition, 47*(Suppl. 2), 352–356.

Doireau, V., Macher, M.A., Brun, P., Bernard, O., & Loirat, C. (1996). Vitamin A poisoning revealed by hypercalcemia in a child with kidney failure. *Archives of Pediatrics, 3*(9), 880–890.

Doweiko, J.P., & Nompleggi, D.J. (1991). The role of albumin in human physiology and pathophysiology, part III: Albumin and disease states. *Journal of Parenteral and Enteral Nutrition, 15*(2), 207–211.

Efron, D.T., & Barbul, A. (1998). Modulation of inflammation and immunity by arginine supplements. *Current Opinion in Clinical Nutrition and Metabolic Care, 1*(6), 531–538.

Ehrlich, H.P., & Hunt, T.K. (1968). Effects of cortisone and vitamin A on wound healing. *Annals of Surgery, 167*(3), 324–328.

Ehrlich, H.P., Tarver, H., & Hunt, T.K. (1972). Inhibitory effects of vitamin E on collagen synthesis and wound repair. *Annals of Surgery, 175*(2), 235–240.

Ehrlichman, R.J., Seckel, B.R., Bryan, D.J., & Moschella, C.J. (1991). Common complications of wound healing: Prevention and management. *Surgical Clinics of North America, 71*(6), 1323–1351.

Elfert, J., & Drees, E. (1999). Case problem: Nutrition issues and wound care in a patient receiving hemodialysis treatment. *Journal of the American Dietetic Association, 99*(12), 1582–1584.

Evans, J.M., Andrews, K.L., Chutka, D.S., Fleming, K.C., & Garness, S.L. (1995). Pressure ulcers: Prevention and management. *Mayo Clinic Proceedings, 70*(8), 789–799.

Fahr, M.J., Kornbluth, J., Blossom, S., Schaeffer, R., & Klimberg, V.S. (1994). H.M. Vars Research Award. Glutamine enhances immunoregulation of tumor growth. *Journal of Parenteral and Enteral Nutrition, 18*(6), 471–476.

Ferguson, M., Cook, A., Rimmasch, H., Bender, S., & Voss, A. (2000). Pressure ulcer management: The importance of nutrition. *Medsurg Nursing, 9*(4), 163–177.

Fernandez-Madrid, F., Prasad, A.S., & Oberleas, D. (1973). Effect of zinc deficiency on nucleic acids, collagen, and noncollagenous protein of the connective tissue. *Journal of Laboratory and Clinical Medicine, 82*(6), 951–961.

Field, J., & Bjarnason, K. (2002). Feeding patients after abdominal surgery. *Nursing Standard, 16*(48), 41–44.

Flaring, U.B., Rooyackers, O.E., Wernerman, J., & Hammarqvist, F. (2003). Glutamine attenuates post-traumatic glutathione depletion in human muscle. *Clinical Science, 104*(3), 275–282.

Food and Nutrition Board. (1997). *Dietary reference intakes for calcium, phosphorus, magnesium, vitamin D, and fluoride.* Washington, DC: National Academies Press.

Food and Nutrition Board. (2000). *Dietary references intakes for vitamin C, E, selenium and carotenoids.* Washington, DC: National Academies Press.

Food and Nutrition Board. (2001). *Dietary reference intakes for vitamin A, vitamin K, arsenic, boron, chromium, copper, iodine, iron, manganese, molybdenum, nickel, silicon, vanadium, and zinc.* Washington, DC: National Academies Press.

Food and Nutrition Board. (2005). *Dietary reference intakes for energy, carbohydrate, fiber, fat, fatty acids, cholesterol, protein, and amino acids (macronutrients).* Washington, DC: National Academies Press.

Fosmire, G.J. (1990). Zinc toxicity. *American Journal of Clinical Nutrition, 51*(1), 225–227.

Fuhrman, M.P. (2003). Wound healing and nutrition. *Topics in Clinical Nutrition, 18*(2), 100–110.

Furnary, A.P., Zerr, K.J., Grunkemeier, G.L., & Starr, A. (1999). Continuous intravenous insulin infusion reduces the incidence of deep sternal wound infection in diabetic patients after cardiac surgical procedures. *Annals of Thoracic Surgery, 67*(2), 352–362.

Galloway, P., McMillan, D.C., & Sattar, N. (2000). Effect of the inflammatory response on trace element and vitamin status. *Annals of Clinical Biochemistry, 37*(Pt. 3), 289–297.

Gastaldelo, K., Vereerstraeten, A., Nzame-Nze, T., Vanherweghem, J.L., & Tielemans C. (1995). Resistance to erythropoietin in iron overloaded hemodialysis patients can be overcome by ascorbic acid administration. *Nephrology, Dialysis, Transplantation, 10*(6), 44–47.

Goetzl, E.J., Wasserman, S.I., Gigli, I., & Austen, K.F. (1974). Enhancement of random migration and chemotactic response of human leukocytes by ascorbic acid. *Journal of Clinical Investigation, 53*(3), 813–818.

Gordillo, G., & Sen, C. (2003). Revisiting the essential role of oxygen in wound healing. *American Journal of Surgery, 186*(3), 259–263.

Gore, D.C., Chinkes, D., Heggers, J., Herndon, D.N., Wolf, S.E., & Desai, M. (2001). Association of hyperglycemia with increased mortality after severe burn injury. *Journal of Trauma, 51*(3), 540–544.

Greaves, M.W., & Skillen, A.W. (1970). Effects of long-continued ingestion of zinc sulphate in patients with venous leg ulceration. *Lancet, 2*(7679), 889–891.

Greenwald, D.P., Sharzer, L.A., Padawer, J., Levenson, S.M., & Seifter, E. (1990). Zone II flexor tendon repair: Effects of vitamins A, E, beta-carotene. *Journal of Surgical Research, 49*(1), 98–102.

Grey, N.J., & Perdrizet, G.A. (2004). Reduction of nosocomial infections in the surgical intensive care unit by strict glycemic control. *Endocrine Practice, 10*(2), 46–52.

Hadley, S.A., & Fitzsimmons, L. (1990). Nutrition and wound healing. *Topics in Clinical Nutrition, 5*(4), 72–81.

Haggard, J., Houston, M.S., Williford, J.H., Meserve, L.A., & Shewokis, P. (1999). Retrospective study of the effects of zinc supplementation in an elderly institutionalized population with decubitus ulcers. *Journal of the American Dietetic Association, 99*(9), A–11.

Hallbrook, T., & Lanner, E. (1972). Serum zinc and healing of various leg ulcers. *Lancet, 2*(7781), 780–782.

Hankenson, K.D., Watkins, B.A., Schoenlein, I.A., Allen, K.G., & Turek, J.J. (2000). Omega-3 fatty acids enhance ligament fibroblast collagen formation in association with changes in interleukin-6 production. *Proceedings of the Society for Experimental Biology and Medicine, 223*(1), 88–95.

Hathcock, J.N., Azzi, A., Blumberg, J., Bray, T., Dickinson, A., Frei, B., et al. (2005). Vitamins E and C are safe across a broad range of intakes. *American Journal of Clinical Nutrition, 81*(4), 736–745.

Havlik, R.J. (1997). Plastic Surgery Educational Foundation DATA Committee. Vitamin E and wound healing. *Plastic and Reconstructive Surgery, 100*(7), 1901–1902.

Haydock, D.A., & Hill, G.L. (1986). Impaired wound healing in surgical patients with varying degrees of malnutrition. *Journal of Parenteral and Enteral Nutrition, 10*(6), 550–554.

Heller, A., & Koch, T. (2000). Immunonutrition with omega-3 fatty acids. Are new anti-inflammatory strategies in sight? *Zentralblatt fur Chirurgie, 125*(2), 123–136.

Hengstermann, S., Fischer, A., Steinhagen-Thiessen, E., & Schulz, R.J. (2007). Nutrition status and pressure ulcer: What we need for nutrition screening. *Journal of Parenteral and Enteral Nutrition, 31*(4), 288–294.

Herbert, V., Shaw, S., & Jayatileke, E. (1995). Vitamin C driven free radical generation from iron. *Journal of Nutrition, 126*(4), 1213S–1220S.

Hornsby-Lewis, L., Shike, M., Brown, P., Klang, M., Pearlstone, D., & Brennan, M.F. (1994). L-glutamine supplementation in home total parenteral nutrition patients: Stability, safety, and effects on intestinal absorption. *Journal of Parenteral and Enteral Nutrition, 18*(3), 268–273.

Hughes, S.J. (2003). Nutrition and healing. *Journal of Clinical Nutrition, 17*(4), 21–26.

Hung, P. (1992). Preoperative fasting of patients undergoing elective surgery. *British Journal of Nursing, 1*(6), 286–287.

Hunt, A.H. (1941). The role of vitamin C in wound healing. *British Journal of Surgery, 28*(111), 436-461.

Hunt, T.K., Ehrlich, H.P., Garcia, J.A., & Dunphy, J.E. (1969). Effect of vitamin A on reversing the inhibitory effect of cortisone on healing of open wounds in animals and man. *Annals of Surgery, 170*(4), 633–641.

Hunt, T., & Hopf, H. (1997). Wound healing and wound infection. What surgeons and anaesthetists can do. *Surgical Clinics of North America, 77*(3), 587–606.

Hurson, M., Regan, M.C., Kirk, S.J., Wasserkrug, H.L., & Barbul, A. (1995). Metabolic effects of arginine in a healthy elderly population. *Journal of Parenteral and Enteral Nutrition, 19*(3), 227–230.

Jacob, R.A. (1999). Vitamin C. In M.E. Shils, J.A. Olson, M. Shike, & A.C. Ross (Eds.), *Modern nutrition in health and disease* (9th ed., pp. 467–483). Baltimore: Williams & Wilkins.

Jenkins, M., Alexander, J.W., MacMillan, B.G., Waymack, J.P., & Kopcha, R. (1986). Failure of topical steroids and vitamin E to reduce postoperative scar formation following reconstructive surgery. *Journal of Burn Care and Rehabilitation, 7*(4), 309–312.

Johnson, L. (1993). Nutrition and wound healing. *Seminars in Perioperative Nursing, 2*(4), 238–242.

Jurado, R.L. (1997). Iron, infections, and anemia of inflammation. *Clinical Infectious Diseases, 25*(4), 888–895.

Kadowaki, M., & Kanazawa, T. (2003). Amino acids as regulators of proteolysis. *Journal of Nutrition, 133*(Suppl. 6), 2052S–2056S.

Kirk, S.J., Hurson, M., Regan, M.C., Holt, D.R., Wasserkrug, H.L., & Barbul, A. (1993). Arginine stimulates wound healing and immune function in elderly human beings. *Surgery, 114*(2), 155–160.

Klimberg, V.S., Souba, W.W., Salloum, R.M., Plumley, D.A., Cohen, F.S., Dolson, D.J., et al. (1990). Glutamine-enriched diets support muscle glutamine metabolism without stimulating tumor growth. *Journal of Surgical Research, 48*(4), 319–323.

Klimberg, V.S., & McClellan, J.L. (1996). Glutamine, cancer, and its therapy. *American Journal of Surgery, 172*(5), 418–424.

Kopple, J.D. (2001). National Kidney Foundation K/DOQI clinical practice guidelines for nutrition in chronic renal failure. *American Journal of Kidney Diseases, 37*(1, Suppl. 2), S66–S70.

Kovacevic, Z., & Morris, H.P. (1972). The role of glutamine in the oxidative metabolism of malignant cells. *Cancer Research, 32*(2), 326–333.

Langkamp-Henken, B., Johnson, L.R., Viar, M.J., Geller, A.M., & Kotb, M. (1998). Differential effect on polyamine metabolism in mitogen- and-superantigen-activated human T-cells. *Biochimica et Biophysica Acta, 1425*(2), 337–347.

Langkamp-Henken, B., Herrlinger-Garcia, K.A., Stechmiller, J.K., Nickerson-Troy, J.A., Lewis, B., & Moffatt, L. (2000). Arginine supplementation is well tolerated but does not enhance mitogen-induced lymphocyte proliferation in elderly nursing home residents with pressure ulcers. *Journal of Parenteral and Enteral Nutrition, 24*(5), 280–287.

Lansdown, A.B. (1996). Zinc in the healing wound. *Lancet, 347*(9003), 706–707.

Lee, M. (1953). An investigation into the value of dl-alpha-tocopheryl acetate (vitamin E) in the treatment of gravitational ulcers. *British Journal of Dermatology, 65*(4), 131–138.

Leininger, S.M. (2002). The role of nutrition in wound healing. *Critical Care Nursing Quarterly, 25*(1), 13–22.

Levenson, S.M., & Demetriou, A.A. (1992). Metabolic factors. In I.K. Cohen, R.F. Diegelmann, & W.J. Lindblad (Eds.), *Wound healing: Biochemical and clinical aspects* (pp. 248–273). Philadelphia: Saunders.

Levenson, S.M., Gruber, C.A., Rettura, G., Gruber, D.K., Demetriou, A.A., & Seifter, E. (1984). Supplemental vitamin A prevents the acute radiation-induced defect in wound healing. *Annals of Surgery, 200*(4), 494–512.

Levine, M., Rumsey, S.C., Daruwala, R., Park, J.B., & Wang, Y. (1999). Criteria and recommendations for vitamin C intake. *JAMA, 281*(15), 1415–1423.

Lewis, S.B., Biondo, C.F., & Page, J.C. (1994). Medical management of the diabetic patient during podiatric surgery. *Journal of the American Podiatric Medical Association, 84*(9), 432–438.

Lewis, B. (2002). Nutrition and wound healing. In L.C. Kloth & J.M. McCulloch (Eds.), *Wound healing: Alternatives in management* (3rd ed., pp. 35–67). Philadelphia: F.A. Davis.

Lown, D. (1998). Wound healing. In L.E. Matarese & M.M. Gottschlich (Eds.), *Contemporary nutrition support practice: A clinical guide* (pp. 583–589). Philadelphia: Saunders.

MacKay, D., & Miller, A.L. (2003). Nutritional support for wound healing. *Alternative Medicine Review, 8*(4), 359–377.

Mann, G.V., & Newton, P. (1975). The membrane transport of ascorbic acid. *Annals of the New York Academy of Sciences, 30*(258), 243–252.

Mathus-Vliegen, E.M.H. (2001). Nutritional status, nutrition and pressure ulcers. *Nutrition in Clinical Practice, 16*(5), 286–291.

McCauley, R., Platell, C., Hall, J., & McCulloch, R. (1991). Effects of glutamine infusion on colonic anastomotic strength in the rat. *Journal of Parenteral and Enteral Nutrition, 15*(4), 437–439.

Meyer, N.A., Muller, M.J., & Herndon, D.N. (1994). Nutrition support of the healing wound. *New Horizons, 2*(2), 202–214.

Mora, R.J. (1999). Malnutrition: Organic and functional consequences. *World Journal of Surgery, 23*(6), 530–535.

National Kidney Foundation, Kidney Disease Outcomes Quality Initiative. (2000). *Clinical practice guidelines for nutrition in chronic renal failure.* Retrieved February 10, 2008, from http://www.kidney.org/professionals/kdoqi/guidelines/doqi_nut.html

Nicosia, R.F., Belser, P., Bonanno, E., & Diven, J. (1991). Regulation of angiogenesis in vitro by collagen metabolism. *In Vitro Cellular and Developmental Biology, 27A*(12), 961–966.

Niu, X.T., Cushin, B., Reisner, A., Levenson, S.M., & Demetriou, A.A. (1987). Effect of dietary supplementation with vitamin A on arterial healing in rats. *Journal of Surgical Research, 42*(1), 61–65.

Norris, J.R., & Reynolds, R.E. (1971). The effect of oral zinc sulfate therapy on decubitus ulcers. *Journal of the American Geriatrics Society, 19*(9), 793–797.

Orgill, D., & Demling, R.H. (1988). Current concepts and approaches to wound healing. *Critical Care Medicine, 16*(9), 899–908.

Park, K.G., Heys, S.D., Blessing, K., Kelly, P., McNurlan, M.A., Eremin, O., et al. (1992). Stimulation of human breast cancers by dietary L-arginine. *Clinical Science, 82*(4), 413–417.

Peng, X., Yan, H., You, Z., Wang, P., & Wang, S. (2005). Clinical and protein metabolic efficacy of glutamine granules-supplemented enteral nutrition in severely burned patients. *Burns, 31*(3), 342–346.

Petry, J. (1999). Nutritional supplements: Good or bad for your surgical patients? *Nursing,* *29*(4), 32hn1–4.

Phillips, J.D., Kim, C.S., Fonkalsrud, E.W., Zeng, H., & Dindat, H. (1992). Effects of chronic corticosteroids and vitamin A on the healing of anastomoses. *American Journal of Surgery,* *163*(1), 71–77.

Phillips, S.J. (2000). Physiology of wound healing and surgical wound care. *ASAIO Journal (American Society for Artificial Internal Organs), 46*(6), S2–S5.

Pories, W.J., Henzel, J.H., Rob, C.G., & Strain, W.H. (1967). Acceleration of wound healing in man with zinc sulphate given by mouth. *Lancet, 21*(7482), 121–124.

Prasad, K.N., Cole, W.C., Kumar, B., & Prasad, K.C. (2001). Scientific rationale for using high-dose multiple micronutrients as an adjunct to standard and experimental therapies. *Journal of the American College of Nutrition, 20*(Suppl. 5), 450S–463S.

Roob, J.M., Khoschsorur, G., Tiran, A., Horina, J.H., Holzer, H., & Winkelhofer-Roob, B.M. (2000). Vitamin E attenuates oxidative stress induced by intravenous iron in patients on hemodialysis. *Journal of the American Society of Nephrology, 11*(3), 539–549.

Ross, A.C. (1999). Vitamin A and retinoids. In M.E. Shils, J.A. Olson, M. Shike, & A.C. Ross (Eds.), *Modern nutrition in health and disease* (9th ed., pp. 305–328). Baltimore: Williams & Wilkins.

Ruberg, R. (1984). The role of nutrition in wound healing. *Surgical Clinics of North America, 64*(4), 705–714.

Ruthig, D.J., & Meckling-Gill, K.A. (1999). Both n-3 and n-6 fatty acids stimulate wound healing in the rat intestinal epithelial cell line, IEC-6. *Journal of Nutrition, 129*(10), 1791–1798.

Salganik, R.I. (2001). The benefits and hazards of antioxidants: Controlling apoptosis and other protective mechanisms in cancer patients and the human population. *Journal of the American College of Nutrition, 20*(Suppl. 5), 464S–472S.

Sandstrom, B. (2001). Micronutrient interactions: Effects on absorption and bioavailability. *British Journal of Nutrition, 85*(Suppl. 2), S181–S185.

Savy, G. (1999). Everything you ever wanted to know about glutamine. *Today's Dietitian, 1,* 52–55.

Schaffer, M.R., Efron, P.A., Thornton, F.J., Klingel, K., Gross, S.S., & Barbul, A. (1997). Nitric oxide, an autocrine regulator of wound fibroblast synthetic function. *Journal of Immunology, 158*(5), 2375–2381.

Scholl, D., & Langkamp-Henken, B. (2001). Nutrient recommendations for wound healing. *Journal of Intravenous Nursing, 24*(2), 124–132.

Selmanpakoglu, A.N., Cetin, C., Sayal, A., & Isimer, A. (1994). Trace element (Al, Se, Zn, Cu) levels in serum, urine and tissues of burn patients. *Burns, 20*(2), 99–103.

Shepherd, A. (2002a). The impact of oral health on nutritional status. *Nursing Standard, 16*(27), 37–38.

Shepherd, A. (2002b). Serum triglycerides and dietary intervention in coronary heart disease. *Complete Nutrition, 2*(1), 37–45.

Stadelmann, W.K., Digenis, A.G., & Tobin, G.R. (1998). Impediments to wound healing. *American Journal of Surgery, 176*(Suppl. 2A), 39S–47S.

Suchner, U., Heyland, D.K., & Peter, K. (2002). Immune-modulatory actions of arginine in the critically ill. *British Journal of Nutrition, 87*(Suppl. 1), S121–S132.

Tarng, D.C., & Huang, T.P. (1998). A parallel comparative study of intravenous iron versus intravenous ascorbic acid for erythropoietin hyporesponsive anemia in hemodialysis patients with iron overload. *Nephrology, Dialysis, Transplantation, 13*(11), 2867–2872.

Taylor, T.V., Rimmer, S., Day, B., Butcher, J., & Dymock, I.W. (1974). Ascorbic acid supplementation in the treatment of pressure-sores. *Lancet, 7*(7880), 544–546.

ter Riet, G., Kessels, A.G.H., & Knipschild, P.G (1995). Randomized clinical trial of ascorbic acid in the treatment of pressure ulcers. *Journal of Clinical Epidemiology, 48*(12), 1453–1460.

Thomas, D.R. (1997). The role of nutrition in prevention and healing of pressure ulcers. *Clinics in Geriatric Medicine, 13*(3), 497–511.

Thomas, D.R. (2001). Issues and dilemmas in the prevention and treatment of pressure ulcers: A review. *Journal of Gerontology, 56A*(6), M328–M340.

Thompson, C., & Fuhrman, M.P. (2005). Nutrients and wound healing: Still searching for the magic bullet. *Nutrition in Clinical Practice, 20*(3), 331–347.

Traber, M.G. (1999). Vitamin E. In M.E. Shils, J.A. Olson, M. Shike, & A.C. Ross (Eds.), *Modern nutrition in health and disease* (9th ed., pp. 347–362). Baltimore: Williams & Wilkins.

Van den Berghe, G., Wouters, P., Weekers, F., Verwaest, C., Bruyninckx, F., Schetz, M., et al. (2001). Intensive insulin therapy in critically ill patients. *New England Journal of Medicine, 345*(19), 1359–1367.

Van den Berghe, G., Wouters, P., Bouillon, P., Weekers, F., Verwaest, C., Schetz, M., et al. (2003). Outcome benefit of intensive insulin therapy in the critically ill: Insulin dose versus glycemic control. *Critical Care Medicine, 31*(2), 359–366.

Vilter, R.W. (1980). Nutritional aspects of ascorbic acid: Uses and abuses. *Western Journal of Medicine, 133*(6), 485–492.

Vinnars, E., Hammarvist, F., von der Decken, A., & Wernerman, J. (1990). Role of glutamine and its analogs in posttraumatic muscle protein and amino acid metabolism. *Journal of Parenteral and Enteral Nutrition, 14*(Suppl. 4), 125S–129S.

Wallace, E. (1994). Feeding the wound: Nutrition and wound care. *British Journal of Nursing, 3*(13), 662–667.

Weiland, R.G., Hendricks, F.H., Amat y Leon, F., Gutierrez, L., & Jones, J.C. (1971). Hypervitaminosis A with hypercalcemia. *Lancet, 1*(7701), 698.

Weisman, K. (1980). Zinc metabolism in the skin 2. In A. Rock & J.A. Savin (Eds.), *Recent advances in dermatology* (pp. 109–129). Edinburgh: Churchill Livingstone.

Wicke, C., Halliday, B., Allen, D., Roche, N.S., Scheuenstuhl, H., Spencer, M.M., et al. (2000). Effects of steroids and retinoids on wound healing. *Archives of Surgery, 135*(11), 1265–1270.

Wiggins, K.L. (1999). *Guidelines for nutrition care of renal patients* (3rd ed.). Chicago: American Dietetic Association.

Wiggins, K.L. (2004). *Renal care: Resources and practical applications: A companion to the Guidelines for Nutrition Care of Renal Patients* (3rd ed.). Chicago: American Dietetic Association.

Williams, J.Z., Abumrad, N., & Barbul, A. (2002). Effect of a specialized amino acid mixture on human collagen deposition. *Annals of Surgery, 236*(3), 369–374.

Williams, L. (2002). Assessing patients nutritional needs in the wound-healing process. *Journal of Wound Care, 11*(6), 225–228.

Wilmore, D. (2001). The effect of glutamine supplementation in patients following elective surgery and accidental injury. *Journal of Nutrition, 131*(Suppl. 9), 2543–2549.

Windsor, J.A., Knight, G.A., & Hill, G.L. (1988). Wound healing response in surgical patients: Recent food intake is more important than nutritional status. *British Journal of Surgery, 75*(2), 135–137.

Winkler, M.F., & Mandry, M.K. (1992). Nutrition and wound healing. *Support Line: A Newsletter of Dietitians in Nutrition Support, 14*, 1–4.

Witte, M.B., & Barbul, A. (2002). Role of nitric oxide in wound repair. *American Journal of Surgery, 183*(4), 406–412.

Worley, C.A. (2004). Why won't this wound heal? Factors affecting wound repair. *Dermatology Nursing, 16*(4), 360–361.

Wu, G., Meininger, C.J., Knabe, D.A., Bazer, F.W., & Rhoads, J.M. (2000). Arginine nutrition in development, health and disease. *Current Opinion in Clinical Nutrition and Metabolic Care, 3*(1), 59–66.

Young, M.E. (1988). Malnutrition and wound healing. *Heart and Lung, 17*(1), 60–67.

Zaloga, G.P. (1994). *Nutrition in critical care*. St. Louis, MO: Mosby.

Zhou, Y.P., Jiang, Z.M., Sun, Y.H., Wang, X.R., Ma, E.L., & Wilmore, D. (2003). The effect of supplemental enteral glutamine on plasma levels, gut function, and outcome in severe burns: A randomized, double-blind, controlled clinical trial. *Journal of Parenteral and Enteral Nutrition, 27*(4), 241–245.

Ziegler, T.R., Benfell, K., Smith, R.J., Brown, E., Ferrari-Baliviera, E., Lowe, D.K., et al. (1990). Safety and metabolic effects of L-glutamine administration in humans. *Journal of Parenteral and Enteral Nutrition, 14*(Suppl. 4), 137S–146S.

Ziegler, T.R., Young, L.S., Benfell, K., Scheltinga, M., Hortos, K., Bye, R., et al. (1992). Clinical and metabolic efficacy of glutamine-supplemented parenteral nutrition after bone marrow transplantation: A randomized, double-blind, controlled study. *Annals of Internal Medicine, 116*(10), 821–828.

CHAPTER 14

Complementary Therapies for Oncology Cutaneous Reactions

Marilyn L. Haas, PhD, RN, CNS, ANP-BC

Introduction

"My body . . . my science."

Oncology patients who are receiving either radiation therapy or chemotherapy can develop skin reactions. Patients undergoing radiation therapy will experience some degree of skin damage, whether visible to the naked eye or only visible at the cellular level. Radiation-induced skin reactions vary from no erythema present to slight erythema and possibly progressing to severe moist desquamation with varying degrees of pain. With newer chemotherapy agents (i.e., epithelial growth factors), skin reactions are becoming more of a challenge for healthcare providers. Practitioners and patients alike continue to search for the best medical evidence to prevent or minimize acute radiodermatitis, skin rashes, infectious lesions, or other problems of the skin.

Over the years, an assortment of prescribed medications has met with various degrees of success. Today, *integrated medicine* is becoming more recognized and accepted, as it combines treatments from conventional medicine and complementary and alternative medicine (CAM). A study of 453 patients with cancer demonstrated that as many as 69% used at least one CAM therapy as part of their cancer treatment (Richardson, Sanders, Palmer, Greisinger, & Singletary, 2000). Dy et al. (2004) found even higher rates in their study of 102 patients enrolled in clinical trials at Mayo Comprehensive Cancer Center; 88% used at least one CAM therapy.

Practitioners may begin to hear "My body . . . my science" as patients begin to search for plant extracts, oils, and herbs to help with the toxicities of therapy. It is extremely important for oncology healthcare professionals to be knowledgeable about CAM products to help to direct patients and address the evidence to support their use (if not already incorporated into clinical guidelines). There is a paucity of data in the literature describing the use of CAM products for cancer therapy–related skin reactions, particularly chemotherapy and biotherapy effects; therefore, this chapter will focus on the most common topical applications for radiation-induced skin reactions. Plant-based extracts will be described along with mechanisms of action, potential side effects, and herbal interactions; evidence-based studies will be discussed if available. Other nontraditional products, such as Chinese herbal ointments and essential oils, will be explored to learn of their potential healing properties.

Plant Extracts

Managing skin problems caused by radiation or chemotherapy is challenging. Prescription medications can prevent or lessen the severity of reactions, yet no established guidelines exist. Interestingly, a number of plant-based products are creeping into traditional medical systems and gaining popularity within the oncology population.

Aloe Vera

The scientific name for aloe vera is *Aloe barbadensis* or *Aloe capensis* (Gruenwald, Brendler, & Jaenicke, 2004). Common names found on the National Institutes of Health National Center for Complementary and Alternative Medicine (NIH NCCAM) Web page are aloe, burn plant, lily of the desert, and elephant's gall (NIH NCCAM, 2008). Aloe vera is derived from the leaves of a plant dating back to the Egyptian civilization. This succulent plant forms a rosette of fleshy basal leaves. The mucilaginous gel comes from the parenchymous tissue in the leaf, whereas the aloe juice is collected from the leaf base of the plant (Yarnell & Meserole, 1996). Many formulations and compounds are used in clinical trials, thus making it difficult to interpret the research studies objectively. Over-the-counter skin care products typically contain both the gel and juice (Roeder, 1994). Although aloe vera also can be ingested, this discussion will focus only on the topical administration.

Some of aloe's purported uses are for burns, cold sores, dry skin, skin inflammation, pain, and pruritus. The topical administration mechanism of action is believed to be an inhibition of bradykinin by contained carboxypeptidase. Also, aloe vera is believed to hinder the formation of thromboxane, which is detrimental to burn wound healing (Foster & Tyler, 1999). Topical administration of aloe vera gel is safe to apply to the skin. It is believed to have a modulating effect by preventing ultraviolet-B sunrays from sensitizing the skin, and it has the ability to penetrate deeply into the skin, thus enhancing the passage of nutrients and rebalance of the pH of the skin (Lee et al., 1997).

Aloe vera dates back almost to the same time as the initiation of radiation as a treatment modality in the early 1900s (Collins & Collins, 1935). While aloe vera may help to reduce radiation-induced skin changes, clinical trials are lacking consistency (Bolderston, Lloyd, Wong, Holden, & Robb-Blenderman, 2006; Heggie et al., 2002; Olsen et al., 2001; Richardson, Smith, McIntyre, Thomas, & Pilkington, 2005; Williams et al., 1996). Of the three recent studies, only one suggested efficacy of applying aloe gel in patients receiving radiation. Williams et al. conducted a randomized, prospective, double-blind evaluation of pure aloe vera gel (98%) compared to a placebo in 194 patients with breast cancer receiving chest wall irradiation. Beginning within three days of the initiation of radiation treatments, the aloe vera gel or placebo was applied twice a day. No statistical difference was seen between the two interventions in relationship to the severity of radiation dermatitis. A second phase of their trial investigated the application of pure aloe vera (98%) compared to observation only. This phase enrolled 107 patients with breast cancer, and again, no statistical significance was found between the two groups. Hence, Williams et al. concluded that aloe vera did not protect against the severity of radiation dermatitis.

Another research trial by Olsen et al. (2001) reported a somewhat different conclusion. They conducted a randomized, blinded, prospective study of 70 patients undergoing radiation therapy. The group consisted of Caucasians (74%) and African Americans (26%), and the ethnic mix was non-Hispanic (65%) and Hispanic (35%). Patients were randomized to prophylactic skin care that included Fruit of the Earth® aloe vera (Fruit of the Earth, Inc.) and mild soap (Dove®, Unilever) versus mild soap alone starting on the first day of radiation therapy. The researchers found no statistical difference at low cumulative radiation doses ($\leq 2,700$ centigray [cGy]), but when higher doses were given ($\geq 2,700$ cGy), a difference occurred when adding aloe to the soap regimen (p = 0.013).

The third major research study was a phase III clinical trial of 225 women with breast cancer after lumpectomy or partial mastectomy who were prescribed postoperative radiation therapy using tangential fields (Heggie et al., 2002). Women were randomized to receive either topical aloe vera gel or topical aqueous cream three times daily at the beginning of treatment and continuing for two weeks after completion of radiation therapy. The researchers concluded that the aloe vera gel did not significantly reduce radiation-induced skin effects, but the aqueous cream was useful in reducing dry desquamation and pain related to radiation therapy.

Two separate systematic reviews supported the same conclusion of the ineffectiveness of aloe vera gel in preventing or minimizing radiation-induced radiodermatitis (Bolderston et al., 2006; Richardson et al., 2005). Richardson et al. (2005) conducted a systematic review of the literature and critically assessed the evidence of effectiveness of aloe vera gel for radiation-induced skin reactions. Their conclusion suggested that no evidence from clinical trials to date indicated the effectiveness of topical aloe vera in preventing or minimizing radiation-induced skin reactions in patients with cancer. Bolderston et al. appraised the literature as well and found insufficient evidence to support or refute specific topical agents for the prevention or management of acute radiation skin reactions.

Possible herb-drug interactions exist with aloe vera gel. According to Brinker (2001), hydrocortisone and aloe together may increase anti-inflammatory effects. No significant side effects have been reported with topical use (NIH NCCAM, 2008). More evidence-based clinical trials are needed to establish the efficacy and possible side effects of aloe vera to guide clinical decision making in the future for practitioners regarding the use of aloe vera during therapy.

Calendula

The scientific name for calendula is *Calendula officinalis*, from the family of *Asteraceae/Compositae* (Gruenwald et al., 2004). Common names include gold-bloom, marigold, marybud, and pot marigold (MedlinePlus Herbs and Supplements, 2008). Calendula is extracted from the flower of the marigold plant. The calendula flower has been used for medicinal purposes since the 12th century. Found in North America, it is also located in Europe and Asia. Calendula is used topically for its wound healing properties and anti-inflammatory effect.

Besides treating radiation side effects, the other purported uses of calendula include (Barnes, Anderson, & Phillipson, 2002)
- Gastrointestinal disorders
- Inflammation
- Menstrual cramps
- Spasms
- Varicose veins
- Conjunctivitis
- Eczema.

Topical applications of calendula are more common in studies, especially in Germany. Reports of quick wound healing are cited because of the rapid increase in blood flow to the affected area (Basch et al., 2006). The active triterpenoids from the calendula have been shown to promote anti-inflammatory activity (Akihisa et al., 1996).

Fresh or dried calendula petals are available in tinctures, liquid extracts, infusions, ointments, and creams. Calendula generally is safe for topical application but should not be applied to open wounds (Bisset, 1994). Calendula's properties of wound healing are based on the formation of granulation tissue, an important process in reepithelialization and healing of wounds (Bisset). The aqueous extract has been shown to induce new blood vessel formation, thus promoting the mechanism of granulation (Patrick, Kumar, Edwardson, & Hutchinson, 1996). Individuals who are sensitive (i.e., develop a skin rash) to the daisy or aster family may develop an allergic reaction to calendula (Schulz, Hansel, Blumenthal, & Tyler, 2004).

The research on calendula in radiation oncology is extremely limited (Basch et al., 2006; McQuestion, 2006; Pommier et al., 2004). The only clinical trial reported in the literature was a phase III randomized trial of *Calendula officinalis* compared to trolamine (Biafine®, OrthoNeutrogena) (Pommier et al.). Because of the difference in texture, color, and smell between the two products, the trial was only single blinded. The trial randomly assigned 254 patients with breast cancer who received postoperative radiation to apply one of the topical agents after each radiation treatment. The occurrence of acute radiodermatitis grade 2 or higher (determined by the acute radiation morbidity scoring criteria from the Radiation Therapy Oncology Group [n.d.]) was significantly lower in the patients who used calendula (p = < 0.0001). Pommier et al. concluded that patients with breast cancer who undergo postoperative irradiation should be offered calendula to prevent acute dermatitis.

Basch et al. (2006) conducted a systematic review of Pommier et al.'s study. Basch et al. graded the level of evidence as "B," representing good scientific evidence. Evidence from this open phase III trial suggested that topical use of calendula may be beneficial for the prevention of dermatitis pain and erythema caused by radiation therapy. However, Basch et al. said the trial should be considered preliminary because of the methodologic limitation and that further testing is required (e.g., double-blind placebo-controlled trial) before a conclusion can be reached.

Chinese Herbal Ointment

Chinese herbal medicine focuses on restoring a balance of energy, body, and spirit to maintain health (American Cancer Society, 2002). There are more than 3,200 herbs, 300 mineral and animal extracts, and more than 400 formulas, which is why replicating herbs can be difficult. Herbal concoctions can be found in herbal "pharmacies" in cities in the United States with a sizable Chinese ethnic community. Some Chinese herbs are used for burns and wound healing; Ching Wan Hung and sea buckthorn will be presented here.

Ching Wan Hung

Ching Wan Hung, also referred to as *Jing Wan Hong*, is a Chinese herbal ointment that treats burns, including radiation burns (Jintu, n.d.). Although not approved by the U.S. Food Drug and Administration (FDA), this ointment is well-known in China and is exported to Singapore, Malaysia, Australia, Japan, and the Americas. Ching Wan Hung is developed by Tianjin Lerentang Pharmaceutical Factory and can be located through the Internet or nature pharmacies that specialize in herbal medicines. Formulations may vary, but the packaging labels list the primary ingredients of lobelia (27.5%), myrrh (17.5%), tang-kuei (12%), borneol (12%), sanguisorba (8.5%), chaenomeles (8.5%), frankincense (8.5%), carthamus (8.5%), and pistacia (8.5%) (Jintu). These ingredients are mixed with an oil base to create the ointment for topical application.

Searching the Web sites of the National Cancer Institute Office of Cancer Complementary and Alternative Medicine (www.cancer.gov/cam/clinicaltrials _list.html) and NCCAM (http://nccam.nih.gov/research/clinicaltrials), no specific clinical trials were offered as of June 2008 for treatment of radiodermatitis or burns with Ching Wan Hung. Although scientific studies are lacking in the United States, there is an interest in cataloging a variety of herbs in the folk pharmacopeias. Of interest are herbs used for burns because ingredients can be isolated (Griffin, 1979). Ching Wan Hung acts to relieve pain, decrease inflammation and infection, and aid in the generation of new tissue (Jintu, n.d.). Ching Wan Hung should be rubbed into the area of the burn and gauze applied to further protect the wound from infection and irritation. The dressings should be changed daily. Care should be taken with Ching Wan Hung; like many Chinese ointments and liniments, it has a red color that can stain clothing (Jintu).

Sea Buckthorn

Sea buckthorn is known scientifically as *Hippophae rhamnoides* (Gruenwald et al., 2004). It often is referred as "shiny horse," which is a traditional Chinese oil containing 190 bioactive components (Aslanov & Novruzov, 1976). Medicinal values can be traced back in European and Asian history. The plant was fed to horses in ancient Greece, where it was found to give a shine to their coats, thus its name. Externally applied, the seed oil provides a one-to-one ratio of omega-3, 6, and 9, and contains linolenic acid. Russian cosmonauts used the oil for protection against radiation burns in space, although this use has not been scientifically proven (Delabays & Slacanin, 1995).

Sea buckthorn oil contains vitamin E, vitamin C (ascorbic acid), beta-carotene, unsaturated fatty acids, essential amino acids, and flavonoids, plus other bioactive compounds. The oil was not abundantly found in herbal pharmacopeias to validate its usage, and only one study was cited on MedlinePlus®. Wang, Luo, and He (2006) reported the therapeutic effects of *Hippophae rhamnoides* oil in managing burns. A total of 151 burned patients were treated by applying the oil to an inner dressing and covering it with a disinfecting dressing. Compared to the control group that used petroleum jelly gauze, patients using sea buckthorn oil expressed relief of pain, an obvious decrease in swelling, and faster epithelial regrowth. Wang et al. concluded that the oil definitely had value in burn patients.

Essential Oils

Essential oils are promoted to enhance quality of life and may not be readily thought of to help with burns. Certainly, there is not a proliferation of literature discussing its use in radiation therapy. Typically, essential oils are used as aromatherapy, but they can be used for their lipophilic and antimicrobial elements (Maddocks-Jennings, Wilkinson, & Shillington, 2005). Essential oils usually are concentrated and contain many different chemical components. Oils are absorbed at different rates into the skin (Buchbauer, 1993). Essential oils have anti-inflammatory and tissue healing properties.

Chamomile is one of the most common essential oils available. The common plant name for chamomile is *German chamomile* or *Roman chamomile.* It comes from the daisy-like family, *Asteraceae* (American Cancer Society, 2002; Decker, 1999). Chamomile extract produced by a cold extraction process is yellow; steam distillation produces the blue essential oil. The oil contains at least 50% alpha-bisabolol, which is found in skin care products. The German- and Hungarian-grown chamomile varieties are the primary plants used in herbal remedies because of their abundance of alpha-bisabolol. The Roman or English chamomile contain similar compounds but are not used as often in herbal medicine because of the lack of bisabolol (Gasic, Lukic, Adamovic, & Canak, 1986).

Chamomile is hypothesized to act as a barrier to prevent water loss from the skin and be soothing. A study conducted by Maiche, Grohn, and Maki-Hokkonen (1991) investigated a chamomile extract called Kamillosan™ (Goldshield) ointment in women receiving radiation therapy. Maiche et al. conducted a randomized controlled trial involving 50 postmastectomy women receiving radiotherapy for breast cancer. The women used either Kamillosan or almond oil *above* their scar twice a day. Physicians blinded to the location of the application were asked to score the skin reaction from 0 (no change) to 3 (moist desquamation). Subjective pain and itching also were recorded. Women in the Kamillosan group developed grade 2 or less toxicity, but neither group was statistically significant. These researchers concluded that more studies are needed to evaluate the efficacy of chamomile oil in radiation therapy.

Other Preparations

Reports on other preparations are sprinkled throughout the literature, many indicating positive effects on irradiated skin. In 1993, researchers conducted a double-blind, randomized, prospective clinical trial to evaluate topical vitamin C solution for the prevention of radiation dermatitis (Halperin, Gaspar, George, Darr, & Pinnell, 1993). The clinical trial was on patients with brain tumors receiving radiation therapy to the head. Blinded to the radiation technologists, the patients would apply the vitamin C lotion on one side of the scalp twice a day throughout therapy and a placebo solution in the same manner to the other side of the scalp. Controlling for age, sex, and total dose of irradiation, no benefit was seen with using ascorbic acid lotion to prevent radiation dermatitis. Additionally, no difference was observed in patient preference or toxicity scores.

Medicinal honey has been cited in the literature to be safe and effective with various wounds, including radiation burns. Researchers in the Netherlands conducted a prospective, controlled, randomized study with adult patients with breast cancer receiving at least 50 gray (Gy) to the chest wall/breast (Moolenaar et al., 2006). Some women received honey gauze (Honey-Soft®, MediProf), and others received the placebo paraffin gauze (Unitulle®, Aventis Pharma Ltd.). Pictures and visual analog scales regarding pain, itching, irritation, odor, and general satisfaction of treatment were measured daily. Only 27 women met the eligibility criteria, of which 24 participated in the trial. Because of the low accrual rate, the clinical trial stopped early. However, the researchers noted a trend toward lower levels of pain, itching, and irritation in patients using the honey gauze dressing.

A pilot study conducted in Australia used wheatgrass extract for the treatment of radiation dermatitis (Wheat, Currie, & Coulter, 2007). The prospective randomized controlled trial used a control group employing current best practice (sorbolene cream) and a treatment group using wheatgrass extract. The researchers enrolled 20 patients with breast cancer who received lumpectomy and postoperative radiation therapy. The experimental group received higher doses of radiation—63.3 Gy versus 59.4 Gy for the control group. There was no statistical significance in acute skin toxicity identified, but there was a significant improvement in the quality of life among the patients who utilized the wheatgrass extract in weeks two ($p = 0.087$), three ($p = 0.092$), five ($p = 0.097$), and six ($p = 0.013$).

Conclusion

As the incidence and survival rates increase among patients with cancer, the use of CAM will likely increase as patients want to control toxicities (reduce side effects or organ toxicity) from radiation and chemotherapy (Frenkel, Ben-Arye, Baldwin, & Sierpina, 2005). No longer can healthcare professionals base their practices on simple tradition and intuition. The "my body . . . my science" statement may become the norm, where patients want to take control of their bodies and use CAM products for healing while undergoing conventional treatment. Today, more evidence exists to suggest benefits from various plant-based treatments, such as calendula cream. Plant-based products, as opposed to prescription steroids, typically do not have side effects; therefore, patients may be more willing to try herbal potions and lotions before seeking traditional products. Oncology healthcare professionals should research evidence to provide accurate information to their patients. Oncology healthcare professionals should also support research on CAM to find ways to help patients to feel better and recover faster from their treatments. Because less is known about the efficacy and safety of CAM products as compared to FDA-approved products, more scientific research is crucial on CAM products and procedures. There is a strong need to replicate some of the aforementioned studies and explore options such as Chinese herbs, essential oils, and other herbal extracts.

References

Akihisa, T., Yasukawa, K., Oinuma, H., Kasahara, Y., Yamanouchi, S., Takido, M., et al. (1996). Triterpene alcohols from the flowers of composite and their anti-inflammatory effects. *Phytochemistry, 43*(6), 1255–1260.

American Cancer Society. (2002). *Complementary and alternative cancer methods handbook.* Atlanta, GA: Author.

Aslanov, S.M., & Novruzov, E.N. (1976). The oil from the pulp residues of Hippohae rhamnoides. *Chemistry of Natural Compounds, 12*(5), 584–585. Retrieved June 20, 2008, from http://www.springerlink.com/content/n2pr7850v4323586

Barnes, J., Anderson, L., & Phillipson, J. (2002). *Herbal medicines.* London: Pharmaceutical Press.

Basch, E., Bent, S., Foppa, I., Haskmi, S., Kroll, D., Mele, M., et al. (2006). Marigold (Calendula officinalis): An evidence-based systematic review by the Natural Standard Research collaboration. *Journal of Herbal Pharmacotherapy, 6*(3-4), 135–159.

Bisset, N. (Ed.). (1994). *Herbal drugs and phytopharmaceuticals: A handbook for practice on a scientific basis.* Boca Raton, FL: CRC Press.

Buchbauer, G. (1993). Molecular interaction: Biological effects and modes of action of essential oils. *International Journal of Aromatherapy, 5*(1), 11–14.

Bolderston, A., Lloyd, N.S., Wong, R.K., Holden, L., & Robb-Blenderman, L. (2006). The prevention and management of acute skin reactions related to radiation therapy: A systematic review and practice guideline. *Supportive Care in Cancer, 14*(8), 802–817.

Brinker, F. (2001). *Herb contraindications and drug interactions* (3rd ed.). Sandy, OR: Eclectic Medical Publications.

Collins, C.E., & Collins, C. (1935). Roentgen dermatitis treated with fresh whole leaf of aloe vera. *American Journal of Roentgenology and Radium Therapy, 33*(3), 396–397.

Decker, G. (Ed.). (1999). *An introduction to complementary alternative therapies.* Pittsburgh, PA: Oncology Nursing Society.

Delabays, N., & Slacanin, I. (1995). Domestication and selection of new plant species of interest to the cosmetics industry. *Revue Suisse de Viticulture—d'Arboriculture-et-d'Horticulture, 27,* 143–147.

Dy, G., Bekele, L., Hanson, L., Furth, A., Mandrekar, S., Sloan, J., et al. (2004). Complementary and alternative medicine use by patients enrolled onto phase I clinical trials. *Journal of Clinical Oncology, 22*(23), 4810–4815.

Foster, S., & Tyler, V.E. (1999). *Tyler's honest herbal: A sensible guide to the use of herbs and related remedies* (4th ed.). New York: Haworth Herbal Press.

Frenkel, M., Ben-Arye, E., Baldwin, C., & Sierpina, V. (2005). Approach to communicating with patients about the use of nutritional supplements in cancer care. *Southern Medical Journal, 98*(3), 289–294.

Gasic, O., Lukic, V., Adamovic, D., & Canak, N. (1986). Variation in the content and the composition of the essential oils in flower heads of Matricaria chamomilla L. during its ontogenetical development. *Acta Pharmaceutica Hungarica, 56*(6), 283–288.

Griffin, R. (1979). Herbal medicine revisited: Science looks anew at ancient Chinese pharmacology. *American Pharmacy, 19*(10), 16–22.

Gruenwald, J., Brendler, T., & Jaenicke, C. (2004). *PDR for herbal medicines* (3rd ed.). Montvale, NJ: Thomson PDR.

Halperin, E., Gaspar, L., George, S., Darr, D., & Pinnell, S. (1993). A double-blinded, randomized, prospective trial to evaluate topical vitamin C solution for the prevention of radiation dermatitis. CNS Cancer Consortium. *International Journal of Radiation Oncology, Biology, Physics, 26*(3), 413–416.

Heggie, S., Bryant, G., Tripcony, L., Keller, J., Rose, P., Glendenning, M., et al. (2002). A phase III study on the efficacy of topical aloe vera gel on irradiated breast tissue. *Cancer Nursing, 25*(6), 442–451.

Jintu. (n.d.). *Ching Wan Hung: Burn ointment.* Retrieved June 20, 2008, from http://www.itmonline.org/jintu/chingwan.htm

Lee, C., Han, S., Mo, Y., Kim, R., Chun, M., Park, Y., et al. (1997). Prevention of ultraviolet radiation-induced suppression of accessory cell function of Langerhans cells by aloe vera gel components. *International Journal of Immunopharmacology, 37*(2-3), 153–162.

Maddocks-Jennings, W., Wilkinson, J.M., & Shillington, D. (2005). Novel approaches to radiotherapy-induced skin reactions: A literature review. *Complementary Therapies in Clinical Practice, 11*(4), 224–231.

Maiche, A., Grohn, P., & Maki-Hokkonen, H. (1991). Effect of chamomile cream and almond ointment on acute radiation skin reaction. *Acta Oncologica, 30*(3), 395–396.

McQuestion, M. (2006). Evidence-based skin care management in radiation therapy. *Seminars in Oncology Nursing, 22*(3), 163–173.

MedlinePlus Herbs and Supplements. (2008). *Calendula (Calendula officinalis L.).* Retrieved June 20, 2008, from http://www.nlm.nih.gov/medlineplus/druginfo/natural/patient-calendula.html

Moolenaar, M., Poorter, R., Van Der Toorn, P., Lenderink, W., Poortmans, P., & Egbers, A. (2006). The effect of honey compared to conventional treatment on healing of radiotherapy-induced skin toxicity in breast cancer patients. *Acta Oncologica, 45*(5), 623–624.

National Institutes of Health National Center for Complementary and Alternative Medicine. (2008). *Herbs at a glance: Aloe vera.* Retrieved June 20, 2008, from http://nccam.nih.gov/health/aloevera

Olsen, D., Bradley, C., Johnson, M., Macias, J., Love, V., & Markoe, A. (2001). The effect of aloe vera gel/mild soap versus mild soap alone in preventing skin reactions in patients undergoing radiation therapy. *Oncology Nursing Forum, 28*(3), 543–547.

Patrick, K.F.M., Kumar, S., Edwardson, P.A.D., & Hutchinson, J.J. (1996). Induction of vascularisation by an aqueous extract of the flowers of Calendula officinalis L the European marigold. *Phytomedicine, 3,* 11–18.

Pommier, P., Gomez, F., Sunyach, M., D'Hombres, A., Carrie, C., & Monthbarbon, X. (2004). Phase III randomized trial of Calendula officinalis compared with trolamine for the prevention of acute dermatitis during irradiation for breast cancer. *Journal of Clinical Oncology, 22*(8), 1447–1453.

Radiation Therapy Oncology Group. (n.d.). *Acute radiation morbidity scoring criteria.* Retrieved March 5, 2009, from http://www.rtog.org/members/toxicity/acute.html

Richardson, J., Smith, J.E., McIntyre, M., Thomas, R., & Pilkington, K. (2005). Aloe vera for preventing radiation-induced skin reactions: A systematic literature review. *Clinical Oncology, 17*(6), 478–484.

Richardson, M., Sanders, T., Palmer, J., Greisinger, A., & Singletary, S. (2000). Complementary/alternative medicine use in a comprehensive cancer center and the implications for oncology. *Journal of Clinical Oncology, 18*(13), 2505–2514.

Roeder, G. (1994). Skin care and aloe vera. *Total Health, 16*(3), 12.

Schulz, V., Hansel, R., Blumenthal, M., & Tyler, V. (2004). *Rational phytotherapy: A reference guide for physicians and pharmacists* (5th ed.). New York: Springer.

Wang, Z.Y., Luo, X.L., & He, C.P. (2006). [Management of burn wounds with Hippophae rhamnoides oil]. *Nan Fang Yi Ke Da Xue Xue Bao, 26*(1), 124–125.

Wheat, J., Currie, G., & Coulter, K. (2007, Summer). Management of acute radiation skin toxicity with wheatgrass extract in breast radiation therapy: Pilot study. *Australian Journal of Medical Herbalism, 19,* 77–81.

Williams, M., Burk, M., Loprinzi, C., Hill, M., Schomberg, P.J., Nearhood, K., et al. (1996). Phase III double-blind evaluation of an aloe vera gel as a prophylactic agent for radiation-induced skin toxicity. *International Journal of Radiation Oncology, Biology, Physics, 36*(2), 345–349.

Yarnell, E., & Meserole, L. (1996). Topical application of botanical medicine: Aloe vera and other medicinal plants for healing. *Alternative and Complementary Therapies, 2*(4), 241–244.

CHAPTER 15

Special Needs of Gero-Oncology Patients

Sarah H. Kagan, PhD, RN, AOCN®

Introduction

Older adults being treated for cancer face an increased risk of skin injury, chronic wounds, and possibly different or worse skin toxicities associated with treatment (Kaya & Saurat, 2007). Normal aging changes and skin pathology common in late life interact with or potentiate effects of cutaneous manifestations of some cancers, skin toxicities of many current therapies, and multi-modality treatment (Baumann, 2007; Brincat, Baron, & Galea, 2005). Health habits such as sun exposure, smoking, and nutritional intake influence skin aging and may contribute to alterations in cutaneous immunity and wound healing (Arnold & Barbul, 2006; Bernhard, Moser, Backovic, & Wick, 2007; Kaya & Saurat). Furthermore, some older adults experience functional limitations that may limit activities of daily life for hygiene, nutrition, and toileting, thus creating or exacerbating skin conditions and wounds (Fleck, 2007; Flood et al., 2006; Rodin & Mohile, 2007; Whitson, Purser, & Cohen, 2007). Oncology nurses are challenged to understand, evaluate, and effectively treat the complex skin conditions experienced by older patients with cancer and to promote self-care and provide caregiver support.

Comprehensive nursing care for older adults with cancer requires understanding of normal and pathologic skin aging. Common skin conditions and chronic wounds commonly overlie skin aging, adding complexity to clinical presentation. As a result, careful and sequential skin assessment is necessary during cancer treatment. Clinical evaluation and management must account for alterations in healing with age as well as the interaction of aging changes and comorbid skin conditions and the cutaneous manifestations of cancer and skin toxicities with specific treatment. However, scant scientific evidence directly addresses the intricate problem of gero-oncology skin care (Kagan, 2004). Evidence-based nursing practice must rely on integrating knowledge of normal aging, common pathology, and care of older people with evidence-based oncology nursing care to create best gero-oncology practices (Kagan).

This chapter outlines considerations in gero-oncology skin care to achieve best practices in nursing. After a review of current and projected demographics, the elements of a framework for skin care for older adults with cancer are explicated. Normal and pathologic aging changes, including delayed wound healing and common skin conditions, are discussed in relation to their impact on skin care for these patients. Aspects of wound healing altered by aging are explored to support clinical management. Clinical management is detailed to describe preventive skin care and wound care as well as psychosocial care and caregiver support. The chapter concludes with a summary of implications for future research and practice to promote evidence-based care.

Framework

The United States, like most economically developed nations, is aging rapidly, and one in five Americans is expected to be older than age 65 by mid-century (Kosmadaki & Gilchrest, 2002). Cancer and many chronic skin conditions such as primary skin cancer, eczematous dermatitis, chronic vascular ulcers, and pressure ulcers are common in older adults (Cohen, 2007; Dewberry & Norman, 2004; Kaya & Saurat, 2007; Kosmadaki & Gilchrest; Norman, 2003; Schneider & Norman, 2004). Clinically, older adults who are treated for cancer may be at risk for or may experience a complex set of skin problems that result from interrelated geriatric, dermatologic, and oncologic etiologies. Clinical management of this patient population can be structured using two principles to understand the interaction of aging changes with pathologic and traumatic conditions, to identify goals of care, and to guide best practices. These principles are *functional reserve* and *skin failure* (Kaya & Saurat; Koroukian, Murray, & Madigan, 2006; Langemo & Brown, 2006; Lunney, Lynn, Foley, Lipson, & Guralnik, 2003; Rodin & Mohile, 2007; Saurat, 2007; Whitson et al., 2007; Worley, 2007).

Functional Reserve

Functional reserve is the extent to which a tissue, organ, organ system, or individual can respond to an insult without change in function (Whitson et al., 2007). It conceptually frames the relationship between aging changes and functional capacity. Declining functional reserve is the clinical manifestation of physiologic, psychological, and social changes with age and is most often seen after a physical injury or disease, psychological problem or emotional event, or a change in social role or relationships (Whitson et al.). Declining functional reserve presents challenges to nurses caring for older adults who may be unable to "bounce back" during cancer treatment and thus exhibit functional limitations or may not return to baseline function without restorative intervention and rehabilitation (Rodin & Mohile, 2007). Functional decline that resists intervention and encompasses global and specific functions is associated with the end of life. Lunney and colleagues identified apparent patterns in such decline associated with death from cancer as opposed those who died suddenly, from organ failure, or who had a marked period of frailty in the last years of life (Lunney et al., 2003; Whitson et al.).

Functional reserve of the skin directly addresses the extent to which the organ can perform its barrier function for the organism: to protect underlying tissues and organs from a variety of threats spanning from microbes to gross physical trauma. For example, skin that has lost keratinized epidermis may allow microbial pathogens to enter, resulting in infections (Fore-Pfliger, 2004). Aged skin in which the epidermal-dermal junction has flattened, resulting in relatively easy traumatic separation, may blister and tear with seemingly incidental trauma (Fore, 2006). Aged skin that is subjected to long-term application of topical corticosteroid preparations may show heightened impairment of cutaneous immune response with more common or severe infections like candidiasis (Fore; Fore-Pfliger). Functional reserve, then, conceptually represents resilience of the skin as an organ to maintain its function in the context of the individual, aging, disease, and environment.

Skin failure is an often neglected case of organ failure, which may provide nurses insight into gero-oncology skin care by revealing the skin conditions that represent complex interactions among aging, age-related disease, cancer, and cancer treatment, and by framing evaluation of those skin conditions for prognosis, therapeutic goals, and intervention (Langemo & Brown, 2006). Kaya and Saurat (2007) and Saurat (2007) noted that because the skin functions as a mechanical and physiologic protective barrier for the entire organism, skin aging should be termed *dermatoporosis*. This term captures the holistic understanding of skin fragility and insufficiencies that are associated with skin aging and that impair the skin's capacity to function as a mechanical and physiologic barrier (Kaya & Saurat; Saurat).

Langemo and Brown (2006) argued that, like any organ, the skin can fail functionally at acute, chronic, and end-stage levels. Fragile skin tissue that insufficiently blocks physiologic and mechanical threats may fail completely. This level of skin failure may be local. *Local skin failure* is easily assessed as an isolated disruption in the organ, seen as a break, ulcer, or other wound. *Generalized skin failure*, although not articulated in the dermatologic, wound, or oncologic literature to date, represents a significant threat to homeostasis for frail gero-oncology patients. Interactions of age-related comorbid disease with cancer and cancer treatment present a greater risk of having fragile skin fail completely. This sort of interaction is posited by Kaya and Saurat (2007) as they outlined the influence of iatrogenesis, typified by steroid use and consequent cutaneous side effects, in dermatoporosis. Kaya and Saurat delineated *secondary dermatoporosis* as an effect of largely iatrogenic forces exacerbating primary photo-aging and intrinsic aging changes that is, therefore, different from primary dermatoporosis.

Langemo and Brown (2006) employed the example of pressure ulcers to illustrate acute, chronic, and end-stage skin failure and to elucidate prognostic expectations, therapeutic goals, and intervention. Their discussion showed how careful, even nuanced, assessment of a clinical problem like pressure ulcers can identify clinically consequential detail that can be added to a comprehensive assessment of the individual and factored into clinical judgment and decision making. Worley (2007) connected skin failure and cancer in clinical judgment when she related the personal and painful story of her mother's death from cancer. Her mother developed a pressure ulcer five days before she died from cancer. Worley and her mother's oncologist differed on whether the pressure ulcer was preventable. Worley felt it was not, as it signified her mother's impending death; Worley used this as an exemplar to summarize her analysis of skin failure.

Langemo and Brown (2006) argued in their review that skin failure is directly related, for the authors who use the term, to hypoperfusion and represents skin death. The portion of the skin that is no longer viable and the overall prognosis and condition of the patient are interrelated and thus interpreted jointly. Therefore, skin failure offers a window into the patient's overall condition and is correlated with the patient's condition. Skin failure helps to frame skin damage conceptually and places it in a context that projects clinical implications. Use of skin failure, in conjunction with functional reserve to outline potential for recovery and rehabilitation, offers clinically relevant structure for gero-oncology skin care.

Aging Skin

Normal Changes

The skin is the largest organ of the body, accounting for about a tenth of the body's weight, and provides essential barrier and homeostatic functions (Barr, 2006; Baumann, 2007; Fore, 2006; Fore-Pfliger, 2004). Skin aging is a result of two processes: intrinsic aging and extrinsic aging. *Intrinsic aging* includes cellular senescence and apoptosis resulting in cellular changes in replication and function that cause cell death and tissue dysfunction (Baumann; Fore). *Extrinsic aging* is the cumulative result of environmental exposure that similarly results in cellular changes, altered tissue structures, impaired replication and regeneration, and tissue dysfunction (Baumann; Fore). Health habits related to interaction with the environment implicate behavior as part of extrinsic skin aging. Use of sun protection and avoidance of tobacco are the best examples of the connections among the individual, behavior, and extrinsic aging. Photo-aging, or the cumulative changes in the skin as a result of ultraviolet light exposure from the sun, represents the majority of visible characteristics of aged skin (Baumann; Fore). Bernhard et al. (2007) proposed that smoking accelerates aging and promotes functional changes in the skin including wrinkles, impaired wound healing, and, potentially, skin cancer. Skin aging also is affected by aging in other organs. Menopause is the most obvious example of this interaction. Physiologically, diminished estrogen after menopause reduces collagen production, water content, and sebaceous secretions, thereby creating drier, more wrinkled, and less resilient skin in postmenopausal women (Brincat et al., 2005).

The functional consequences of aging skin are manifold although challenging to summarize, as they stem from multiple changes in the structure of the skin (Fore, 2006). Essentially, with age, the skin becomes less strong and is not as elastic as younger skin; the epidermis and dermis are more easily separated; the dermis thins and becomes less vascular. As a result, the skin is more easily injured by trauma including stretching, pulling, and blunt forces. Injuries more common among older adults are skin tears, traumatic purpura, blistering, and pressure ulcers (Fleck, 2007; Fore; Saurat, 2007). The keratinized epidermis is more fragile in older adults and the sebaceous glands produce less sebum, while the hair follicles atrophy and produce less hair. As a result of these changes and alterations in the dermis, thermoregulation and the physical barrier functions of the skin are impaired (Kaya & Saurat, 2007; Saurat). In addition to reduced mechanical barrier performance, cellular changes in immune cell subsets and melanocytes result in altered physiologic protection from the sun and microbes. Viral, fungal, and bacterial skin infections may be more common among older adults (Fore). Older adults may have more melanocytic nevi and more nonmelanoma skin cancers because of decreased photo-protection (Baumann, 2007; Dewberry & Norman, 2004). Declining cell replication in general results in delayed or frankly impaired wound healing (Baumann; Fore; Kaya & Saurat) (see Figure 15-1).

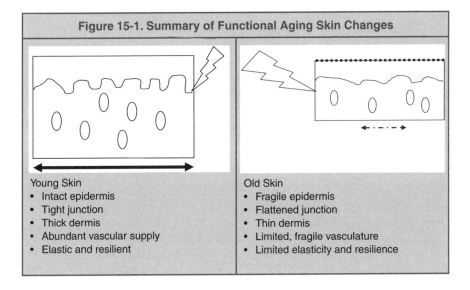

Figure 15-1. Summary of Functional Aging Skin Changes

Young Skin
• Intact epidermis
• Tight junction
• Thick dermis
• Abundant vascular supply
• Elastic and resilient

Old Skin
• Fragile epidermis
• Flattened junction
• Thin dermis
• Limited, fragile vasculature
• Limited elasticity and resilience

Common Skin Conditions

Several skin conditions and diseases common to older adults result from the intersection of aging skin with environmental risk and cumulative exposure to irritants and pathogens. These skin problems can be classified, for purposes of this discussion, to project implications for care and the need for specialized consultation, into the following categories.

- Benign conditions and minor injury
- Eczema and irritant dermatitis
- Skin infections
- Common chronic wounds
- Nonmelanoma skin cancers

More rare and complex skin disorders, such as *bullous phemphigoid* and *pyoderma gangrenosum*, are beyond the scope of this chapter and require specialized dermatology consultation and management. Nurses, in addition to relying on the expertise of the physician and advanced practice nurse colleagues in dermatology, can turn to texts such as *Skin and Aging Processes* (Gilchrest, 1984) and to authors like Norman and colleagues for clinically relevant geriatric dermatology references (Norman, 2003; Schneider & Norman, 2004).

Understanding the pathology and standard management of common skin conditions aids in considering potential interactions with cutaneous manifestations of cancer or cancer therapies. Knowledge of common skin conditions also helps in selection of therapeutic interventions for cutaneous complaints. Benign conditions such as dry skin, known as *xerosis*, and minor injuries such as skin tears are often troubling to the older person and yet are easily managed with consistent, evidence-based treatment that relies on avoiding further drying agents or other injury and restoring the physical integrity and lipid barrier functions of the skin, using few, if any, drugs or advanced wound care products. Pruritic conditions other than xerosis, including eczema and irritant dermatitis, may require the use of topical corticosteroids and antipruritics for comfort, in addition to essential identification and removal of causative agents. However, the use of topical corticosteroids, as Kaya and Saurat (2007) noted in describing secondary dermatoporosis, can be risky for older adults. Topical corticosteroids accentuate aging changes, risking further thinning of the skin and cutaneous immune impairment resulting in new or worse skin infections. Common skin infections such as candidiasis, cellulitis, and scabies are predicated on the interface of the individual's skin with the immediate environment and exposure to pathogens. Thus, for example, candidiasis easily occurs when urinary incontinence is unmanaged, given the presence of *Candida albicans* as normal skin flora. Management of skin infections incorporates environmental risk reduction, avoiding or limiting pathogen exposure, and optimizing immune and barrier function, in addition to the use of antimicrobial agents in topical or systemic form.

Chronic wounds include pressure ulcers and vascular ulcers, as well as those resulting from cancer (e.g., fungating malignant wounds) or cancer treatment (e.g., late radiation necrosis). Principles that guide chronic wound management may be successfully employed to create individualized care that acknowledges the underlying pathology of the wounds themselves. Interdisciplinary team management is essential, and oncology nurses are instrumental in coordinating the team for older adults with cancer. Careful systematic assessment of underlying systemic disease and the wounds themselves clarify the goal for therapy—whether healing by primary, secondary, or tertiary intent or relying on palliative maintenance—and ground the treatment plan. Diabetic neuropathic foot ulcers that limit ambulation and self-care and worsen on an antineoplastic therapy (e.g., cetuximab) are a prime exemplar of chronic wounds that influence function and overall health during cancer treatment and are worsened by the cancer therapy (Schneider & Norman, 2004). Attention to control or cure of systemic disease and correction of related conditions such as malnutrition undergirds any local wound care (Norman & Bock, 2003; Schneider & Norman). In addition to the strength of the interdisciplinary team to the coordinated delivery of often complex care, oncology nurses may also rely on texts that guide evidence-based non-oncologic wound management, such as *Acute and Chronic Wounds: Current Management Concepts* (Bryant & Nix, 2007).

Finally, older adults who are being treated for cancers may, in the presence of risk factors such as cumulative lifetime occupational, recreational, and incidental sun exposure, simultaneously have nonmelanoma skin cancers as well as melanoma (Dewberry & Norman, 2004). Although nonmelanoma skin cancers often are viewed as less aggressive and worrisome than other solid tumors or lymphomas and leukemias, they require special attention during therapy for other cancers. Immune impairment may result in aggravation and worsening of existing lesions. Focus on the treatment of primary cancers that are not cutaneous may change health behaviors that result in additional sun exposure, neglect of sun protection, or trauma to advancing nonmelanoma skin cancer lesions. Comprehensive cancer treatment plans thus merit cautious periodic skin assessment and conservative treatment of these lesions in addition to education about and coaching for self-care.

Considerations in Clinical Management

Clinical management of skin problems related to cancer, cancer treatment, and the interactive effects of comorbid disease in older adults merges principles and evidence for care employed for any adult with considerations that adapt that care to the unique needs of older adults. The current evidence of specific skin problems in cancer treatment such as external beam radiation reactions or the acneform rash toxicity of epidermal growth factor receptor inhibitors offers sharply limited insight into how older adults' physiologic, functional, and psychosocial responses are different from those of their younger counterparts. A search of the current literature via MEDLINE® and *Cumulative Index to Nursing and Allied Health Literature* (*CINAHL*®) at the time of this writing returned no citations specific to this comparison that adapts evidence-based guidelines for older adults based on measured differences. Thus, best practices in management rely on interpolation of two different bodies of literature and consideration of adjusting intervention to meet individual learning needs, functional capacity, and resources, including family support and financial status.

For example, skin care management for prevention of radiation reactions, including toxicity and recall, must account for changes in keratinized epidermis and delay in healing with age and radiation, as well as sensitivities (Brincat et al., 2005; Fore, 2006; Fore-Pfliger, 2004). Selection of products and protocols that maintain moisture and address xerosis and pruritus for older patients with cancer undergoing radiation, however, may not look different from those used for younger patients as the clinical issues are similar, although possibly not of the same magnitude. Explicit acknowledgment of aging changes and the potential exacerbation of reaction, differential perception of symptoms, and prolonged healing are imperative to successful, comprehensive skin care. Such care anticipates and obviates problems related to the cancer and cancer therapy and identifies concurrent conditions to obtain treatment that will limit influence on cancer treatment by promoting function and limiting skin failure.

Similarly, wound care must fuse principles of chronic wound care with the response of the older adult and caregiver to the chronic wound and the resources available to achieve care. Goal setting for patients who have chronic wounds always acknowledges the underlying pathology and the degree to which it can be corrected to select primary, secondary, or tertiary intent if healing is possible, and palliative maintenance if it is not. Goals for older adults must account for delayed wound healing and contributions of comorbid diseases such as diabetes mellitus and cumulative effects of health habits such as smoking (Ayello, 2005; Bernhard et al., 2007; Fore, 2006). Evidence-based interventions, as with younger patients, should be readily available and easy to use. Older adults may require adaptation of aspects of the treatment plan that aggravate effects of aging changes or psychosocial ramifications of being older. For example, because skin tears are more common among older adults as the epidermal-dermal junction flattens, dressings must be secured atraumatically and with devices that do not employ strong adhesives, when possible. Likewise, wound care devices and dressing materials should be selected with consideration of both caregiver availability and function, and of Medicare and other insurance reimbursement. Older adults who have cancer and comorbid disease may not be able to complete wound care without the support of an informal or paid caregiver. As a result, any home wound-care protocols should trigger evaluation for home nursing. Concomitant analysis of costs and financial resources also is warranted, as older adults are more likely to have higher healthcare expenditures and risk of out-of-pocket costs while on fixed incomes.

Finally, psychosocial care and support for older patients with cancer and informal family or friend caregivers is a part of any plan for skin care. As the skin visibly ages during later life, the older person's identity and sense of self and being frequently are affected. These changes are gradual and generally allow for accommodations in the perceptions of their meaning for both older adults and those around them. However, the overlay of cutaneous manifestations of cancer and its treatment often dramatize or accentuate those aging changes and their implications in understanding what it is to be older and have cancer. Cutaneous manifestations are, by their nature, visible and can symbolize being older and being ill, in general, and having cancer, specifically. The visibility and symbolic aspects of these manifestations engender concerns and questions, as well as symptoms and care needs that may overwhelm the older person's function and resources. As a result, special consideration to the information needs and questions from older adults and their caregivers should be given in patient education. Routine assessment of skin pain and other symptoms, such as pruritus; ongoing patient and caregiver education including review of the goals of skin and wound care; and review of care needs, caregiving support, and caregiver burden are essential elements of psychosocial care that ensure comprehensiveness and support concordance and adherence.

Implications for the Future

Evidence and interventions to optimize the quality of daily life for older people who have cancer and comorbid disease are vital to oncology nursing practice and will become more so as the United States and other economically developed nations experience progressive aging of their populations, advances in treatment for cancer and other chronic diseases, and consequent extension of the life span. Skin problems can limit function and generally diminish the quality of daily living for any patient but are doubly troubling to older patients, whose risk of skin conditions, diseases, and symptoms is greater than their younger counterparts. Oncology nurses can face the challenge of threats to their patients' experiences by recognizing that most people with cancer are older and that knowledge of aging changes and age-related pathology enhances care of older patients with cancer. Oncology nurses further must pursue, in their practice and research, comparative, focal knowledge of how older adults react and respond to cutaneous manifestations of cancer and cancer treatment, in addition to evaluating the utility and efficacy of interventions for skin problems with older adults.

Conclusion

Older adults with cancer have an increased risk of skin injury, chronic wounds, and possibly treatment-related skin toxicities. Furthermore, skin changes with aging, skin conditions common in late life, and cutaneous manifestations of comorbid disease may interact with the cutaneous effects of cancer and cancer treatment to present complex skin conditions. Declining functional reserve and skin failure, or dermatoporosis, conceptually frame the understanding of skin problems in older patients with cancer. Major functional skin aging changes include epidermal fragility; flattened epidermal-dermal junction and increased susceptibility to shearing trauma; decreased thickness, elasticity, and resilience; diminished and more fragile vascular supply; and impaired cutaneous immune response and delayed wound healing. Clinical management of skin problems for older patients with cancer merges oncologic evidence with geriatric evidence to create best practices and individualized care. Additionally, advancement of oncology nursing practice requires recognition that most people with cancer are older and that more research is needed to optimize nursing practice and quality of daily living for older patients, as it is influenced by the cutaneous manifestations of cancer and cancer treatment.

References

Arnold, M., & Barbul, A. (2006). Nutrition and wound healing. *Plastic and Reconstructive Surgery, 117*(Suppl. 7), 42S–58S.

Ayello, E.A. (2005). What does the wound say? Why determining etiology is essential for appropriate wound care. *Advances in Skin and Wound Care, 18*(2), 98–111.

Barr, J.E. (2006). Impaired skin integrity in the elderly. *Ostomy/Wound Management, 52*(5), 22–24.

Baumann, L. (2007). Skin ageing and its treatment. *Journal of Pathology, 211*(2), 241–251.

Bernhard, D., Moser, C., Backovic, A., & Wick, G. (2007). Cigarette smoke—an aging accelerator? *Experimental Gerontology, 42*(3), 160–165.

Brincat, M.P., Baron, Y.M., & Galea, R. (2005). Estrogens and the skin. *Climacteric, 8*(2), 110–123.

Bryant, R.A., & Nix, D.P. (Eds.). (2007). *Acute and chronic wounds: Current management concepts* (3rd ed.). St. Louis, MO: Elsevier Mosby.

Cohen, H.J. (2007). The cancer aging interface: A research agenda. *Journal of Clinical Oncology, 25*(14), 1945–1948.

Dewberry, C., & Norman, R.A. (2004). Skin cancer in elderly patients. *Dermatologic Clinics, 22*(1), 93–96.

Fleck, C.A. (2007). Preventing and treating skin tears. *Advances in Skin and Wound Care, 20*(6), 315–320.

Flood, K.L., Carroll, M.B., Le, C.V., Ball, L., Esker, D.A., & Carr, D.B. (2006). Geriatric syndromes in elderly patients admitted to an oncology-acute care for elders unit. *Journal of Clinical Oncology, 24*(15), 2298–2303.

Fore, J. (2006). A review of skin and the effects of aging on skin structure and function. *Ostomy/Wound Management, 52*(9), 24–37.

Fore-Pfliger, J. (2004). The epidermal skin barrier: Implications for the wound care practitioner, part I. *Advances in Skin and Wound Care, 17*(8), 417–425.

Gilchrest, B. (1984). *Skin and aging processes.* Boca Raton, FL: CRC Press.

Kagan, S.H. (2004). Gero-oncology nursing research. *Oncology Nursing Forum, 31*(2), 293–299.

Kaya, G., & Saurat, J.H. (2007). Dermatoporosis: A chronic cutaneous insufficiency/fragility syndrome. Clinicopathological features, mechanisms, prevention and potential treatments. *Dermatology, 215*(4), 284–294.

Koroukian, S.M., Murray, P., & Madigan, E. (2006). Comorbidity, disability, and geriatric syndromes in elderly cancer patients receiving home health care. *Journal of Clinical Oncology, 24*(15), 2304–2310.

Kosmadaki, M.G., & Gilchrest, B.A. (2002). The demographics of aging in the United States: Implications for dermatology. *Archives of Dermatology, 138*(11), 1427–1428.

Langemo, D.K., & Brown, G. (2006). Skin fails too: Acute, chronic, and end-stage skin failure. *Advances in Skin and Wound Care, 19*(4), 206–211.

Lunney, J.R., Lynn, J., Foley, D.J., Lipson, S., & Guralnik, J.M. (2003). Patterns of functional decline at the end of life. *JAMA, 289*(18), 2387–2392.

Norman, R.A. (2003). Geriatric dermatology. *Dermatologic Therapy, 16*(3), 260–268.

Norman, R.A., & Bock, M. (2003). Wound care in geriatrics. *Dermatologic Therapy, 16*(3), 224–230.

Rodin, M.B., & Mohile, S.G. (2007). A practical approach to geriatric assessment in oncology. *Journal of Clinical Oncology, 25*(14), 1936–1944.

Saurat, J.H. (2007). Dermatoporosis. The functional side of skin aging. *Dermatology, 215*(4), 271–272.

Schneider, J.B., & Norman, R.A. (2004). Cutaneous manifestations of endocrine-metabolic disease and nutritional deficiency in the elderly. *Dermatologic Clinics, 22*(1), 23–31.

Whitson, H.E., Purser, J.L., & Cohen, H.J. (2007). Frailty thy name is . . . phrailty? *Journals of Gerontology. Series A, Biological Sciences and Medical Sciences, 62*(7), 728–730.

Worley, C.A. (2007). Skin failure: The permissible pressure ulcer? *Dermatology Nursing, 19*(4), 384–385.

Index

The letter f after a page number indicates that relevant content appears in a figure; the letter t, in a table.

E

F

G

National Center for Complementary and Alternative Medicine (NCCAM), 298, 302

National Comprehensive Cancer Network (NCCN)
distress management guidelines, 94–95, 263
skin toxicity management, 159

National Council on Aging, 267

National Institutes of Health (NIH), National Center for Complementary and Alternative Medicine (NCCAM), 298, 302

necrosis/necrotic tissue, 25–26, 48*t*

negative pressure wound therapy (NPWT), 90, 111

nervous tissue, 8–10

neuroglial cells, 8–10

neurons, 8

neuropathic pain, 92, 238–239, 240*t*, 252–253

Neutrogena Norwegian Formula®, 161–162

neutropenia, 23, 61–62

neutrophilic eccrine hidradenitis, 48*t*

nevirapine, cutaneous reaction from, 43*t*

Nicolau syndrome, 48*t*

nitric oxide, 274, 276

nitrogen, 270, 273

nitrogen mustard. *See* mechlorethamine

nitrous oxide/oxygen, for pain management, 93

nociceptive pain, 92, 238, 240*t*, 247*t*–249*t*, 247–252

nodular lesions, 58*t*

nodules, 36*t*

nonimmunologic drug reactions, 35. *See also* cutaneous drug reactions

nonmelanoma skin cancers, in older adults, 315

nonsteroidal anti-inflammatory drugs (NSAIDs)
for pain management, 93, 248*t*, 250–251
skin reactions from, 34, 37, 43*t*, 201

nonvesicant agents, 154*f*

nucleoside analogs, radiation recall with, 149

Numeric Pain Intensity Scale (NPIS), 240*t*, 241

nummular eczema-like eruption, 48*t*

nursing history, 52

nutritional assessment, 268–269

nutrition, effect on healing process, 20, 201–202, 267

O

obesity. *See* overweight/obesity

occlusive dressings, 133–134

ochronosis, exogenous, 48*t*

oculocutaneous albinism (OCA), 69–70

odor control, of malignant fungating wounds, 84–89, 105

oil glands, 5

older adults, 309–310
functional reserve in, 310–311
management considerations for, 315–317
normal skin aging in, 312–313, 313*f*
skin conditions in, 314–315

omega-3 fatty acids, 276–277

omega-6 fatty acids, 276–277

Oncology Nursing Society (ONS)
Acute Skin Toxicity Scale, 124
CAM position, 55
Patient Outcomes Survey (2004), 241
Radiation Therapy Patient Care Record, 125

onycholysis, 151

opioids
for pain management, 92, 248*t*–249*t*, 250–251
patient education on, 252
skin reactions from, 37

opportunistic mold infections, 61

Oral Assessment Guide, 228

oral candidiasis, 227–228

Oral Mucosa Rating Scale, 228

oral mucositis, 54

Oral Mucositis Assessment Scale, 228

Oral Mucositis Index, 228

organ failure, 202

ornithine, 274

overlap cGVHD, 188. *See also* chronic graft-versus-host disease

overweight/obesity, 21–22, 209–210, 269

oxaliplatin
hypersensitivity reactions from, 153
as irritant agent, 154*f*, 156*t*

oxycodone, for pain, 248*t*–249*t*, 251

oxygen therapy
for pain management, 93
for wound healing, 111–112

P

Pacinian corpuscles, 4

paclitaxel